Labour Ward Manual

Edited by

David T Y Liu MPhil MB BS DM MBA FRCOG FRANZCOG

Nottingham University Hospital NHS Trust, Nottingham, UK

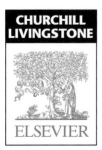

CHURCHILL
LIVINGSTONE

ELSEVIER

EDINBURGH LONDON NEW YORK OXFORD PHILADELPHIA ST LOUIS SYDNEY TORONTO 2007

CHURCHILL
LIVINGSTONE
ELSEVIER

An imprint of Elsevier Limited

© Butterworth-Heinemann 1985
© Butterworth-Heinemann 1991
© Elsevier Science Limited 2003
© 2007, Elsevier Limited. All rights reserved.

First edition 1985
Second edition 1991
Third edition 2003
Fourth edition 2007

ISBN-13: 978-0-443-10252-3
ISBN-10: 0-443-10252-X

British Library Cataloguing in Publication Data
A catalogue record for this book is available from the British Library

Library of Congress Cataloging in Publication Data
A catalog record for this book is available from the Library of Congress

Notice
Neither the Publisher nor the Editor assume any responsibility for any loss or
injury and/or damage to persons or property arising out of or related to any use
of the material contained in this book. It is the responsibility of the treating
practitioner, relying on independent expertise and knowledge of the patient, to
determine the best treatment and method of application for the patient.

The Publisher

Working together to grow
libraries in developing countries

www.elsevier.com | www.bookaid.org | www.sabre.org

ELSEVIER | **BOOK AID** International | Sabre Foundation

ELSEVIER | your source for books,
journals and multimedia
in the health sciences

www.elsevierhealth.com

The
publisher's
policy is to use
**paper manufactured
from sustainable forests**

Printed in China

Contents

Contributors and mentors   vii
Comment   ix
Preface   xi
Acknowledgements   xii

1. Attitudes and conduct   1
   Author: David T Y Liu

2. Legal considerations   5
   Author: Andrew Parsons

3. Maternal and perinatal mortality   13
   Author: David T Y Liu
   Mentor: Charles Rodeck

4. The birthing environment   19
   Authors: Amanda Sullivan, Carol McCormick

5. Admission to labour ward   23
   Author: David T Y Liu

6. Admission emergencies   35
   Author: David T Y Liu
   Mentors: Khaled Ismail, Mark Kilby

7. Normal labour and delivery   45
   Authors: David T Y Liu, Pamela M Thwaites

8. Intrapartum nutrition and electrolytes   55
   Authors: Paul Tomlinson, David T Y Liu

9. Analgesia and anaesthesia   59
   Author: David M Levy

10. Intrapartum fetal surveillance   73
    Author: David T Y Liu
    Mentors: Rosemary Buckley, Toby Fay

11. Episiotomy and tears   85
    Author: David T Y Liu

12. The newborn   91
    Author: David A Curnock

13. Preterm labour and preterm premature rupture
    of membranes   101
    Author: David T Y Liu
    Mentor: Ronald Lamont

14. Abnormal labour   109
    Author: David T Y Liu
    Mentor: Martin Whittle

15. Induction and augmentation of labour   117
    Author: David T Y Liu
    Mentors: Sam Mukhopadhyay,
    Sabaratnam Arulkumaran

16. Assisted vaginal delivery and shoulder
    dystocia   127
    Author: David T Y Liu
    Mentor: George S. H. Yeo

17. Caesarean section   145
    Author: David T Y Liu
    Mentor: Alexander Omu

18. Emergencies in the immediate
    puerperium   155
    Author: David T Y Liu
    Mentor: Charles Rodeck

19. Malpresentation and malpositions   163
    Author: David T Y Liu

20. Breech 171
Author: David T Y Liu
Mentor: Pamela Loughna

21. Twins and multiple deliveries 181
Author: David T Y Liu

22. Medical complications 187
(i) Haematological, coagulation, respiratory and neurological disorders 188
Author: Lucy Kean

(ii) Endocrine disorders 192
Author: Renée Page

(iii) Cardiac disease 195
Author: Philip Baker

(iv) Infections 199
Author: Christine A Bowman

(v) Psychiatric illness 204
Author: David Liu

23. Fetal and maternal misadventure 207
Author: David T Y Liu
Mentor: Charles Rodeck

24. Obstetric emergencies: training with skills drills 213
Author: Andrew Simm

Index 219

Contributors and mentors

CONTRIBUTORS

Philip Baker DM MRCOG
Professor and Director, Maternal and Fetal Health Research Centre, St Mary's Hospital, Manchester, UK

Christine A Bowman BM BCh MA FRCP
Consultant Physician Genito-urinary Medicine, The Hallamshire Hospital, Sheffield, UK

David A Curnock MB Bchir FRCP FRCPCH DCH D Obst. RCOG
Consultant Paediatrician, Nottingham University Hospitals NHS Trust, Nottingham, UK

Lucy Kean DM MA MRCOG
Sub-specialist in Maternal-Fetal Medicine, Nottingham University Hospitals NHS Trust, Nottingham, UK

David M Levy FRCA
Consultant Anaesthetist, Nottingham University Hospitals NHS Trust, Nottingham, UK

David T Y Liu MPHIL MB BS DM MBA FRCOG FRANZCOG
Consultant Obstetrician and Gynaecologist/Clinical Tutor, Nottingham University Hospitals NHS Trust, Nottingham, UK

Carol McCormick BSc (Hons) RM RGN PDL ADM
Consultant Midwife, Nottingham University Hospitals NHS Trust, Nottingham, UK

Renée Page BSc MD FRCP
Consultant Endocrinologist, Nottingham University Hospitals NHS Trust, Nottingham, UK

Andrew Parsons LLB
Solicitor of the Supreme Court, RadcliffesLeBrasseur, Westminster, London, UK

Andrew Simm MB ChB MRCOG
Consultant Obstetrician, Nottingham University Hospitals NHS Trust, Nottingham, UK

Amanda Sullivan PhD BA (Hons) PGDip RGN RM
Consultant Midwife, Nottingham University Hospitals NHS Trust, Nottingham, UK

Pamela M Thwaites SRN SCN NNEB
Community Midwife, Nottingham, UK

Paul Tomlinson FRCA
Consultant Anaesthetist, Nottingham University Hospitals NHS Trust, Nottingham, UK

MENTORS

Sabaratnam Arulkumaran MD PhD MRCS Eng FRCS Ed MRCOG
Professor and Head of Department of Obstetrics and Gynaecology, St George's Hospital Medical School, London, UK

Rosemary Buckley BSc RGN RM
Senior Audit Midwife, Nottingham University Hospitals NHS Trust, Nottingham, UK

Khaled Ismail MD MRCOG
Clinical Lecturer, Keele University, Consultant in Obstetrics and Gynaecology, North Staffordshire Combined Healthcare Trust, Stoke on Trent, UK

Mark Kilby MD MBBS MRCOG
Professor and Consultant in Fetal Medicine, Birmingham Women's Hospital, Birmingham, UK

Toby Fay MD FRCOG
Consultant Obstetrician, Nottingham University Hospitals NHS Trust, Nottingham, UK

Ronald Lamont BSc DM FRCOG
Consultant Obstetrician and Gynaecologist/Honorary Reader, Northwick Park and St Marks NHS Trust, Middlesex, UK

Pamela Loughna MBBS MD FRCOG MRCGP
Consultant Obstetrician/Honorary Senior Lecturer, Nottingham University Hospitals NHS Trust, Nottingham, UK

Sam Mukhopadhyay MD DMB MRCOG
Consultant Obstetrics and Gynaecology, Department of Obstetrics and Gynaecology, Norwich and Norfolk Hospital, Norfolk, UK

Alexander Omu FRCOG
Professor and Chairman, Department of Obstetrics and Gynaecology, Faculty of Medicine, Kuwait University, Kuwait

Charles Rodeck DSc FRCOG FRCPath
Professor and Head of Department, Royal Free and University College Medical School, London, UK

Martin Whittle MD FRCOG FRCP
Professor and Head of Division of Reproductive and Child Health, Birmingham Women's Hospital, Birmingham, UK

George S Yeo MBBS FAMS (Singapore) FRCOG
Chief of Obstetrics, Head and Senior Consultant, Department of Maternal Fetal Medicine, KK Women's & Children's Hospital, Singapore

Comment

As the mother of four wonderful children all born at the City Hospital under the careful caring professionalism of Mr Liu, I feel well qualified to recommend this book. I have first-hand knowledge of the efficient way in which the labour ward is managed. Giving birth is one of the most moving and memorable times of any woman's life; her confidence comes from the team that supports her and creates calm surroundings for her. It is true to say that those memories will stay with her all her life.

Thank you to Mr Liu and his team for fulfilling all those needs.

Emma Rutland
Duchess of Rutland

Preface

The first edition of the *Labour Ward Manual* was published in 1985, the second in 1991, followed by a third in 2003. Each edition, including this, the fourth edition, emphasises significant changes in concepts and approaches to our care for women in labour. The principles and fundamental steps of operative procedures as taught by generations of skilled clinicians have altered little over four editions, but contemporary research has introduced modifications to ensure evidence-based practice.

Publications from the Department of Health and Royal Colleges (such as *Changing Childbirth: Report of the Maternity Group EMG* (1993), *A First Class Service: Quality in the New NHS* (1998) and *The New NHS: Modern, Dependable* (1997)), together with guidance from *Towards Safer Childbirth: Minimum Standards for the Organisation of Labour Wards, Report of a Joint Working Party* (RCOG Press 1999), *Clinical Negligence Scheme for Trusts, Maternity: Clinical Risk Management Standards* (National Health Service Litigation Authority 2005) and *Seven Steps to Patient Safety: The Full Reference Guide* (National Patients Safety Agency 2004) all promote the ethos of the woman as central to the process of care, with her safety as the paramount concern. Effective and appropriate systems and processes must be in place to facilitate communication, learning and exercise of governance.

These publications further emphasise the advantages of devolvement of uncomplicated pregnancies to the care of midwives and general practitioners while obstetricians deploy their specialised skills to the increasing numbers of complex situations encountered within the labour ward.

To enable women to have flexibility of choice and confidence in the continuity of their care, teamwork is essential between obstetricians, midwives, neonatologists, anaesthetists and when necessary, specialists from other disciplines. The offer of choice determines the need for a process of negotiation, after an informed discussion of options together with consequences and outcomes. Consent to accept care necessitates an understanding of the available choices (*Obtaining Valid Consent*. Clinical Governance Advice Number 6, London, RCOG, 2004; *Consent Implementation Guide: Consent to Examination or Treatment*, London, Department of Health, 2001). The negotiated outcome incorporates the ingredients of informed choice, safety, dignity and evidence-based practice.

The editor welcomes these progressive changes within obstetric practice and has ensured they have been taken into account in this new edition. An international team of specialists continues to participate either as contributors to chapters, or as mentors, to ensure contents of the text remain contemporary and representative. The enduring fundamental aim of the *Labour Ward Manual* is for all women to receive optimum care at this important time, thus safeguarding the health of the family and the next generation.

David T Y Liu

Nottingham, 2006

Acknowledgements

This book remains dedicated to all those mothers who have taught us so much about how we can look after mothers even better in the future. The continuing efforts of health providers in their search to improve care are not forgotten. I am grateful for the support of my contributors and mentors who share the vision of the need for such a text. My thanks to Anne Whitchurch who coordinated the contributions, and to my family.

Chapter 1

Attitudes and conduct

David T Y Liu

Childbirth is a physiological function. It is natural that women should want to perform this function in the way that they consider most appropriate. Individual preconceived ideas, the media, and social and cultural background all contribute in varying degrees to the expectations of the woman in labour. Safety of the woman and fetus or newborn must be the prime objective. However, the birth of a baby should also be remembered as a happy and enriching experience. Labour can only be deemed to have been successfully conducted when these ideals are satisfied.

Attendant medical personnel may have views of their own about the conduct of labour. However, the outcome is unlikely to be considered a success unless medical staff feel they have achieved good rapport with the parturient woman and conducted the labour to enhance the ideals discussed above. The following guidelines may benefit those who have not appreciated the importance of correct attitudes and conduct as salient measures of proper labour ward management.

- A congenial atmosphere should be maintained to emphasise the concept that labour and delivery are not illnesses. This should not lead us to believe that a degree of professionalism is not respected by women or their attendant partners. Anxiety is associated with childbirth. Modesty is not automatically relinquished merely because a woman is in labour. Decorum and suitable attire enhance this rapport.

- The shift system for staffing means it is seldom possible for the same medical team to attend for the whole course of labour, although supervision remains the prerogative of the obstetrician in charge. All attendants should have a thorough knowledge of the woman's history and preferences.

This will avoid inadvertent comments which prejudice rapport and undermine confidence.

- Modern technology is used in the labour ward to enhance the safety of the woman and fetus. When the reasons for its use and the value of its application are explained, these instruments and special equipment will be viewed by parents as ancillary aids rather than an intrusion. For example, showing the woman and her partner the pattern of some basic fetal heart rate recordings can invite a sense of additional involvement and commitment.

- For women with their own preferences for the conduct of labour, ascertain the type of antenatal preparation she has had. Within reason, support the concepts and practices she expects. Introduction of alternative practices or procedures at this late stage can confuse, with the resultant loss of confidence. Special preferences which may endanger the woman and fetus should be fully discussed, preferably during the antenatal period, so that risk can be explained and minimised. Flexibility in the attitude of the attendant staff is all important, but it is an indictment against our training and values if we jeopardise the welfare of our charges by subscribing without comment to fashionable idiosyncrasies that we believe may put them at risk of possible medical hazards.

- Husbands or partners are encouraged to stay with the women throughout labour. Demanding or aggressive behaviour on their part may reflect feelings of helplessness in the perceived situation or guilt because they have subjected their partner to the traumas of childbirth. Ensure a woman is comfortable, and if needed there is ready access to analgesia. Ask after the woman's comfort when her partner is present so that he can be verbally reassured by her. If a woman is obviously overreacting, explain in the presence of the partner that such behaviour is not conducive to an atmosphere of calm for the birth of their baby. This direct approach reinforces communication between the partners to benefit all concerned.

- Husbands or partners are there to provide support and encourage the ethos of participation by both in the birth of their offspring. This role must be emphasised during operative procedures when a reassuring voice or quiet hand clasp can assist maternal relaxation and control.

- Caesarean section performed under regional anaesthesia may be better accepted if the partner attends to support the woman. There is no justification for the partner's presence if general anaesthesia is used. Minors should not attend labours. Their mother's natural reactions may be misconstrued and frighten or create anxiety.

- Tact is all important when dealing with women whose expectations are not realised. Women who approach labour convinced that all things natural are beneficial may be disappointed. Nature is often cruel and capricious and has not endowed all women with the means to easy childbirth. Realisation that they are not one of Nature's fortunates can come as an unpleasant surprise. Full explanation helps to dispel some of the feelings of guilt and failure when an assisted delivery is anticipated.

- Women who are used to positions of responsibility in society may have difficulty in accepting advice or the 'dictates' of labour ward staff whom they may consider more junior. Rapport and confidence is enhanced if these women can observe the efficiency and obstetric training exhibited by their attendants.

- A normal obstetric situation can develop rapidly into an emergency. Anticipation by thorough knowledge of the woman's history and an appreciation of the significance of that history by the woman and her partner is important. Equally important is knowledge of the correct procedures to be followed when an emergency arises. Regular drills for emergencies to familiarise all staff with emergency procedures are essential. A professional and calm approach reduces anxiety and psychological stress.

All of us who attend labouring women must learn to appreciate the limitations of our individual expertise and that of the 'system' in which we work. If we maintain the welfare of the woman and fetus as our prime objective, there should be no reluctance to seek help from more experienced colleagues when required.

Labour is a reminder of Nature's insistence on survival of the fittest. The role of the obstetric team should be to allow what is physiological to continue, but to intervene where appropriate to counter Nature's indiscretions.

Expectations are, however, exceptionally high and when these are not realised the trend is ready resort to legal redress. The challenge is to provide the highest quality of service within the constraints of both fiscal and human resource. Safe delivery for woman and baby becomes a fundamental expected right while quality is measured in terms of

Box 1.1   Guideline for women with special requirements

High expectations and intolerance of any complication mean that a woman may seek legal redress whenever the outcome is unexpected or untoward. Special requirements or wishes to dictate management must be fully discussed, and risk and likely outcome explained. These exchanges should then be carefully documented. Verbal consent for special procedures such as induction of labour should be notated. The woman's signature is required for surgical procedures such as caesarean section or sterilisation. Additional considerations are:

- Women are encouraged to indicate their requirements by 'birth plans'. Discuss their contents and ability to comply before onset of labour.
- Find out reasons behind their requests, for example social and cultural needs or anxiety after previous obstetric experience. Detailed explanation and reassurance may suffice to correct misconceptions.
- Communication is all important. Inadequate communication is the basis of many legal proceedings. Avoid unprofessional loose remarks.
- If a woman's request is difficult to accept discuss care with a colleague or legal representative if negotiation cannot achieve a compromise.

Informed consent
Women's rights and wishes must be a priority. Current guidelines are given in detail in Chapter 2. Specifically note:

- Obtaining and providing consent is a process in which a woman's mental competence and

understanding must be ensured and her right to change is recognised.

- Refusal of treatment must be explored fully to exclude inadequate information or misconception. Document discussions. Obtain the woman's signature or disclaimer form to release medical attenders and hospital from responsibility. Notify relevant authorities.
- Parents cannot override consent provided by a child (under 16 years of age) who is assessed as competent (Gillick competent). However, parents can obtain legal sanction to provide consent if a competent child refuses treatment which can benefit.

Satisfaction with care
This is best achieved when medical carers are welcoming and helpful, when women participate in decision making and pain relief is well managed.

Specific risk factors requiring attention
The latest Confidential Enquiry into Maternal and Child Health (*Why Mothers Die, 2000–2002*) drew attention to need for special requirements for minority ethnic groups, e.g. black African women and asylum seekers, the socially disadvantaged, among whom domestic violence and substance misuse may be more likely, and those with medical histories, e.g. severe psychiatric history, cardiac diseases and body mass index of 35 or more.

satisfaction and the softer paraphernalia around the delivery process. This is best achieved by what I describe as negotiated care when the informed recipient (woman) and providers (medical carers) enter into a dialogue to determine within the boundaries of risk the acceptable option for all. Expectations are underlined at the outset leaving medical carers to focus effort on the process and incorporate issues for quality.

Some women will have special requirements and these are set out in Box 1.1.

Chapter 2

Legal considerations

Andrew Parsons

CHAPTER CONTENTS

Consent   5
  General principles   5
    Informed consent   5
  Obstetric cases   5
    Special types of patient   6
  Capacity   6
    The Common Law (until 2007)   6
    Is the patient mentally competent? (The
      capacity test)   6
    Advance directives (also known as
      living wills)   6
    Treatment without consent   7
  The Mental Capacity Act 2005   7
    Principles relating to capacity   7
    Capacity test   7
    Best interests   7
    Additional matters covered by the Mental
      Capacity Act   8
    Applications to the court to authorise
      medical treatment   8
    Guidelines for court applications   8
Surrogacy   9
Termination of pregnancy   9
Confidentiality   10
  When confidential information may be
    passed on   10
Registration of births and stillbirths   10
Negligence   10
Medical records   11
Human Rights Act   11
Issues of clinical governance   11

Litigation as a result of medical treatment is increasing. This chapter provides guidance on some of the most common issues likely to arise in the labour ward. However, it is only a brief summary of the law in England and Wales, and in cases of any doubt legal advice must be obtained.

CONSENT

General principles

A patient has the right under common law to give or withhold consent to medical examination or treatment. The courts have ruled that a mentally competent person has an absolute right to refuse to consent to medical treatment for any reason, rational or irrational, or for no reason at all, even where the decision may lead to the patient's own death. Until the Mental Capacity Act comes into force in April 2007 (see below), no one else (even next of kin) can consent on behalf of an adult patient (whether competent or not): it is a widely held misconception that a family can consent on behalf of the patient – *they can not*. The different types of consent are outlined in Box 2.1.

Informed consent

Patients are entitled to receive sufficient information in the way that they can understand about proposed treatments, possible alternatives and any significant risks (which may be special in kind or magnitude or special to the patient), so that they can make a balanced judgement. Box 2.2 lists the essential features of informed consent.

Obstetric cases

A woman who is mentally competent to make a treatment decision may choose not to have medical

---

Box 2.1   Types of consent

Implied: Consent not discussed but implied by action. An example is offering arm for venepuncture.

Verbal: Consent is sought and verbal permission for procedure is obtained. Documentation of this is advised.

Written: Documentation must be obtained if procedure or treatment carries risks or has side effects.

Box 2.2   Essential for informed consent

- Document discussions and treatments in detail, particularly when consent is not available or refused.
- Give information in language which is sensitive and at appropriate level for easy understanding. Allow time for questions and reflection.
- Information must be balanced and in adequate detail to allow meaningful choice of options.
- Consent must be obtained by the person who will perform or is able to perform the procedure. The person or team performing the procedure must be disclosed.
- Separate or additional consent must be obtained for further procedures – unless treatment is immediately necessary in the patient's best interests when consent cannot be obtained.
- Where training is involved, the level of experience and supervision must be indicated.

---

intervention, notwithstanding the risk to her health, and even though the consequences may be the death or serious handicap of the child she bears or her own death. It is the patient's right to make such a decision and medical staff have no power to override this. Furthermore, in such cases the court does not have jurisdiction to declare medical intervention lawful.

Special types of patient

Children (i.e. under 18 years)   Those over 16 years can consent to treatment on their own behalf. For those under 16, the person(s) with parental responsibility has the power to make treatment choices for the child, unless the child is 'Gillick competent', in which case the child can consent. The wellbeing of the child is paramount. Application may be made to the court (as part of its inherent jurisdiction or under the Children's Act as a specific issue order) to provide legal sanction for a specific action when doubt or dispute arises.

Psychiatric patients   Patients with mental illness or disability have the same rights as other patients. Mental illness (even detention under the Mental Health Act) does not of itself render them incompetent to make treatment choices unless their illness is so severe so as to mean that they are unable to make a treatment choice and are thus incompetent (see below). However, patients detained under the Mental Health Act can be treated without consent under the direction of their resident medical officer (RMO) if the treatment is for their mental disorder (section 63 Mental Health Act).

Jehovah's Witnesses   Such patients absolutely refuse the transfusion of blood and blood products even where life is put at risk. Alternative treatment should be considered. It is essential to establish the views held by each Jehovah's Witness patient as some transfusion treatments may be acceptable (such as blood salvage techniques, haemodilution, haemodialysis, cardiopulmonary bypass, albumin, immunoglobulin, clotting factors). To administer blood in the face of refusal may be unlawful. Mentally competent adult patients are entitled to make such a refusal even if others may percieve this to be unwise. This may be by advance directive (which may be oral or written). Treatment of the children of Jehovah's Witnesses may require application to the court for an order.

Capacity

The Common Law (until 2007)
Is the patient mentally competent?
(The capacity test)
In determining if a patient is mentally competent, and therefore whether she has capacity to consent to, or to refuse treatment, the patient must be assessed as being able to:

1. understand and retain the treatment information
2. believe it
3. weigh it in the balance to make a choice.

Only if the patient can do all this is she capable of consenting. This test relates to the patient's *ability* to make a decision but is not concerned with the rationality of it – a capable patient is entitled to make a wholly irrational decision.

Advance directives (also known as living wills)
Advance directives are decisions made while a person has the necessary mental capacity, intended to give effect to wishes as to how treatment or care should be provided in the event they lose capacity.

Advance directives are recognised by English law. They are potentially valid instructions as to which medical treatment that person would or would not be prepared to accept if she should subsequently lose the capacity to decide. However, clinicians are not legally bound to provide treatment if it conflicts with their professional judgement about the most appropriate treatment. Nevertheless the patient's wishes should be taken into account in deciding the appropriate course of action. An advance directive cannot authorise a doctor to do anything that is illegal. They may express preferences between treatment options or list an individual's values as a basis for others to reach decisions. They can be in writing or oral.

Healthcare proxies (i.e. the purported delegation to a third party of the right to make a decision to consent to or refuse medical treatment) are not recognised currently in English Law.

Treatment without consent

Only if the patient is *not* mentally competent can treatment proceed without consent. In which case the following must also apply:

1. The proposed treatment must be necessary to save the patient's life or prevent deterioration in her physical or mental health.
2. The proposed treatment must be in her best interests. (Note: the best interests of the fetus – save to the extent that delivery of a healthy child is in the woman's best interests – does not form part of this test.)
3. The treatment must be such as would be accepted as appropriate by a responsible body of medical opinion.

The Mental Capacity Act 2005

In 2007 the law relating to adults who lack capacity will be changed and governed by the Mental Capacity Act 2005. It provides a statutory framework for assessing whether a person has capacity and a regime for making decisions on their behalf. It has wide ranging applicability covering both financial affairs and personal welfare (including healthcare decisions).

Principles relating to capacity

The Mental Capacity Act is underpinned by five key principles:

- A presumption that every adult has capacity unless it is proved to the contrary.
- A right for individuals to be supported to make their own decisions and given all appropriate help to do so.
- The right to make what may be seen to be unwise decisions.

- Anything done for or on behalf of an individual without capacity must be in their best interests.
- Anything done for or on behalf of the person who lacks capacity should be the least restrictive of their basic rights and freedoms.

Capacity test

The Act defines incapacity as an inability to make a particular decision because of an impairment of, or a disturbance in the functioning of, the mind or the brain. Capacity is issue specific: an individual may have capacity to undertake some decisions but lack capacity in respect of more important ones. Capacity cannot be established merely by reference to a person's age, appearance or any condition or aspect of a person's behaviour which might lead to unjustified assumptions about capacity.

Capacity is to be assessed using a statutory test. This specifies that an individual is lacking capacity if they are unable to make decisions due to:

- The individual is unable to understand the information relevant to the decision.
- The individual is unable to retain that information.
- The individual is unable to use or weigh that information as part of the process of making the decision.
- The individual is unable to communicate a decision.

Best interests

If an individual is assessed as lacking capacity, everything that is done for or on behalf of that person must be in the person's best interests. The Act defines best interests and provides a checklist of factors that must be considered when deciding when to act in a person's best interests. An individual may put their wishes and feelings into a written statement in advance, which should be taken into account. The Best Interests Check-List includes the following:

- The period of incapacity and the possibility of regaining capacity in the future.
- The individual should be encouraged to participate as much as possible in decision making and information provided to them in the best practical way to assist them in doing so.
- The individual's past and present feelings, beliefs and values should be taken into account.
- A list of Statutory Consultees[1] should be consulted if practicable and their views taken into account.

[1]The list includes the following: 1. anyone named by the individual to be consulted 2. anyone caring for the person or interested in his welfare 3. any holder of an LPA 4. any court deputy

- Any relevant statement made when the person had capacity should be taken into account.
- Actions must not be motivated by a desire to bring about the person's death when the issue relates to life sustaining treatment.

When care or treatment are being provided for an individual who lacks capacity, the healthcare professional will not incur legal liability if this is undertaken in the individual's best interests. However, restraint[2] is only permitted if the person using it reasonably believes it is necessary to prevent harm to the incapacitated person and it is proportionate to the likihood and seriousness of harm.

Additional matters covered by the Mental Capacity Act

1. Lasting Powers of Attorney.

The Act creates a new role, allowing an individual to appoint an attorney to act on their behalf if they lose capacity in the future. The Lasting Power of Attorney (LPA) replaces the current Enduring Power of Attorney. An LPA can be used to appoint an individual to make decisions for a person who lacks capacity relating to their welfare and finances, as well as healthcare. This therefore permits an individual to appoint a Healthcare Proxy. Where a Healthcare Proxy is appointed under the terms of the LPA, that individual has all the rights to make decisions as to the healthcare of that individual that the incapacitated person would be able to make themselves if they had capacity. Where expressly granted, this can include decisions regarding life sustaining treatment.

2. Court Appointed Deputies

The Court of Protection can appoint a deputy. This will replace the current system of receivership. Deputies will be able to make financial decisions as before, but will also be able to make decisions on welfare and healthcare.

3. Independent Mental Capacity Advocates.

Where a person lacks capacity and, amongst other circumstances, serious medical treatment is proposed, an IMCA must be instructed. The IMCA makes representations about the person's wishes, feelings, beliefs and values and acts as an advocate for that person. They cannot make decisions on behalf of the incapacitated individual.

4. Advance Decisions.

The Common Law previously recognised Advance Directives (see above). The Act provides statutory rules for Advance Decisions. However, there are no formal requirements, nor does an Advance Decision need to be in writing, unless the Advance Decision relates to life sustaining treatment. Where it does, the Advance Decision must be in writing, signed and witnessed, and must expressly address the issue of life sustaining treatment.

5. Criminal Offence

The Act introduces a new Criminal Offence where an individual ill-treats or neglects a person who lacks capacity.

6. Research.

The Act provides a detailed regime where research is undertaken involving individuals who lack capacity.

7. Code of Practice.

The Mental Capacity Act is intended to provide a legal framework for all issues relating to those who lack capacity. A Code of Practice is to be published (publication is currently awaited) providing guidance and information on the implementation of the Act and advice on good practice. Unless there is good reason to depart from the provisions of the Code, its guidance should be followed.

Applications to the court to authorise medical treatment

If the patient's competence is unclear, the court can be asked to consider this. If the court finds that the patient is incompetent it can declare that a proposed treatment is lawful, even if the patient does not consent. Such declarations should be sought before treatment and can be obtained urgently at short notice.

Guidelines for court applications

1. Competent adult patients can refuse treatment.

2. Such a refusal should be recorded in writing by the patient or, if the patient refuses to do so, this should be entered and counter-signed in the medical records.

3. If the patient is definitely mentally incompetent, she should be treated in accordance with her best interests.

4. Treat in accordance with any advance directive – if the reliability of this is in doubt, apply to the court.

5. Identify concerns over capacity early (e.g. in antenatal clinics).

---

[2]Defined as the use or threat of force or the restriction of liberty

6. Obtain a psychiatric opinion on mental capacity.

7. Ensure that the patient has legal representation (if patient is unable to instruct solicitors, contact The Official Solicitor, tel: 0207 936 6000).

8. Take account of the criteria in Re MB 1997:
   a. Every person is presumed to have capacity to consent to or refuse medical treatment unless and until this presumption is rebutted.
   b. A competent woman who has sufficient capacity to decide can choose not to have medical intervention even though the consequence might be death or serious handicap of the fetus, or her own death.
   c. The graver the consequences of the decision the commensurately greater the level of competence required to take the decision.
   d. A patient can lack capacity if some impairment or disturbance of mental functioning renders the person unable to make a decision whether to consent or to refuse treatment. This might include temporary factors such as confusion, shock, fatigue, pain or drugs which might erode capacity. However, clinicians must be satisfied that such factors are operating to such a degree.
   e. Panic induced by fear might paralyse the will and thus destroy the capacity to make a decision.

SURROGACY

Surrogacy is an arrangement made before conception for a woman to hand over her child to another person.

- Surrogate agreements do not affect the child's legal parentage – therefore the birth mother and her partner remain parents until the genetic parents obtain a parental responsibility or an adoption order from the court.

- A surrogacy arrangement is not illegal itself. A woman can lawfully accept payment of her expenses.

- Medical staff assisting in the delivery of a child subject to a surrogacy arrangement is not unlawful.

- Consent to treatment for the surrogate mother remains her right and she retains all such rights in respect of the fetus/child (i.e. this is not a right of the genetic parents). Genetic parents can only obtain a parental responsibility order 6 weeks after birth. Until this time, parental responsibility remains with the birth parents. Be aware of the possibility of breaching the birth mother's medical confidentiality.

- Surrogacy arrangements are not enforceable contracts – if the birth mother changes her mind and wishes to keep the baby she is entitled to do so.

- The birth certificate will have the name of the birth mother, not the genetic mother.

TERMINATION OF PREGNANCY

Termination of pregnancy (TOP) may only be undertaken by a registered medical practitioner in accordance with the provisions of section 1 of the Abortion Act 1967. Otherwise any termination will be unlawful. The Abortion Act requires:

1. Two medical practitioners must agree:
   a. the pregnancy does not exceed 24 weeks and continuance would involve risk greater than if it were terminated of injury to the physical or mental health of the mother or existing children; or
   b. termination is necessary to prevent grave permanent injury to the physical or mental health of the woman; or
   c. continuance of the pregnancy would involve risk to the life of the pregnant woman greater than if the pregnancy were terminated; or
   d. there is a substantial risk that if the child were born it would suffer from such physical or mental abnormalities as to be seriously handicapped.

2. In determining a or b account may be taken of the woman's actual or foreseeable environment.

3. TOP must be carried out in a National Health Service (NHS) hospital or in a place approved by the Secretary of State for terminations.

4. The requirement for the opinion of two registered medical practitioners and for TOP to take place in a hospital is not required if the termination is immediately necessary to save the life or prevent grave permanent injury to the physical or mental health of the woman.

5. Notification of TOP is required to the Chief Medical Officer at the Department of Health.

6. Staff may not be compelled to take part in TOP and may exercise a conscientious objection to participation in such treatment – save that this exception does not affect any duty to participate in treatment necessary to save the life or to prevent grave

permanent injury to the physical or mental health of a woman.

7. Anything done to procure a miscarriage is unlawful unless authorised by the Abortion Act provisions referred to above.

8. Assisting in suspected illegal abortion can constitute a criminal offence as can procuring, administering or using drugs or instruments otherwise to procure an abortion.

CONFIDENTIALITY

Patient information may not be used for a different purpose or passed to anyone else without the consent of the patient. 'Patient information' applies to all personal information held in whatever form. It includes medical details and a patient's name and address, financial and domestic circumstances, etc. A patient should be informed of the uses to which information about them may be put. (Note that the use of personal data is restricted by the Data Protection Act.)

When confidential information may be passed on

A patient's healthcare information is held under legal and ethical obligations of confidentiality and should not be used or disclosed without consent. There are however exceptions to this rule that apply in certain specific circumstances.

A patient should be informed of the likely use and disclosure of their information associated with their healthcare. They should also be made aware of the choices that they have (and the implications of those choices) as to how information may be used and shared. Thereafter explicit consent is not usually required for use of the information for the purposes described and within the ambit of the consent given. Even then healthcare information should only be shared among the healthcare team on a 'need to know' basis.

There are however uses for information that are not directly associated with healthcare that individuals receive: research, public health, health service management, clinical audit. Specific consent should be obtained from the patient before patient information is used in connection with these.

Disclosure of information is restricted by a wide range of legal obligations including the Common Law of Confidentiality, the Data Protection Act 1998, the Human Rights Act 1998 and a further specific legislation that is beyond the ambit of this chapter (such

as the restriction on information related to sexually transmitted diseases including HIV under the NHS Trusts and Primary Care Trusts (Sexually Transmitted Diseases) Directions 2000).

In the absence of consent from the patient, confidential information may only be disclosed:

• where required by law, or

• where disclosure is ordered by a Court, or

• where disclosure is in the public interest in order to prevent and support the detection, investigation and punishment of serious crime and/or to prevent abuse or serious harm to others where they judge, on a case by case basis, that the public good that would be achieved by the disclosure out-weighs both the obligations of confidentiality to the individual patient concerned and the broader public interest in the provision of a confidential service. (Department of Health 2003.)

REGISTRATION OF BIRTHS AND STILLBIRTHS

It is the duty of the father or mother to notify within 42 days the Registrar for the Sub-District in which the birth takes place. If the father or mother are unable to do this the duty falls on the hospital authority in which the child is born.

For stillborn births, the information to be provided to the Registrar is a written certificate that the child was not born alive. The certificate must be signed by the registered practitioner or midwife in attendance at the birth or the person who has examined the body. A stillborn child is one born after 24 weeks of pregnancy who did not breathe after birth.

If an abandoned baby is found, the obligation to notify the Registrar falls on the person finding the child.

For adopted children, the obligation falls on the natural mother and father.

All births (in hospital or at home) must be notified by a doctor or midwife attending at the birth to the district medical officer within 36 hours.

NEGLIGENCE

Medical staff owe patients a duty of care. The standard of care is to act in accordance with practice that would be accepted by a responsible body of similar practitioners (Bolam v Friern 1957).

There is no breach of the standard of care if:

• you act in accordance with practice accepted by your peers and this was appropriate in this case

Table 2.1   Common situations leading to litigation – and how to avoid them

Complaint	Prevention
Patient did not consent	Ensure a patient has full information and consents to any treatment
Shoulder dystocia	Ensure senior staff are involved in delivery and carry out drill procedures
Cardiotocograph tracing shows ominous fetal heart rate patterns	Call for prompt medical assistance
Delay in proceeding to caesarean section in an emergency	Ensure all staff are aware of warning signs for the need to proceed to operative delivery and put in place necessary protocols to ensure this is achieved quickly (decision to delivery in 30 minutes)
Fetus delivered too early 'by dates'	Double-check dates at each antenatal appointment
Damage to the perineum	Experienced staff to follow established protocols

- there is no accepted body of opinion for this situation but what you did was reasonable in all the circumstances
- you did not follow accepted practice but what you did was reasonable in the circumstances.

Table 2.1 presents some common situations that may lead to litigation with suggestions as to how to avoid them.

MEDICAL RECORDS

Clear and detailed medical records enable communication between members of the clinical team. As such medical records are an important part of ensuring the quality of patient care. They also provide the best defence for staff when matters go wrong. Full and detailed notes should be made in all cases and clearly signed by the member of staff making them. A failure to do so may make a claim for compensation indefensible, or the fact that notes are incomplete can give rise to a breakdown in communication and thus poor patient care.

Therefore, record all important steps and decisions on patient care as contemporaneously and fully as possible, timing the entry and the time the event occurred. Sign, print name and indicate grade.

HUMAN RIGHTS ACT

The European Convention on Human Rights is now part of English Law (Human Rights Act 1998). Public authorities (such as NHS hospitals) must not act in a way that is incompatible with an individual's rights under the Convention including:

- Article 2 – everyone's right to life shall be protected by law.
- Article 3 – inhuman or degrading treatment is prohibited.
- Article 5 – all individuals have the right to liberty and security of their person, save where this is sanctioned by law (e.g. lawful detention of psychiatric patients).
- Article 8 – everyone has the right to respect for their private and family life, home and correspondence.
- Article 12 – men and women of marriageable age have the right to marry and found a family.

Where issues arise regarding an individual's human rights, legal advice should be sought.

ISSUES OF CLINICAL GOVERNANCE

Clinical governance is the organisations' concept of total quality management mapped across medical

---

Box 2.3   Essentials of risk management

- There is awareness of evidence-based practice and its relevance.
- Procedures and advice are dispensed by medical carers with the right level of experience.
- There is continuous audit and there are education programmes, such as for shoulder dystocia drill and cardiotocograph interpretation.
- There is good communication between medical carers and between medical carers and expectant mothers and their families. Loose talk and inadvertent comments are frequent sources for complaints.
- There is thorough and detailed review of events and outcomes surrounding every untoward incident.
- Encouragement of a no-blame culture to reinforce learning from mistakes and correct discrepancies.

practice. It is defined as a framework of practice where there is continuous improvement in service quality in an environment which encourages excellence in clinical care.

Well-trained staff involved in regular audit and risk assessment form the cornerstones for quality care.

Regular appraisal of staff to determine competency, proper supervision and continuing education will maintain high standards of clinical capability. Constant audit of process and procedures ensure improvement of service. Steps which will contribute to minimise clinical risk are listed in Box 2.3.

Bibliography

Abortion Act 1967. HMSO, London

Association of Anaesthetists of Great Britain and Ireland 1999 Information and Consent for Anaesthesia. Association of Anaesthetists of Great Britain and Ireland, London

Bolam v Friern Hospital Management Committee 1957 2 All ER 118 1 WLR 582 Judgement of Mr Justice McNair

British Medical Association 2003 Consent Toolkit, 2nd edn. BMA, London

Department of Health 2001 Reference Guide to Consent for Examination or Treatment. HMSO, London

Department of Health 2003 Confidentiality: NHS Code of Practice November 2003. HMSO, London

General Medical Council 2001 Guidance: Intimate Examinations. GMC, London

General Medical Council 2002 Ethical Guidance. GMC, London

HC(90)22 A Guide to Consent for Examination or Treatment

HSG(92)32 Patient Consent to Examination or Treatment Model Forms

Human Rights Act 1998. HMSO, London

Medical Defence Union 1992 Consent to Treatment. Available from the Medical Defence Union (MDU). Tel: 0207 486 6181

Medical Research Council 2001 Human Tissue and Biological Samples for Use in Research. MRC, London

Mental Health Act 1983. HMSO, London

National Collaborating Centre for Women's and Children's Health 2004 Caesarean Section. Clinical Guideline. RCOG Press, London

Re MB 1997 2 FLR 426

Royal College of Obstetricians and Gynaecologists 2002 The Care of Women Requesting Induced Abortion, Guideline. Setting standards to improve women's health. RCOG, London

Section 124 NHS Act 1977. HMSO, London

Chapter **3**

Maternal and perinatal mortality

David T Y Liu
Mentor: Charles Rodeck

CHAPTER CONTENTS

Maternal mortality   14
   Cause of maternal mortality   14
   Pulmonary thromboembolism and
      thrombosis   14
   Haemorrhage   15
   Hypertensive disorders   15
   Amniotic fluid embolism   15
   Sepsis   15
   Genital trauma – uterine rupture   16
   Anaesthesia   16
Perinatal mortality   16

Reports from the Confidential Enquiries into Maternal Deaths in the UK have appeared every 3 years since 1952 and are the first example of audit by the medical profession. The Department of Health document *A First Class Service – Quality in the New NHS* (1998) states that all health workers are required to participate in these enquiries. Information and case notes must be made available for enquiry assessors and reports completed within 9 months of the death. The 1994–1996 triennia audit emphasised awareness of social and public health issues. These issues include advice for seatbelt usage, identification and coordinated care for psychiatric disorders especially postnatal depression, impact of social sequestration from access to help and contribution from domestic violence.

These enquiries have led to substantial improvement in care and safety for childbirth. The direct maternal death rate for the 1994–1996 triennium is 6.1 per 100 000 maternities (total of 12.2 per 100 000 maternities). Women older than 40 years, high parity, thromboembolism, pregnancy hypertension, amniotic fluid embolism, sepsis, haemorrhage and uterine rupture remain as salient but often avoidable causations. There is no room for complacency. In the 2000–2002 triennium the direct death rate is 3.5 per 100 000 maternities. In the past 6 years indirect causes have exceeded direct causes of maternal deaths, emphasising the need for coordinated multidisciplinary care when a woman has an existing psychiatric or medical condition. Inadequate contribution and support from experienced senior obstetricians, and inappropriate delegation and treatment emphasise the need for protocols, teamwork and drills to address emergencies. The continuing challenge is to achieve year on year improvement in the safety and satisfaction of childbirth, using evidence-based practice.

MATERNAL MORTALITY

Maternal mortality is defined by the *International Classification of Diseases, Injuries and Causes of Death – Ninth Revision* (ICD9; World Health Organization (WHO) 1993) as 'death of a woman while pregnant or within 42 days of termination of pregnancy from any cause related to or aggravated by the pregnancy or its management, but not from accidental or incidental causes.' This is further subdivided into the following in which maternities are defined as pregnancies which result in a live birth at any gestation or a stillbirth occurring at or after 24 completed weeks' gestation. (Note statement for twin pregnancies.)

- Direct obstetric death results from obstetric complications of the pregnancy state.

- Indirect obstetric death is where existing or pregnancy precipitated medical disorders led to or is associated with maternal mortality, for example following diabetes mellitus, cardiac diseases, vascular aneurysm, epilepsy or suicides.

- Fortuitous obstetric death is when pregnancy is incidental to the causation, for example road traffic accident, murder or unrelated malignancies.

- Late obstetric death. The *ICD10* revision (WHO 1993) introduced inclusion of direct and indirect deaths 'occurring between 42 days and one year after abortion, miscarriage or delivery.' The last two Confidential Enquires included late deaths in their figures.

Cause of maternal mortality

Only direct and indirect deaths are counted for the Confidential Enquiries. The denominator is registered live or stillbirths and not total pregnancies as exact numbers of pregnancies are not known. International comparison is not reliable as not all countries use the same inclusion criteria. The increase in the maternal mortality figures for the 1994–1996 triennium reflected alterations in the baseline with inclusion of extra cases. Salient causes of death relevant to the labour ward remained similar for 2000–2002 and included pulmonary thromboembolism, hypertensive diseases, amniotic fluid emboli, sepsis and uterine rupture. Deaths due to anaesthesia and haemorrhage increased.

Substandard care continues as a contributory factor (over 50%). Steps for improvement include:

- Awareness of your limitations. Seek advice when there is uncertainty or doubt.
- Ensure delegation is appropriate for the level of competency.

- Consultants or experienced seniors must attend to assist or supervise where complications are anticipated.
- Become familiar with protocols, evidence-based practice and drills for emergencies. A team approach with inclusion of relevant disciplines is essential for complex situations or emergencies.
- Where possible identify potential risk in the antenatal period (e.g. risk assessment charts).

The lowest mortality is in the second pregnancy while age more than 40 remains a risk factor. Socially isolated ethnic groups, for example new immigrants with communication difficulties, need particular attention. The 2000–2002 Enquiry included the socially disadvantaged, the obese (body mass index (BMI) 35 or more) substance misuse, domestic violence and limited antenatal care as risk factors for maternal deaths. Psychiatric disorders were the leading cause of indirect maternal mortality for 1997–1999 and remained so in the 2000–2002 triennium.

Pulmonary thromboembolism and thrombosis

In the UK the rate of pulmonary embolism is between 1 and 2.1 per 100 000 maternities and remains the major direct cause of maternal mortality. Most women survive if thromboembolism is treated. Failure to provide prophylaxis, to diagnose the condition or consider possibility of diagnosis continues to place mothers at risk. The following steps should be taken to reduce risk:

- Identify family or personal history of thrombosis. Screening for thrombophilia and antiphospholipid antibody, for example cardiolipin, Leiden factor V mutation and anti-lupus anticoagulant may be appropriate to plan prophylaxis. Antenatal classification into low, moderate or high risk is helpful for focusing attention.

- Women older that 35 years weighing over 80 kg (BMI 35 or more), and after having four babies require some form of prophylaxis. Consider prophylaxis after 4 days of bed rest when there is pre-eclampsia, dehydration and major medical illness or infection.

- In addition to stockings, heparin prophylaxis in adequate doses must be prescribed when there is a personal or family history of thrombosis, thrombophilia or when major surgery is being contemplated.

- When there is a suspicion or there are symptoms suggestive of venous thrombosis or pulmonary embolism perform a duplex ultrasound examination or ventilation–perfusion lung scan.

- Neither unfractionated nor low molecular weight heparin cross the placenta. Where risk is high prescribe unfractionated heparin 7500 units every 12 hours or equivalent (e.g. Clexane 20 mg or 2000 units for moderate risk and 4000 units for high risk 2 hours before surgery). Appropriate doses must be prescribed.

- Continue prophylaxis for 5 days or until mobilised. Women with a history of thromboembolism need prophylaxis for 6 weeks.

- In contemporary practice all caesarean sections are covered by prophylaxis for thromboembolism.

Haemorrhage

Death due to severe haemorrhage has fallen to 5.5 per 1 000 000 maternities. Haemorrhage occurs in 1 in 1000 deliveries, and the management of this complication can be improved by:

- appropriate delegation for difficult caesarean sections such as placenta praevia, particularly when the placenta is sited anterior with a previous caesarean section scar

- frequent drills to familiarise staff with protocols for severe haemorrhage, including test communication with blood banks. Recruit help from haematologists and anaesthetists. Postpartum haemorrhage (loss of 500 ml or more of blood) occurs in 1% of deliveries. Correct estimation of blood loss and being aware of clotting defect is important

- early resort to hysterectomy if bleeding continues despite simple procedures

- transfer of care to a tertiary unit when risk of haemorrhage is considered to be high

- consider agreeing on a management plan for women who decline blood products.

Hypertensive disorders

The following are suggested to improve care:

- Educate medical staff and women about the significance of complications, need for prompt attention or delivery, and benefit of a team approach in a referral centre where senior expertise is available. Proteinuria and/or hypertension can present alone before the full clinical picture.

- Clear guidelines and protocols must be in place for management of pre-eclampsia and eclampsia.

- Mortality due to hypertension ranges between 9 and 12 per 1 000 000 maternities. Mothers younger than 25 years are at particular risk. The risk also increases with age (>35), severe obesity and a family history of pre-eclampsia.

- An average of 6 days separate normality at antenatal review and subsequent onset of hypertension. Ensure close liaison with general practitioners and community midwives as the complication can arise between antenatal visits.

- Monitor severity and progression of pre-eclampsia by full blood count, uric acid, electrolytes, and liver and renal function tests. Fluid overload with pulmonary oedema and acute respiratory distress syndrome (ARDS) is a frequent cause of death. Cerebral pathology, particularly infarction and haemorrhage, is also significant.

- Administer antihypertensive drugs early to prevent high systolic blood pressure – a risk for intracerebral haemorrhage.

Amniotic fluid embolism

Sudden collapse (hypotension and cardiac arrest), respiratory distress, and cyanosis followed rapidly by death is suggestive of this complication but lung autopsy showing presence of squames and hair is needed for confirmation. Prevention is difficult but note the following:

- Strong uterine contractions, fetal distress and severe haemorrhage due to coagulopathy are other clinical features. Avoid uterine over-stimulation and delay in resolving obstructed labour.

- Complications increase with age (over 35 years) and high parity. Although classically associated with polyhydramnios and induction of labour with oxytocics, other obstetric complications can contribute. It is not common in a totally straightforward pregnancy but amniotic fluid embolism can present before onset of labour.

- Early transfer for intensive care is important when complication presents.

Sepsis

Puerperal sepsis has increased in the UK and remains the fourth major cause of maternal mortality. This is associated with increased virulence in streptococcal infections. To reduce the risk:

- Note history of infection especially haemolytic streptococcal infections. Exclude infections in complications such as prolonged membrane rupture or presence of a cervical suture.

- Investigate promptly any pyrexia. (Pyrexia may be absent especially in severe sepsis.) Check full blood count. Note presence of thrombocytopenia. Obtain blood culture. Recruit help from microbiologist for severe infection. Do not wait for culture results before instigating broad-spectrum antibiotics.
- Prescribe prophylactic antibiotics where indicated. This is routine for caesarean section in contemporary practice.

Genital trauma – uterine rupture

Death rate due to uterine rupture is between 1.3 and 2.3 per 1 000 000 maternities. For further details see Chapter 14 and note the following when there is a uterine scar:

- An experienced obstetrician must assess suitability for vaginal delivery. Exclude risk of disproportion and pelvic anatomical deformities.
- Conduct delivery in an equipped unit with full maternal and fetal surveillance. An experienced obstetrician must supervise care.
- Emphasise again care with oxytocic usage for induction of labour and recognition of signs and symptoms of uterine rupture (Chapters 15 and 17).

Anaesthesia

The rate of death due to anaesthesia has dropped to 0.5 per 1 000 000 maternities (it was about 1.4 per 1 000 000 between 1997 and 1999). Between 2000 and 2002 there were 6 instead of 3 deaths all due to general anaesthesia with inadequate supervision of junior anaesthetists. Good communication within a multidisciplinary team, availability of consultant advice and support, prompt appropriate decisions and ready access to intensive care units will continue to reduce the contribution from anaesthesia to maternal mortality. The labour ward is not suitable for high dependency care. The following should be noted:

- Adrenaline is the drug of choice for severe anaphylaxis.
- All medical personnel should be aware of resuscitation techniques and airway maintenance.
- Identify at risk mothers antenatally for assessment by consultant anaesthetist.

PERINATAL MORTALITY

Perinatal mortality is defined as a stillbirth from 24 weeks onwards or the death of a liveborn baby at any gestational age within 7 days of birth (early neonatal death). Death of one twin delivered after 24 weeks is considered a stillbirth. Some countries accept the range from 20 weeks' gestation to 28 days after birth hence comparisons must take the definition into consideration. In England and Wales the perinatal mortality is about 9 per 1000. Factors associated with perinatal mortality include:

- congenital and inherited abnormalities
- perinatal mortality is increased after the third birth, in multiple pregnancies and when birth weight is low such as preterm births and fetal growth restriction
- perinatal mortality is increased when women have obstetric and medical complications.

Discuss mode of delivery with women and their partners. If vaginal delivery is appropriate close surveillance is mandatory. The process of labour can exert hypoxic stress. If there is much fetal compromise deliver by caesarean section.

More important than mortality is maternal and fetal morbidity, for which we have no detailed statistics.

References

Department of Health 1998 A First Class Service – Quality in the New NHS. London, Department of Health

World Health Organization 1993a International Classification of Diseases, Injuries and Causes of Death – Ninth Revision. WHO, Geneva

World Health Organization 1993b International Classification of Diseases, Injuries and Causes of Death – Tenth Revision. WHO, Geneva

Bibliography

CESDI 2000 The Fetal and Infant Postmortem. Maternal and Child Health Consortium 2000. CESDI, London

Department of Health 1998 Why Mothers Die. Report on Confidential Enquiries into Maternal Deaths in the United Kingdom 1994–1996. TSO, London

Duley L, Gulmezoglu AM Henderson-Smart DJ 2000 Anticonvulsants for women with pre-eclampsia. Cochrane Database of Systematic Reviews (2): CD000025. Update in: Cochrane Database of Systematic Reviews 2003 (2):CD000025

Drife J 1997 Management of primary post partum haemorrhage. British Journal of Gynaecology 104: 275–277

Holme SE 1996 Invasive group A streptococcal infections. New England Journal of Medicine 335: 590–591

Polkinghorne J 1989 Review of the Guidance on the Research use of Fetuses and Fetal Material. HMSO, London

Royal College of Obstetricians and Gynaecologists 2005 Why Mothers Die 2000–2002. The sixth report of the Confidential Enquiries into Maternal and Child Health (CEMACH) in the United Kingdom. RCOG Press, London

Royal College of Obstetricians and Gynaecologists 1995 Report of a Working Party on Prophylaxis against Thrombo-embolism in Gynaecology and Obstetrics. RCOG Press, London

Scottish Office Department of Health 1998 Acute Services Review Report. SODH, Edinburgh

The Welsh Office 1998 Quality Care and Clinical Excellence. The Welsh Office, Cardiff

Chapter 4

The birthing environment

Amanda Sullivan, Carol McCormick

CHAPTER CONTENTS

Hospital birthing rooms   19
Support in labour   20
Use of water immersion for labour and birth   20
   Guidelines for water birth   21
Home birth   21
Psychological requirements for the place of
   birth   22

A labouring woman's sense of safety and privacy influences the birth process (Buckley 2004). This fundamental and life-changing event should therefore take place in an optimum environment. The environment for birth should take account of new developments in attitudes and practice while remaining mindful of safety for all concerned (Royal College of Obstetricians and Gynaecologists (RCOG) and Royal College of Midwives (RCM) 1999).

HOSPITAL BIRTHING ROOMS

The importance of creating a home-like birth environment was shown in a systematic review by Hodnett et al (2005) which found that home-like settings significantly reduce the need for intrapartum analgesia, and increase spontaneous vaginal birth and maternal satisfaction.

Birthing rooms should be comfortable, decorated in a homely style and contain, or have access to, equipment that allows mobility and position change such as beanbags and floor mats. It is important to match facilities with workload and work within national guidelines. For example a cardiotocograph (CTG) must be used in conjunction with fetal blood sampling (National Institute for Clinical Excellence (NICE) 2001).

Towards Safer Childbirth (RCOG and RCM 1999) specifies the requirements for equipment in the case of emergency, which was supplemented on the basis of local experience. The full list of equipment is shown in Box 4.1.

There should be guidelines in place for pathways of care and prompt access to high-dependency facilities such as adult and neonatal high-dependency unit/intensive care. An ultrasound scanner should be

Box 4.1 Equipment for hospital birthing rooms

Fetal assessment
- Two to four CTG machines per 1000 births (with facilities for monitoring twins)
- Pinard stethoscope/Doppler/hand held electrical auscultation device
- Access to fetal blood sampling

Neonatal resuscitation
- Flat surface with a heat source (radiant or/and mattress)
- Clock
- Suction
- Oxygen/air mix with variable regulated flow mix and adjustable pressure relief valve including positive end-expiratory pressure (PEEP) and neonatal size Ambu bag
- Neonatal laryngoscopes
- Endotracheal tubes
- Umbilical catheterisation pack, syringes scissors
- Drugs including surfactant

Maternal resuscitation
- Bed available for prompt resuscitation
- Oxygen and suction
- Equipment for intravenous access and resuscitation
- Drugs including oxytocics, and drugs for cardiac resuscitation and anaphylaxis
- Defibrillator

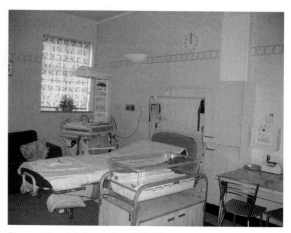

Figure 4.1   A fully equipped birthing room.

available for use by staff trained in its use. Beds should be easily adaptable for assisted birthing and be effortlessly mobile so in an emergency the woman can be transported while in her bed to a dedicated obstetric theatre. Emergency equipment should be out of view (for example in purpose-built cupboards) from the labouring woman and her partner or companion (Figure 4.1).

SUPPORT IN LABOUR

An appropriate birthing environment must be accompanied by a philosophy which encourages only necessary and evidence-based interventions. The atmosphere created by staff is equally a vital part of the environment. Staff should be kind and supportive, open and honest. Privacy and confidentiality must be respected. Staff must behave in a way that is as unobtrusive as possible. Most women will request the presence of a birth companion for support. Positive effects, including reduction in the rates of caesarean

sections have been demonstrated when this birth companion is a doula (a laywoman experienced in providing continuous emotional, informational and physical support in labour). If a doula is not available, evidence suggests that support from a significant other or midwife also leads to a more positive childbirth experience.

USE OF WATER IMMERSION FOR LABOUR AND BIRTH

In the UK, water immersion labour and birth is now an option in both hospital and community settings. This option is offered only to women with a normal obstetric history and a problem-free spontaneous labour at term. Women with complicated pregnancies requesting this option will need individual assessment. Research findings concerning the safety and efficacy of the option remain inconclusive. However, both RCM (1995) and RCOG (2001) have issued position statements and guidelines as most maternity units in the UK now have purpose-built rooms (Figure 4.2) for a water birth (Box 4.2).

The potential benefits of a water birth include:

- Woman's choice – for relaxation
- Reduced need for pharmacological analgesia
- Shorter labour
- Cost effective

Potential hazards include:

- Delay in instigating emergency interventions
- Increased incidence of postpartum haemorrhage
- Increased maternal and neonatal infection

Women should be given balanced information to enable them to make an informed choice.

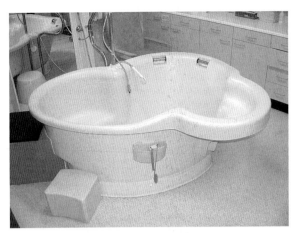

Figure 4.2   Equipment for a water birth.

Box 4.3   Equipment for home birth (in addition to equipment for any other birth)

- Phone
- Warm environment
- Entonox or intramuscular pain relief of woman's choice
- Suturing equipment and lidocaine
- Light source
- Scales
- Birth notification forms
- Emergency kit containing equipment for intravenous access, catheterisation, and maternal and fetal resuscitation
- Oxytocin (Syntocinon)

Box 4.2   Requirements for a water birth

Infection control
- Liquid soap to wash pool after use – pool should be completely dry when not in use.
- Safe tap water should enter and exit water drain out through separate apertures.

Maternal and fetal wellbeing/health and safety
- Manual handling training for staff.
- Awareness of how to act in an emergency – shoulder dystocia, maternal collapse.
- Equipment (reinforced net) and guideline for emergency lift out of pool.
- Non-slip floor.
- Any electrical equipment used must meet the standard for bathrooms.
- Besides equipment as for any other birth, a water thermometer is required to check the pool temperature hourly.

Guidelines for water birth

- The use of water must be at the woman's request.
- There should be no known or envisaged obstetric problem.
- Labour must not be pre or post term. Labour should have commenced between 37 and 41 weeks' of gestation.
- An admission fetal heart trace, CTG, is not compulsory but the fetal heart rate should be recorded prior to the use of the pool.
- The presentation must be cephalic.
- All maternal observations must be within normal limits.

- No sedatives should have been administered for at least 4 hours.
- If there are any abnormalities such as raised blood pressure, the midwife must seek the advice of an obstetrician.
- The woman and her partner must agree to leave the pool if requested to do so by the midwife.

HOME BIRTH

Although some areas in the UK have a 10% home birth rate (Office of National Statistics 2003) the national rate across England is about 2% (Department of Health (DoH) 2003). The *National Service Framework for Children, Young People and Maternity Services* (DoH 2004) recommends that women be given the choice for the most appropriate place to give birth, which includes delivery at home and midwifery-led units, provided there are facilities for rapid transfer to a hospital if complications arise.

Some women may prefer to deliver at home because of the convenience of being in their own environment, reduced interference in labour and less restriction. Planned home birth is only advisable for low-risk pregnancies, but what constitutes a low-risk pregnancy is difficult to anticipate. Robust and clear guidelines for transfer to hospital should problems arise must be in place (RCOG and RCM 1999). The midwife must recognise when transfer is necessary and act accordingly.

A midwife attending home births must be proficient in managing emergencies and able to initiate resuscitation of both the mother and baby in the home. The midwife must accompany the mother during transfer. This statement also applies for transfer from midwifery-led delivery units. The equipment required for home delivery is listed in Box 4.3.

PSYCHOLOGICAL REQUIREMENTS FOR THE PLACE OF BIRTH

Although the physical environment is important for the safety and wellbeing of those involved with a birth, as stated at the beginning of this chapter the atmosphere created by staff is also vital. Carers should be pleasant and relaxed while remaining as unobtrusive as possible. Women and their chosen companions must be allowed to share the birth experience with maximum privacy and dignity. Teaching hospitals require students to gain experience, but the wishes of the woman should be paramount. At times, gender issues may arise and women and their partners may request female attendants. Where possible, the wishes of parents should be respected. Good working relationships between members of the multidisciplinary team involved in a woman's care are essential. A spirit of collaboration and clear lines of communication between staff can significantly enhance women's perceptions of their birth environment in a positive light.

References

Buckley S 2004 Undisturbed birth – nature's hormonal blueprint for safety, ease and ecstasy. MIDIRS Midwifery Digest 14(2):203–209

Department of Health 2003 Report to the DoH Children's Taskforce from the Maternity and Neonatal Workforce Group. Part 1: the nature of care during pregnancy and childbirth. DoH, London

Department of Health 2004 National Service Framework for Children, Young People and Maternity Services. Standard 11. The Stationery Office, London

Hodnett ED, Downe S, Edwards N et al 2005 Home like versus conventional institutional settings for birth. Cochrane Database of Systematic Reviews, Issue 1

National Institute for Clinical Excellence 2001 The Use of Electronic Fetal Monitoring. NICE, London

Office of National Statistics 2003 Birth Statistics: Births and Patterns of Family Building. England and Wales. ONS, London

Royal College of Midwives 1995 The Use of Water During Birth – Position Statement. RCM, London

Royal College of Obstetricians and Gynaecologists 2001 Birth in Water, RCOG Statement No 1. RCOG, London

Royal College of Obstetricians and Gynaecologists and Royal College of Midwives 1999 Towards Safer Childbirth. Minimum Standards for the Organisation of Labour Wards, Report of the RCOG/RCM working parties. RCOG/RCM, London

Bibliography

Chamberlain G, Wraight A, Crowley P 1997 Home Births. The Report of the 1994 Confidential Enquiry by National Birthday Trust Fund. Parthenon, USA

Charles C 1998 Fetal hyperthermia risk from warm water immersion. British Journal of Midwifery 6:152–156

Cluett E, Pickering RM, Getliffe K et al 2004 Randomised controlled trial of labouring in water compared with standard of augmentation for management of dystocia in the first stage of labour. BMJ 328:314–318

Geissbuehler V, Stein S, Eberhard J 2004 Waterbirths compared with land births: an observational study of nine years, Journal of Perinatal Medicine 32(4): 308–314

Nicum R, Karoo R 1998 Expectations and opinions of pregnant women about medical students being involved in care at the time of delivery. Medical Education (32)3:320–324

Olsen O, Jewell MD 1993 Home versus hospital birth. Cochrane Database of Systematic Reviews, Issue 3

Stockton A 2003 Doulas – the future guardians of normal birth? MIDIRS Midwifery Digest 13(3):347–350

Tarkka MT, Paunonen M 1996 Social support and its impact on mothers' experience of childbirth. Journal of Advanced Nursing 23:70–75

Woodward J, Kelly SM 2004 A pilot study for a randomised controlled trial of waterbirth versus land birth. British Journal of Obstetrics and Gynaecology 111:537–545

Yogev S 2004 MIDIRS Midwifery Digest 14(4):486–492

Chapter 5

Admission to labour ward

David T Y Liu

CHAPTER CONTENTS

Admission for labour   23
    Organisational requirements   24
    Requirements for quality care   24
Assessment following admission   24
    Presentation   24
    Lie   24
    Engagement   25
    Auscultation   25
    Examination of abdomen and pelvis   25
    Cervical examination   27
    Vaginal examination   27
    Pelvic examination   28
        Contracted pelvis   28
        Routine for pelvic examination   30
        Erect lateral pelvimetry (ELP)   31
Subsequent management   32

ADMISSION FOR LABOUR

The modern labour ward subserves many functions. It is a place where women can self-admit or are referred for assessment and reviewed by a well-equipped obstetric team when there are anxieties or complications associated with their pregnancy, for example suspected preterm labour, membrane rupture or abdominal pain.

Requirements for care are:

- Take a detailed history. Review the obstetric and gynaecological history.
- If appropriate, consult colleagues in other medical disciplines.
- Perform a thorough examination of the woman and fetus. This can include a cardiotocograph record and an ultrasound scan for reassurance.
- Reassure and allow home if there is no evidence of complication. Where necessary arrange follow-up appointments to ensure continuity of care.
- Admit to the antenatal ward for observation or treatment if there are medical or obstetric reasons. There is a place for admission to promote a caring attitude when a woman's anxieties are not resolved.

The labour ward is also a place for emergency care of expectant mothers. Reasons for admission include medical emergencies, for example status asthmaticus or myocardial infarction, and obstetric complications, for example antepartum haemorrhage or eclampsia. When an emergency situation arises:

- Address the emergency. Stabilise the woman's condition.
- Recruit support from appropriate colleagues such as anaesthetists, haematologists, physicians or

surgeons. Where possible consult colleagues with particular interest in obstetrics.

- Address obstetric emergencies (see Chapter 6).
- Document clearly in detail all steps undertaken. This retrospective record is made as soon as possible when memories of events are still fresh in the mind.
- Keep partners and accompanying persons fully informed.
- Any emergency is a frightening situation. Efficient professionalism contributes much to a calm atmosphere and reduces anxiety.

Organisational requirements

The various functions of the labour ward demand a sound organisational structure to provide effective care. Requirements include:

- A lead clinician with particular interest in the labour ward and a lead midwife coordinator.

- A labour ward forum which meets on a regular basis (for example weekly) to encompass audit, teaching, health and safety and risk management issues.

- Close liaison with neonatologists.

- Frequent drills and regular updating to anticipate emergencies, for example shoulder dystocia or haemorrhage, to ensure provision of evidence-based care. Ability to interpret cardiotocograph traces is essential.

- Levels of staffing must be adequate. A robust process for induction of new staff of all levels, regular appraisal and continuing education programmes must be in place.

- A senior obstetrician supervises and must be readily available to advise and support. The ideal is a move towards consultant-based care for complicated pregnancies whereas midwives will attend to normal deliveries.

Requirements for quality care

Cultural changes prompted by better information, national (for example 'Changing childbirth' (Brown and Lumley 1998)) and international (for example National Health and Medical Research Council (NHMRC) 1996) directives, and surveys indicate women and their partners expect quality and satisfaction in addition to safe delivery. There is evidence to show the following contribute to perceived quality and satisfaction:

- Rapport and satisfaction during antenatal care.
- A welcoming attitude at the time of admission.
- Good communication. Women and partners kept well-informed at all stages and encouraged to participate in care decisions.
- Reassurance, encouragement and good pain relief. These steps are essential if active labour unexpectedly extends beyond 12 hours.
- Limiting the number of people in the delivery room at any one time. Respect the need for privacy.
- Ensuring continuity of care expectations even if the carer changes. Not all personal midwives can stay for the whole duration of labour.
- Being as helpful as possible.
- Taking note of the choice of language used for communication.
- Limiting use of episiotomy.
  Labour is the most common reason for admission.
- Ascertain detailed history to determine diagnosis for onset of labour, the state of the fetal membranes and the presence of mucoid show.
- Consider the differential diagnosis for intermittent abdominal pain, vaginal bleeding and leakage of fluid from the vagina (e.g. urinary incontinence or infection).
- Review the antenatal history. Knowledge of antenatal history is particularly important when women ring in for advice. Document main points of conversation.
- Reassure once the correct diagnosis of labour has been established.

ASSESSMENT FOLLOWING ADMISSION

Presentation

This describes the fetal part presented or nearest to the cervix, e.g. cephalic presentation.

Lie

This defines the relation between the longitudinal axis of the fetus and that of the mother (Figure 5.1).

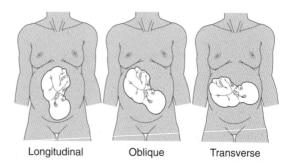

Longitudinal   Oblique   Transverse

Figure 5.1   Longitudinal, oblique and transverse lie.

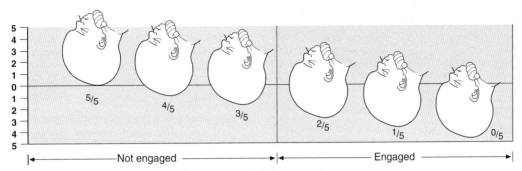

Figure 5.2   Engagement described in fifths: left, non-engaged; right, engaged.

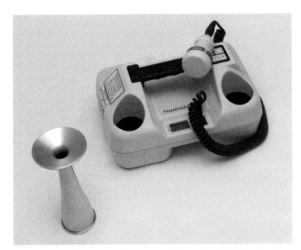

Figure 5.3   Pinard stethoscope and Doppler fetal heart rate detector.

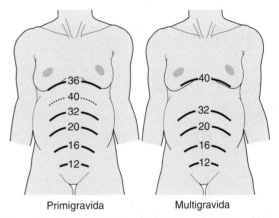

Figure 5.4   Fundal height in primigravida and multigravida.

Engagement

This occurs when the biparietal (vertex) or bi-ischial (breech) diameters descend below the pelvic brim. Descent of the fetal head into the pelvis is usually described as if the head is divided into five segments. The head would be engaged if less than three-fifths were palpable above the pelvic brim (Figure 5.2).

Auscultation

Auscultate with a Pinard stethoscope (Figure 5.3). The position of the anterior shoulder is further from the midline in the occipito-lateral and posterior positions.

Examination of abdomen and pelvis

* Place the woman on her back, with her head on a single pillow, her hands by her side and both knees slightly bent. The bladder should be empty. Use the semi-recumbent position if supine hypotension troubles.
* Note the general health and clinical condition, for example generalised oedema. Record temperature, pulse, blood pressure, and examine urine for presence of protein, ketones, sugar and blood.
* Observe and note the shape and contour of the abdomen.
* Note the frequency, duration and intensity of uterine contractions.
* Stand on the woman's right side, maintain rapport by conversation and watch her facial expression as a guide to inadvertent cause of discomfort during palpation.
* Warm hands and palpate the abdomen gently to estimate the gestational age by fundal height, approximate fetal size, lie, presentation, amount of liquor and engagement of the presenting part.
* Place hand on the fundus or measure to estimate fundal height. Percuss if there is difficulty locating upper limit of uterus. Fundal height is only a rough guide to gestational age (Figure 5.4).

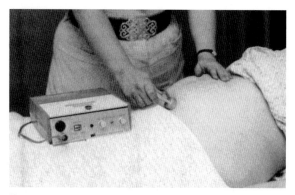

Figure 5.5   Detection of fetal heart rate by Doppler technique.

Many physical features, such as the woman's stature, affect estimation of gestation by fundal height. Take into account the weight of the woman and her partner, when they were born and the size of the previous babies. A reduction in fundal height in primigravidae near term is due to engagement of the presenting part.

- Auscultate with the Pinard stethoscope or Doppler fetal heart rate heart detector (Figure 5.3). Fetal heart sound is loudest over the anterior fetal shoulder (Figure 5.5). Listen through a contraction to exclude late fetal heart rate deceleration.

- Perform speculum examination (Box 5.1) if indicated.

Box 5.1   Speculum examination

Pass the speculum (Figure 5.6) with full aseptic precautions to examine the cervix.

Step 1
Explain the need for examination, cleanse the vulval area and indicate your intention before insertion of the instrument.

Cusco's speculum: Step 2
Insert the speculum with the blades closed and in line with opening of the introitus for 3–4 cm, rotate so the handle is towards the sacrum. Warn the woman of the sensation of pressure as the speculum is opened.

Step 3
Advance speculum to locate cervix.

Sim's speculum: Step 2
Place the woman in Sim's position. Insert the speculum 3–4 cm, maintaining direction towards the sacrum. Warn the woman of sensation of pressure as speculum is gently pulled backwards to view cervix (Figure 5.7).

Step 3
Consider the position of the fourchette to be 6 o'clock. Move the speculum through an arc between 5 and 7 o'clock to obtain a better view. Displace the anterior vaginal wall with sponge forceps if necessary.

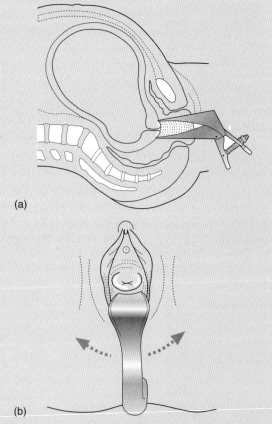

(a)

(b)

Figure 5.7   Illustrating use of (a) Cusco's and (b) Sim's speculum.

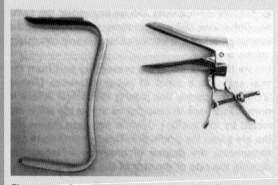

Figure 5.6   Speculums in common use: Sim's (left) and Cusco's (right).

- If the membranes are ruptured, note the colour of the amniotic fluid and whether meconium or blood staining is present. Take samples for culture if the membranes have been ruptured for more than 6 hours.

- Note application of the presenting part of the fetus to the cervix. Exclude cord prolapse.

Cervical examination

- The cervix dilates in concentric circles from a diameter of less than 1 cm to full dilatation of 10 cm. Estimate cervical dilatation (Figure 5.8).

- The cervix is essentially a thick cylinder of collagen. Before dilatation can occur a process of thinning and shortening, or effacement, must take place. During pregnancy and early labour physiological changes are directed towards softening of the cervix (Figure 5.9).

   Effacement reflects the existence of uterine activity and indicates the ease and readiness of the cervix to dilate. Once the effaced cervix can no longer resist uterine contractions, dilatation begins.

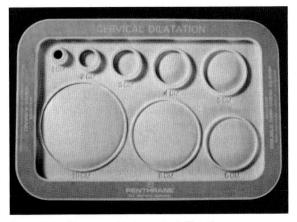

Figure 5.8   Plate as guide to cervical dilatation.

- Before removal of the speculum check for normality of the cervix, for the presence of vaginal infection and for evidence of varicosities. When indicated take cervical swabs. Learn to recognise presence of active herpes infection.

Vaginal examination

- Use full aseptic precautions (speculum examination only if membranes have ruptured).

- Warn the woman of what to expect.

- Insert the index and, if that is tolerated, the middle finger through the introitus.

- Palpate around the fornices and sense the proximity of the presenting part of the fetus to the examining finger. A spongy feel interposed between the finger and the presenting part warns of the possibility of undiagnosed placenta praevia.

- Confirm observed cervical dilatation. The number of fingers accommodated by the cervix can be used as a measure, e.g. four fingers indicates full dilatation (one finger-breadth is approximately 1.5 cm).

- Feel for fetal membranes. If the membranes are ruptured exclude cord prolapse. If the membranes are intact palpate to exclude pulsations due to cord presentation or vasa praevia. When active labour is present and the cervix is 4 cm or more dilated the membranes can be ruptured to facilitate labour. A scalp 'clip' for electronic fetal heart rate monitoring can be applied at the same time. Determine the presentation, application of the presenting part of the fetus, and length and consistency of the cervix.

- Estimate the distance of the presenting part from the ischial spine as a point of pelvic reference (Figure 5.10). The imaginary line joining the ischial spines is station 0. Positions in centimetres above the spine are denoted by the prefix '−' and posi-

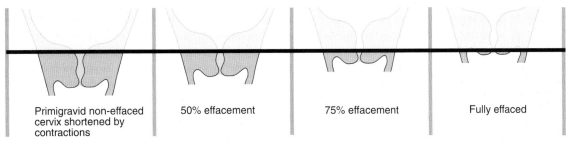

Primigravid non-effaced cervix shortened by contractions   50% effacement   75% effacement   Fully effaced

Figure 5.9   Cross-section of cervix to illustrate the degree of effacement.

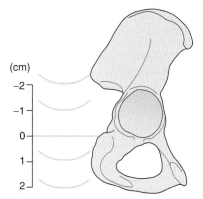

Figure 5.10   Pelvic landmarks as rough guides to level of presenting parts.

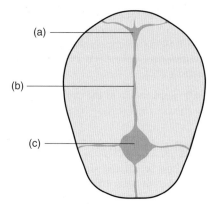

Figure 5.11   (a) Posterior fontanelle, (b) sagittal suture and (c) anterior fontanelle.

Table 5.1   Modified Bishop's cervical score

Cervix	Score			
	0	1	2	3
Dilatation (cm)	Closed	1–2	3–4	>5
Length (cm)	3	2	1	0
Consistency	Firm	Medium	Soft	
Position	Posterior	Middle	Anterior	
Station of head (cm)	–3	–2	–1 to 0	+1 to +2

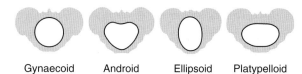

Gynaecoid   Android   Ellipsoid   Platypelloid

Figure 5.12   The four basic pelvic types.

tions below the spine are given the prefix '+'. This nomenclature can communicate the amount of progress in labour by indicating the rate of descent of the presenting part.

Information acquired at this stage of examination can be expressed collectively as a score, which was first introduced by Bishop (Table 5.1). A score of more than 5 reflects ease of cervical dilatation.

- In cephalic presentation, locate and note direction of the sagittal suture. Identify the anterior and posterior fontanelles (Figure 5.11). The posterior fontanelle dimples in the shape of a 'V' where the three sutures meet, whereas the anterior fontanelle is larger, the surrounding bones feel less firm, and can be followed out to four sutures. A readily palpable anterior fontanelle indicates poor head flexion. Identification of sutures is made more difficult by oedema of the fetal scalp or caput succedaneum.

Pelvic examination

Develop a routine for examination which is thorough, gentle and quick. During examination bear in mind the following:

- The four basic pelvic types: gynaecoid, android, ellipsoid and platypelloid (Figure 5.12). With experience combinations of these basic types can be identified.
- The various pelvic planes (Box 5.2). The plane of least pelvic diameter describes the narrowest part of the pelvis.
- The two narrowest diameters are the inter-ischial (10.5 cm) and the transverse diameter of the outlet (11.5 cm).
- Any diameter which is less than 9.5 cm is not adequate for a normal full-term fetus. Absolute disproportion is present.
- Knowledge of the length of the examiner's fingers and width of the knuckles is useful.
- There are ethnic differences. All pelvic diameters in women of smaller stature may be reduced by 0.5–1 cm.

The average diameters of the normal pelvis are given in Table 5.2.

Contracted pelvis

This is suspected when any of the above diameters is reduced by more than 1 cm. Take into consideration ethnic differences and gestation. Suspicion should be aroused when:

- a congenital skeletal defect is present
- the woman is of short stature

Box 5.2   Pelvic planes

Diameters of pelvic planes are shown in Figure 5.13. Anteroposterior diameters of the pelvis are shown in Figure 5.14.

(a) True conjugate = promontory to innermost posterior surface of symphysis (measured in erect lateral pelvimetry)
(b) Diagonal conjugate = promontory to lower border of symphysis pubis (measured clinically)
(c) Anteroposterior diameter of outlet = lower border of symphysis pubis to end of sacrum (measured clinically and radiologically)

Pelvic planes are shown in Figure 5.15.

(a) Brim or inlet = upper border of symphysis pubis, iliopectineal line, sacrum
(b) Mid-cavity or greatest pelvic diameter = mid-point of posterior symphysis upper aspect of sacrosciatic notch, junction of second and third sacral vertebrae. This is above plane of least diameters
(c) Least-pelvic diameters = mid-symphysis pubis, ischial spines, sacrospinous ligament and tip of sacrum. This is the narrowest part of the pelvis.
(d) Outlet = this plane is made up of two segments angled at the intertuberous diameter. Lower border of the symphysis, pubic arch, ischial tuberosity, sacrotuberous ligament and tip of coccyx.

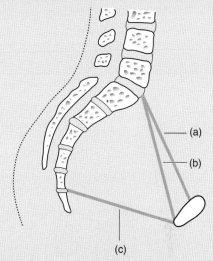

Figure 5.14   Anteroposterior diameters of the pelvis, (a) true conjugate (b) diagonal conjugate, and (c) anteroposterior diameter of outlet.

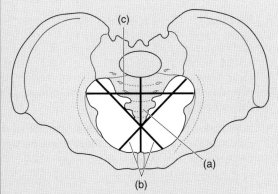

Figure 5.13   Pelvic diameters (a) anteroposterior, (b) oblique, and (c) transverse. In each case the widest diameter is chosen.

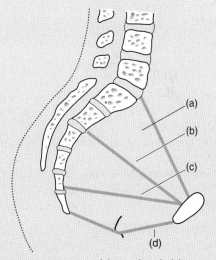

Figure 5.15   Pelvic planes (a) brim (inlet); (b) mid-cavity (greatest pelvic diameter); (c) least pelvic diameters; and (d) outlet.

Table 5.2 Average diameters of the normal pelvis (cm)

	Anteroposterior	Transverse	Oblique
Brim	12	12	12
Cavity	12	12	12
Outlet	12	11.5	12

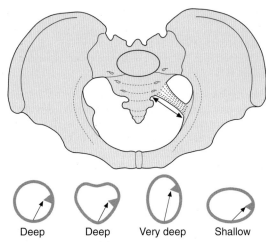

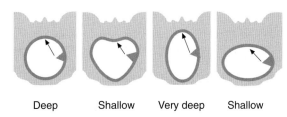

| Deep | Deep | Very deep | Shallow |

Figure 5.17 Ischial spine and length of sacral spinous ligament.

| Deep | Shallow | Very deep | Shallow |

Figure 5.18 Width of the sacrosciatic notch.

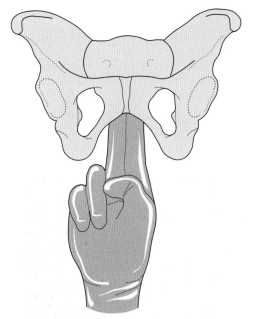

Figure 5.16 Subpubic angle.

- there is history of pelvic trauma (e.g. road traffic accident)
- there is evidence of dietary or medical diseases affecting bone formation (e.g. tuberculosis or osteomyelitis).

Routine for pelvic examination
A useful routine for pelvic assessment is given below.

1. Tell the woman of your intent and warn her that some pressure may be felt.

2. Introduce your fingers through the introitus and press against the subpubic arch (Figure 5.16). If the arch accommodates two fingers comfortably (more than 90°) then the pelvis is likely to be gynaecoid or platypelloid.

3. Locate the ischial spines, note their prominence and depth from the symphysis to the anterior half of the pelvis (Figure 5.17).

4. Keeping the third finger in contact with the ischial spine, move the index finger along the sacrospinous ligament and gauge the width of the sacrosciatic notch (Figure 5.18). The notch, which indicates the depth of the posterior half of the pelvis, is wide if the sacrum is 3 cm or more from the ischial spine.

5. Repeat this procedure on the opposite side of the pelvis. Make a mental note of the distance between the spines.

6. Determine whether the promontory is palpable. It is not necessary to touch the promontory if the length of the examining finger is known. An engaged presenting part prevents examination but signifies an adequate inlet (Figure 5.19).

7. Sweep the fingers along the sacral curve. Note any reduction in curvature or protrusion of the sacrum into the pelvic cavity.

8. Test the mobility of the coccyx.

9. Withdraw the fingers. Clench them and measure the intertuberous diameter with the knuckle of the

hand. Take into account the shape of the pubis. Note the distance from the tuberosity to the tip of the sacrum. This distance indicates the room available in the outlet if the subpubic arch is narrowed (Figure 5.20).

The above procedure need take no more than 1 minute and provides a comprehensive picture of pelvic diameters. What is not known is the mobility of the pelvic at the lumbosacral and symphysial joints.

Table 5.3 summarises the four basic pelvic configurations.

Erect lateral pelvimetry (ELP)

When disproportion is suspected an upright lateral X-ray (Figure 5.21) or magnetic resonance (MR) image (Figure 5.22) of the pelvis provides additional information.

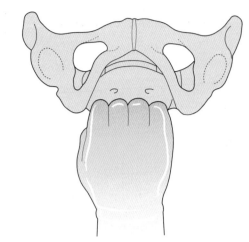

Figure 5.20   Intertuberous diameter.

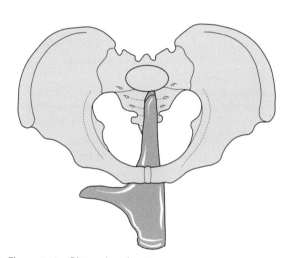

Figure 5.19   Diagonal conjugate.

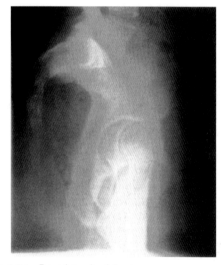

Figure 5.21   Erect lateral pelvimetry.

Table 5.3   Summary of the four basic pelvic configurations

Type	Gynaecoid	Android	Ellipsoid	Platypelloid
Incidence	50 per cent	20 per cent	25 per cent	5 per cent
Geometrical shape	◯	▽	◯	⬭
Subpubic angle	>90°	<90°	<90°	>90°
Ischial spines	Not prominent	Prominent	Usually not prominent	Can be prominent
Sacrosciatic notch	Wide	Narrow	Wide	Wide
Interspinous diameter	Wide	Narrow	Narrow	Wide
Pelvic walls	Parallel	Convergent	Parallel	Divergent
Intertuberous diameter	Wide	Reduced	Reduced	Wide

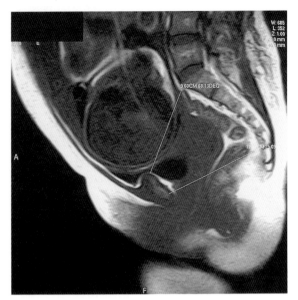

Figure 5.22   Magnetic resonance image of the pelvis.

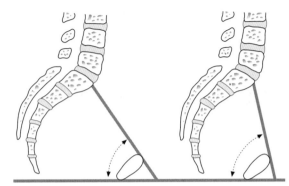

Figure 5.23   Increased inclination presents a less favourable angle for entry to the pelvis.

signifies the possibility of a longer labour (Figure 5.23). The angle of inclination is formed by the angle made by the line joining the promontory, the upper border of the symphysis and the horizontal plane.

- ELP assesses adequacy of the pelvis in one plane only. The width of the pelvis must be determined before adequacy is pronounced. An MR image provides three-dimensional measurements.

For interpretation of an ELP or MR image of the pelvis, the following should be carried out:

- Check that the femoral trochanters are aligned.

- Check the presentation and position of the fetus. Density of the fetal bones gives an indication of their maturity.

- Count the number of sacral vertebrae. Note the degree of curvature of the sacrum and the length of the coccyx. Sacralisation of the fifth lumbar vertebrae (inclusion of the fifth lumbar vertebra into the sacrum) increases the depth of the pelvis and impedes engagement.

- Measure the true conjugate and the anteroposterior diameter of outlet. Pelvic convergence is readily identified.

- Inclination of the pelvis is normally 55° (range 40–60°). The greater the angle of inclination the more difficult it is for engagement to take place, hence

SUBSEQUENT MANAGEMENT

When complications have been excluded and further labour is safe, note the following:

- If labour is in its early stages and the cervix is less than 3 cm dilated, the bowels can be emptied with suppositories. Women usually feel more comfortable after this procedure and there is less risk of faecal contamination. If there is no contraindication the woman can remain ambulant.

- The perineum is seldom shaved nowadays.

- Women in active labour frequently prefer to lie in bed.

- Safety must dictate choice for alternative mode of delivery, e.g. in water.

References

Brown S, Lumley J 1998 Changing childbirth: Lessons from an Australian Survey of 1336 women. British Journal of Obstetrics and Gynaecology 105:143–155

National Health and Medical Research Council 1996 Report on options for effective care in childbirth. NHMRC, Canberra

Bibliography

Carr-Hill R 1992 The measurement of patient satisfaction. J Public Health Medicine 14:236–249

Department of Health. 1998 Why Mothers Die. Report on Confidential Enquiries into Maternal

Deaths in the United Kingdom 1994–1996. TSO, London

Expert Maternity Group 1993 Changing Childbirth: The Report of the Expert Maternity Group (Cumberlege Report). HMSO, London

House of Commons Select Committee on Health 1992 Second Report on Maternity Services (Winterton Report). HMSO, London

Ince JGH, Young MD 1940 The bony pelvis and its influence on labour. Journal of Obstetrics and Gynaecology of the British Empire 47:130–190

Morrison JJ, Sinnatamby R, Hackett GA et al 1995 Obstetric pelvimetry in the UK: an appraisal of current practice. British Journal of Obstetrics and Gynaecology 102:748–750

Royal College of Obstetricians and Gynaecologists 1998 Pelvimetry – Clinical Indications. Guideline No 14. RCOG, London

Royal College of Obstetricians and Gynaecologists and Royal College of Midwives 1999 Towards Safer Childbirth, Minimum Standards for the Organisation of Labour Wards. RCOG/RCM, London

Chapter 6

Admission emergencies

David T Y Liu
Mentors: Khaled Ismail, Mark Kilby

CHAPTER CONTENTS

Management of imminent delivery with or without
     fetal compromise   35
Specific problems   36
     Cord presentation or prolapse   36
          Cord presentation   36
          Cord prolapse   36
     Major obstetric haemorrhage   37
          Management   37
     Antepartum haemorrhage   37
          Important points to remember about vaginal
               bleeding in pregnancy   38
          General guidelines for management   38
     Placental separation (abruption)   38
          Diagnosis   38
          Management   39
     Placenta praevia   40
          Grading of placenta praevia   40
          Management   40
     Fits   40
     Eclampsia   41
          Guidelines for management   41
     Suspected fetal death   43
     Cardiac arrest and cardiopulmonary resuscitation
          in the obstetric woman   43
     Myocardial infarction   43
          Management   43

When emergencies occur a well-rehearsed approach facilitates efficient teamwork and ensures that all correct steps are taken. Availability of clear, updated protocols is crucial for immediate management by staff on the labour ward.

Training protocols or drills for staff (doctors, midwives, anaesthetists, paediatricians and theatre assistants) are encouraged for improving performance and outcome in emergencies.

MANAGEMENT OF IMMINENT DELIVERY WITH OR WITHOUT FETAL COMPROMISE

The following procedures should be adopted if delivery is imminent.

- Determine at once whether vaginal delivery is **feasible** and **safe**.

- **Reassurance**. These women are often agitated and distressed on admission to hospital. Reassurance and supportive care are necessary. Discourage pushing until vaginal examination is performed.

- Transfer the woman to the delivery room if vaginal delivery is safe. If fetal distress is present, expedite delivery and anticipate the need for neonatal resuscitation.

- If there is indication for or need for recurrent caesarean section proceed to immediate delivery by caesarean section. For uncomplicated cephalic presentation when the fetal head is on the perineum a short period of close observation is acceptable, but anticipate assisted delivery if there is delay or onset of compromise.

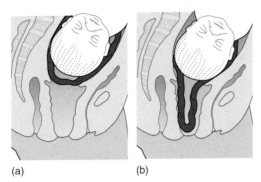

(a)   (b)

Figure 6.1   (a) Cord presentation and (b) cord prolapse.

SPECIFIC PROBLEMS

Cord presentation or prolapse

Always **confirm gestational age** before planning any further management.

Cord presentation

This occurs when the cord is in front of the presenting part of the fetus behind intact membranes. When the membranes are not ruptured, palpate through them with the tip of the fingers to exclude the presence of pulsation due to cord presentation or vasa praevia (Figure 6.1a). The diagnosis can also be made using ultrasound and colour flow Doppler, and is useful in circumstances such as an unstable breech presentation. Variable fetal heart rate decelerations may be evident.

Management
- Cord presentation during labour and before full cervical dilatation necessitates delivery by caesarean section.
- If the cervix is fully dilated, the presenting part is below the ischial spines and the pelvis is adequate, rupture the membranes, displace the cord and deliver by forceps or ventouse.

Cord prolapse

Following membrane rupture the cord may prolapse through the cervix, may remain in the vagina or be expelled through the introitus (Figure 6.1b).

Cord prolapse occurs in approximately 0.2% of all births.

Risk factors for cord prolapse
- Amniotomy.
- Low birth weight (<2.5 kg).
- Premature birth/preterm prelabour rupture of membranes.
- Malpresentations/(flexed or footling, breech).

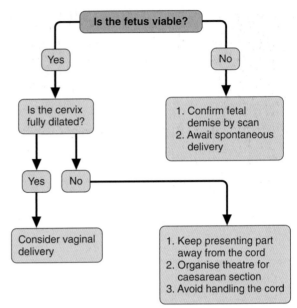

Figure 6.2   Steps in the management of cord prolapse.

- Second twin.
- High presenting part/disproportions/placenta praevia grade I or II.
- Polyhydramnios and uncontrolled rupture of membranes.
- Anencephaly and other congenital malformations with a potential for cephalopelvic disproportion.
- Long cord or abnormal cord insertion.

Points to remember in management   Figure 6.2 presents an algorithm for management of cord prolapse.

- Anticipate in the presence of risk factors.

- Note suspicious or abnormal cardiotocographic changes.

- Inform the woman of the situation and the need for urgency (if fetus is alive).

- If fetal demise is suspected confirm by scan and manage as for stillbirth. It has been reported that fetal activity could be visualised in cases of inaudible fetal heart tones and absent cord pulsation.

- Check the presence of pulsation, replace the cord in the warmth of the vagina and determine dilatation of the cervix.

- Maternal oxygen, intravenous access and group and save.

- Deliver by forceps or ventouse if cervix is fully dilated and vaginal delivery is considered to be safe.

- If the cervix is not fully dilated, displace the presenting part of the fetus away from the cervix with examining digits to prevent cord compression (most effective). This manoeuvre is made easier if the mother is placed in Trendelenburg's or knee-chest position. Some authors advocate a temporary measure by inserting a number 16 Foley catheter to fill the bladder with 500 ml of saline using a standard infusion set. Bladder filling raises the presenting part of the fetus away from the cord. (Digital elevation of presenting part is more effective.)

- Avoid handling the cord because this will cause spasm of the vessels and fetal bradycardia.

- Request assistance and organise a theatre for caesarean section if vaginal delivery is not considered safe. Fetal resuscitation is often required.

Major obstetric haemorrhage

- Haemorrhage remains one of the leading causes of maternal mortality in the world. It is the leading cause of maternal mortality in developing countries.

- It is defined as the loss of more than 500 ml of blood, either antepartum or postpartum.

- Accurate measurement of blood loss is difficult hence a definition based on volume alone has shortcomings. Tachycardia (>120 beats per minute), hypotension (systolic below 100 mmHg), peripheral vasoconstriction and decreased urine output are important signs.

- Underestimation of blood loss may delay steps to prepare for or prevent further bleeding. Check haemoglobin and haematocrit levels as objective guides to blood loss.

Management
- Clear guidelines must be available for haemorrhage. These will include details for contact of senior obstetric staff, anaesthetists and haematologist.

- Adequate tissue perfusion is essential to preserve organ function.

- Hypotension-mediated endothelial damage may trigger disseminated intravascular coagulation (DIC).

- Basic resuscitation includes:
  - Minimising effects of aortocaval compression (left lateral tilt or wedging 5–15°).
  - Administering a high concentration of oxygen to the woman regardless of her oxygen saturation.

- Assess **A**irway and **B**reathing effort. Intubation may be indicated if the mother has depressed conscious level due to hypotension (near arrest scenario).
- Establish two 14 G intravenous lines and take 20 ml of blood for diagnostic test (full blood count, urea and electrolytes, coagulation screen and cross matching).
- Maintain the **C**irculation by normal/saline or Hartmann's solutions and colloid until blood is available.

- Monitor pulse, blood pressure (direct or indirect), respiratory rate, oxygen saturation, urine output and fluid balance.

- Central venous pressure monitoring is recommended. Use antecubital fossa and long line, as safer when coagulopathy threatens. Fluid warmers and high pressure infusers are helpful in these situations. If CVP is more than 5 mmHg maintenance fluid volume is sufficient.

- Delegate one member of staff to record time, drugs given and fluids used.

- Identify and treat the cause of bleeding.

- A well-drilled multidisciplinary team of anaesthetists, haematologists, and maternity staff will achieve best results. Observe in high-dependency unit after resuscitation.

Box 6.1 gives details of blood component therapy.

Antepartum haemorrhage

- This is vaginal bleeding after a gestational age of 24 weeks.

- Bleeding is due to:
  - placental abruption or separation of the placenta, which is normally situated in the upper uterine segment
  - placental praevia or separation of the abnormally situated placenta which lies in or encroaches onto the lower uterine segment
  - non-placental causes secondary to trauma, infection or neoplasms
  - vasa praevia. Bleeding is associated with rupture of blood vessels in the fetal membranes. Fetal blood is lost. Abnormal cord insertion or succenturiate placenta is commonly found. The Apt test can be used if bleeding of fetal origin is suspected. The basis of this test is that fetal haemoglobin is alkaline stable, whereas adult haemoglobin is not.

Box 6.1   Blood component therapy

- O negative blood should be available on the delivery suite. This carries a small risk of sensitisation to 'c' antigen.

- Full infection screen is necessary for fresh whole blood.

- After 48 hours storage, platelet numbers and function of important clotting factors (V and VIII) are reduced.

- Full cross-match of blood may take up to an hour.

- Fresh frozen plasma (FFP) is separated from whole blood within 6 hours of donation and stored for up to 1 year at −20°C to −30°C. FFP provides all necessary clotting factors. Give 1 unit after 8 units of rapidly transfused blood. Use coagulation screen as guide.

- Cryoprecipitate contains more fibrinogen than FFP but lacks antithrombin III (coagulation inhibitor), which is depleted in obstetric related coagulopathies. Cryoprecipitate is useful for hypofibrinogenaemia.

- Platelet packs have a limited shelf life of 5 days and should be given through a platelet filter. Rarely indicated above a platelet count of 50 × 10^9/l.

- In the presence of maternal antibodies, blood should be cross-matched before onset of labour or caesarean section.

- Use blood warming equipment.

Important points to remember about vaginal bleeding in pregnancy

- A show is diagnosed only when blood-stained mucus is noted, usually in association with contractions. Presence of pure blood is not a show.
- A high presenting part or malpresentation on abdominal examination may be due to placenta praevia (irrespective of an early pregnancy ultrasound scan).
- A tense contracted tender uterus is one of the signs of placental abruption.
- Vaginal examination is contraindicated until placenta praevia is excluded.
- The fetus can contribute to the bleeding hence the real risk of exsanguination.
- Bleeding is often more extensive than that observed.

- Increased uterine activity can produce or follow placental separation.
- Anti-D for rhesus negative mothers – use Kleihauer's test.
- Anticipate postpartum haemorrhage.
- Ultrasound scan may detect retroplacental collection of blood.
- Placental damage and thromboplastin release can cause coagulation defect.

General guidelines for management

1. Apply general rule for resuscitation (**A**irway, **B**reathing and **C**irculation + **O**$_2$)
2. Ensure intravenous access (at least 16 G, preferably 14 G).
3. Perform full blood count, group and cross-match blood (number of units required depends on amount of bleeding).
4. Exclude placenta praevia by ultrasound scan. Check fetal viability.
5. Perform speculum examination (if no placenta praevia) to exclude local causes for bleeding.
6. Take vaginal swab to screen for infection.
7. Commence cardiotocography to assess fetal well-being. Further placental separation can occur. Do not stop monitoring too early.
8. Note presence or absence of uterine activity.
9. Clot lysis suggest activation of fibrinolytic system. Correct coagulopathy (present in up to 30%) before caesarean section.
10. Epidural anaesthesia is contraindicated if the mother is hypotensive or coagulopathy is present.
11. Consider peritoneal and abdominal wound, drain if oozing is present.
12. Keep uterus contracted by intravenous oxytocin (Syntocinon) infusion after delivery to prevent postpartum haemorrhage.
13. A neonatologist must attend delivery. Fetal blood loss (asphyxia pallida) will require urgent resuscitation.

Note: Modify guidelines for degree of antepartum haemorrhage.

Placental separation (abruption)

Presentation depends on the amount of bleeding (Table 6.1).

Diagnosis

- A careful history should be taken to define obstetric complications, the site of pain and if coitus had taken place.

Table 6.1 Placental separation: presentation and consequences

Bleeding	Pain	Uterus	Cardiovascular system	Fetus	Mother
Slight	Mild	Irritable	Unchanged	Unaffected	Well
Moderate	Moderate/labour	Labour	Compensation	Distressed	Distressed
Severe	Severe/labour	Hard/labour	Compensation/decompensation	Death	Shocked

- Exclude differential diagnosis.
- If pain is not localised to the placental site concealed haemorrhage is less likely.
- Note the presence of uterine activity.
- Ultrasound examination is helpful for assessing fetal wellbeing, placental localisation and identifying retroplacental haematoma.
- A negative scan does not exclude the diagnosis of abruption.
- Major placental separation produces the classic picture of shock, a rock-hard uterus, coagulation defects and fetal death (in 50% of cases).
- Uterine tenderness and rigidity may be absent if the placenta is posterior.
- Haematuria may be present.
- There is an association with pre-eclampsia (2%).

Management

This is governed by the amount of bleeding, whether bleeding continues, the status both of the mother and fetus, the gestational age of the pregnancy and previous obstetric history.

Placental abruption can occur at any gestational age. Follow the general guidelines of management of antepartum haemorrhage. Placental abruption is usually treated actively by delivery, by caesarean section if the fetus is alive and viable but vaginally if the fetus is dead. Close monitoring throughout labour is essential. Caesarean section might be required if labour is prolonged to decrease the risk of severe coagulopathy.

Severity of bleeding is a useful guide for management.

Mild bleeding

- Admit and observe after instituting general procedures.
- If the woman is in labour and the fetus is mature, rupture the membranes to check the state of liquor and provide access to the fetus for direct fetal heart rate monitoring.
- Close observation is mandatory. This includes extended cardiotocography if conservative management is adopted. Further placental separation can occur.

Moderate bleeding

- Replace blood loss.
- Carry out coagulation screen and correct defects.
- Rupture the membranes, administer oxytocics if labour is delayed.
- Perform caesarean section for fetal distress. Coagulation defects must first be excluded.
- An indwelling drain for the abdomen and wound after caesarean section is advised.
- An experienced obstetrician and anaesthetist are required.
- Ensure strict fluid balance and monitor the renal output (>20 ml/h).
- Epidural anaesthesia is contraindicated if the mother is hypotensive or there is evidence of coagulopathy (up to 30%).
- Presence of pre-eclampsia requires close watch for blood pressure fluctuations, renal shut down and electrolyte disturbances. These women are best observed on the labour ward until clinically stable.
- Keep uterus contracted by intravenous Syntocinon infusion after delivery.
- A neonatologist must attend delivery. Fetal blood loss (asphyxia pallida) will require urgent resuscitation.

Severe bleeding See Major obstetric haemorrhage above.

- Fetal death is usual. The aim is to resuscitate and evacuate the uterus.
- Correct coagulation defects.
- Blood transfusion is required.
- Control fluid replacement by use of a central line (exclude coagulopathy).
- Rupture the membranes and encourage labour.
- Watch closely for blood pressure changes and onset of coagulopathy.
- Labour usually supervenes or follows Syntocinon infusion. If not, caesarean section is justified if condition is stable, the cervix is unfavourable and there is no coagulation defect. Delay allows further decompensation of the situation and risks onset of coagulopathy.
- Keep uterus contracted after delivery to prevent risk of postpartum haemorrhage. The Couvelaire uterus may not contract well.

Placenta praevia

- This describes a placenta inserted partially or wholly in the lower uterine segment.
- Characteristically presents with unprovoked painless bleeding. Occasionally, bleeding may be provoked by sexual intercourse. Note evidence of uterine activity.
- It is discovered following clinical or ultrasound examination. Unstable lie or high presenting part should alert to this condition. Transvaginal scanning is safe and more accurate.

Grading of placenta praevia

Not clinically useful for predicting severity of antepartum haemorrhage.

I. The placenta is in the lower uterine segment but the placental edge does not reach the internal os.
II. The lower edge of the placenta reaches but does not cover the internal os.
III. The placenta covers the internal os asymmetrically.
IV. The placenta covers the internal os symmetrically.

Management

Management depends on the gestational age, the amount of blood loss, fetal position and the placental site (in cases of minor placenta praevia).

- Apply the general guidelines for antepartum haemorrhage.
- Consider expectant management if the gestational age is less than 37 weeks when bleeding is mild. Close observation is mandatory.
- It is safer to avoid tocolytics in cases of antepartum haemorrhage. However, in a tertiary setting for selected situations prolonged gestation can be achieved with no increase in mortality or morbidity.
- Ensure cross-matched blood is available at all times.
- For moderate bleeding after 36 completed weeks or if bleeding is severe or continues after 24 weeks, caesarean section should be performed. Additional cross-matched blood must be available. A senior obstetrician and anaesthetist should be available to assist or advise especially where placentation is anterior. Placenta praevia, particularly in women with a previous uterine scar, may be associated with uncontrollable uterine haemorrhage at delivery and caesarean hysterectomy may be necessary. A consultant must be in attendance.

Box 6.2   Examination in theatre: requirements

- Blood must be available in theatre.
- No fetal distress.
- Prepare the woman for caesarean section.
- Lithotomy position.
- Palpate around fornices. Interposing placenta distant present parts.
- Locate the cervix and examine with a single digit in enlarging circles. The placenta has a spongy feel.
- Brisk bleeding indicates the need for immediate delivery.

For grade I anterior placenta praevia, rupture the membranes and attempt vaginal delivery. Close surveillance is mandatory. All other grades of placenta praevia necessitate caesarean section.

- Remember placenta accreta in an anterior placenta with a previous caesarean section scar.
- Examination in theatre is acceptable when diagnosis is uncertain or when there is a grade I anterior placenta praevia (see Box 6.2).
- Choice of anaesthetic technique must be made by the anaesthetist.
- Placenta accreta, increta and percreta: there is a strong association between these abnormal placentations and placenta praevia and presence of a uterine (caesarean section) scar. Ultrasound scanning and magnetic resonance imaging can forewarn. Apply drill for massive haemorrhage. Consider hysterectomy early rather than late.

Fits

Pregnancy can aggravate an existing tendency to fits (epilepsy), or convulsions can complicate pre-eclampsia (eclampsia). The presence of hypertension, proteinuria and generalised oedema and past history of epilepsy are important points that need to be considered in this situation. Close monitoring of the woman's condition, the fetus (by cardiotocography) and laboratory results (e.g. blood count, urea, electrolytes, clotting screen and liver function) are mandatory.

Two-thirds of eclampsia occur before and a third after delivery, sometimes 3 or more days post partum (12%). Eclampsia is associated with up to 14% direct maternal deaths in the UK (Confidential Enquiries into Maternal Deaths in the United Kingdom 2004).

Eclampsia

Prevention and anticipation are important measures. Note symptoms (hyper-reflexion, clonus, headaches, photophobia, epigastric pain, flashing lights) elevated transaminases, creatinine, urea, proteinuria (>1 g/24 h or 3 plus) platelets below $100 \times 10^9/l$ or prolonged clotting times.

Guidelines for management

- Clear, written management protocols for severe pre-eclampsia should guide initial and ongoing treatment in hospital.

- Established intravenous access and inserted bladder catheter.

- Stop/prevent fitting. **Give** intravenous magnesium sulphate (4 g over 15 minutes).

- Reduce blood pressure. **Give** hydralazine/labetalol/nifedipine. (Care should be taken when combining magnesium sulphate and nifedipine. This combination is best avoided (calcium chelator and calcium blocker).) Both drugs can have a synergistic effect which can cause significant hypotension.

- Management protocols should recognise the need to avoid very high systolic blood pressures associated with the risk of intracerebral haemorrhage.

- Automated blood pressure recording systems can systematically underestimate blood pressure in pre-eclampsia, to a serious degree.

- Anticipate complications. Review the woman frequently and monitor closely in a high-dependency unit with senior staff involvement.

- Deliver the baby. There is no place for continuing the pregnancy if eclampsia occurs. Consider induction of labour or caesarean section. A major complication is fetal or maternal mortality.

- There should be early engagement of consultant obstetricians and intensive care specialists in the care of women with severe pre-eclampsia.

- Ensure detailed documentation of drugs, fluids and observations.

Magnesium sulphate

- This drug is used for seizure prophylaxis. This is the current drug of choice in eclampsia (dispensed in 50% W/V solutions with 1 g in 2 ml).
- There must be a protocol for magnesium sulphate administration.
- After the loading dose (4–5 g given slowly over 15–20 minutes) infuse 1–2 g/h for maintenance

(20 ml magnesium sulphate in 250 ml normal saline at 50 ml/h).
- Adjust therapeutic levels by increasing or decreasing infusion.
- Infusion should be continued for 24 hours. Post partum ensure tendon reflex is present, note urine output (should be 30 ml/h or 100 ml/4 h).
- The first sign of toxicity is loss of the knee reflex. Check serum magnesium levels 1 hour after loading dose and then every 6 hours to ensure therapeutic levels of 2–3 mmol/l.
- Calcium gluconate 10% intravenously is given as antidote (require 10–20 ml).
- Continuous monitoring of oxygen saturation is required.
- Magnesium sulphate increases sensitivity to muscle relaxants (non-depolarising). Reduce infusion if blood pressure <110/70 mmHg and respiratory rate is below 16 per minute.
- Use clinical findings as guide to duration of infusion.
- If fits continue give diazepam 5 mg/min (up to 20 mg) intravenously.

Fluid balance

- Insert an indwelling urinary catheter and keep a strict input/output chart with hourly running totals. Aim for 100 ml/h total fluid input.

- Maintenance fluids should be given as crystalloid (85 ml/h). Beware of fluid overload.

- Colloids may be required prior to vasodilatation (with epidural anaesthesia).

- Diuretics are only indicated for women with confirmed pulmonary oedema.

- Central venous pressure monitoring might be required.

- Oliguria (urine output <30 ml/h persists) follows renal vessel spasms, renal failure precipitated by haemorrhage and hypotension or fluid deficit. Check urea, creatinine and electrolytes (test by 200 ml bolus of crystalloid over 30 minutes and review urinary output).

- Total fluid intake should not exceed 2.5 l over 24 hours. Colloids can be used with caution for fluid challenges (200 ml) if the urine output is decreased.

- Furosemide is used for pulmonary oedema, in the presence of overhydration, particularly with heart failure or with impending renal failure.

Antihypertensives (see Boxes 6.3 and 6.4) A blood pressure of 160 mmHg systolic over 110 mgHg

Box 6.3 Hydralazine treatment

Mode of action
- Direct acting vasodilator
- Can cause sodium and fluid retention
- Plasma half life 2–3 hours

Contraindications
- Known hypersensitivity
- Systemic lupus erythematosus
- Tachycardia
- High output state (thyrotoxicosis)
- Aortic or mitral stenosis
- Isolated right ventricular failure due to pulmonary hypertension

Cautions
- Renal impairment
- Ischaemic heart disease
- Surgery can exaggerate hypertension

Side effects
- Tachycardia, palpitations, flushing hypotension, anginal symptoms, oedema, heart failure
- Headache dizziness, peripheral neuritis, hyper-reflexion
- Arthralgia rash
- Proteinuria, increased plasma creatinine, haematuria, renal failure
- Gastrointestinal disturbances, abnormal liver function
- Agitation, anxiety
- Dyspnoea

Compatibility
- Incompatible with dextrose
- Use following magnesium sulphate or other anti-hypertensives can cause precipitous fall in blood pressure

Acute treatment
- 5 mg by slow (1 mg/min) intravenous bolus (up to 10 mg)
- Check blood pressure (BP) every 5 minutes for 30 minutes, or until BP is stable at <100 mmHg diastolic, then every 15 minutes for further 60 minutes
- Repeat bolus if blood pressure is not controlled after 30 minutes

Maintenance
- 40 mg hydralazine in 40 ml 0.9% saline (via syringe pump) giving 1000 µg/ml solution

Start	40 µg/min	(2.4 ml/h)
30 min	80 µg/min	(4.8 ml/h)
60 min	120 µg/min	(7.2 ml/h)
90 min	160 µg/min	(9.6 ml/h)

Do not increase if pulse is >140 or if target BP is reached. Reduction by 10–20 µg/min every 30 minutes.

Prolonged use (more than 24 hours) of hydralazine results in tachycardia and loss of antihypertensive effect. If required consider adding a β-blocker.

Box 6.4 Labetalol treatment

Cautions
- Asthma
- Heart failure
- Cardiogenic shock
- Atrio-ventricular block

Side effects
- Postural hypotension
- Tiredness, weakness, headache, rashes, scalp tingling
- Difficulty in micturition
- Epigastric pain
- Nausea, vomiting
- Rarely lichenoid rash

Oral therapy
- 200 mg oral loading then 200 mg oral three times daily
- Increase to a maximum of 600 mg four times daily

Intravenous therapy
- Acute: bolus dose for acute therapy, 10–20 mg intravenously slowly (5–10 min), effective within 5 minutes and lasts for 6 hours (repeat if needed to maximum of 100 mg)
- Intravenous infusion solution: 5 mg/ml (200 mg in 40 ml) as alternative to repeat bolus
  Set a target BP. Increase infusion as stated until target BP is reached
  Start at 20 mg/h (=4 ml/h)

At 30 min	40 mg/h
At 60 min	80 mg/h
At 90 min	160 mg/h

To reduce, decrease by 10 mg/h every 30 min as required. Convert to oral therapy by giving 200 mg orally 1 hour prior to stopping infusion, followed by 200 mg three times daily.

diastolic requires urgent treatment to prevent cerebral haemorrhage. Aim for a diastolic of 90–95 mmHg to ensure adequate placental perfusion. Monitor maternal blood pressure (5–10 minutes intervals) and fetal heart rate (cardiotocography).

Suspected fetal death

Any mother presenting with diminished fetal movements must be examined at once.

- Check for fetal heart rate.

- Reassure mother if the fetal heart is heard. Obtain a 30-minute external cardiotocographic trace of the fetal heart for inspection.

- Discharge if the antenatal history suggests no cause for concern. Admit and investigate if obstetric complications are present.

- Perform ultrasound scan if fetal heart is not heard. If fetal death is confirmed after ultrasound scan as a double check, inform the woman and partner immediately. Transfer to a quiet room for natural expression of grief. Discuss openly possible reasons for the tragedy but protect them from any feeling of guilt.

- At a convenient time discuss the proposed course of further action.

- Suppress lactation.

- Counsel the couple about the different levels of post-mortem examination (see Box 23.2).

- Provide administrative support and aid to parents for registration of the stillbirth.

- Provide a follow-up appointment for further counselling when results such as post-mortem findings are available.

Cardiac arrest and cardiopulmonary resuscitation in the obstetric woman

- Cardiac arrest in late pregnancy or during delivery is a rare event. It usually accompanies major complications (e.g. amniotic fluid embolism). The physiological changes in late pregnancy often hamper effective cardiopulmonary efforts.

- Some causes include:
  - total spinal anaesthetic
  - local anaesthetic toxicity from unintentional intravascular injection
  - trauma
  - pulmonary embolism
  - amniotic fluid embolism.

- Physiological changes in pregnancy relevant to cardiopulmonary resuscitation (CPR) include:
  - women become hypoxic more readily (20% decrease in their functional residual capacity and 20% increase in their resting oxygen consumption)
  - the enlarged uterus can decrease compliance during controlled ventilation
  - aortocaval compression in the supine position necessitate lateral tilt.

- Tilt the uterus to the left side. A member of the team should be instructed to act as a 'human wedge' by kneeling down (both knees). The woman is placed across the wedge of the bent knees.

- CPR should begin immediately after establishing airway. Follow advanced cardiac life support programme.

- If CPR is not successful after 5 minutes, caesarean delivery must be performed.

- CPR should be continued throughout the procedure.

Myocardial infarction

Myocardial infarction associated with labour or need for delivery is not a common situation (6.2 per 100 000 maternities). In pregnancy the majority of infarcts are transmural involving the anterior rather than posterior myocardium. The cause is usually coronary artery thrombosis where pre-existing arteriosclerosis or aneurysm of the artery may exist. Coronary artery spasm is also a possibility. Haemodynamic changes during labour and delivery more often precipitate myocardial infarcts in the primigravida in the postpartum period whereas infarct in multigravid mothers is usually an antepartum event. Maternal mortality (7.3%) and fetal mortality is high.

Management
- Note risk factors for myocardial infarction, e.g. longstanding hypertension, family history, hypercholesterolaemia.

- Intensive care requires a multidisciplinary team of cardiologists, anaesthetists and obstetricians.

- Vaginal delivery if considered appropriate requires close monitoring of fetus with cardiotocography and continuous electrocardiographic surveillance of the woman; epidural anaesthesia to reduce pain and thus the adverse effects of catecholamines release and appreciation of effects associated with haemodynamic changes. Ergometrine should not be used. Oxytocin reduces coronary blood flow when levels exceed 4 mm/L.

- Elective caesarean section should be considered for myocardial infarction at term to allow better control of the situation and haemodynamic changes.

References

Confidential Enquiries into Maternal Deaths in the United Kingdom 2004 Why Mothers Die. The Sixth Report of

Confidential Enquiries into Maternal Deaths in the United Kingdom 2000–2002. London, CEMACH

Bibliography

Altman D, Carolli G, Duley L et al 2002 Do women with pre-eclampsia, and their babies benefit from magnesium sulphate? The Magpie Trial: a randomised placebo-controlled trial. Lancet 2002; 359:1877–1890

Andra H, James MD, Margaret G et al 2006 Acute myocardial infarction in pregnancy. A United States population based study. Circulation 113:1564–1571

Baldwin KJ, Johanson RB, Anthony J 1997 The acute management of severe hypertensive illness in pregnancy. In: O'Brien S (ed) The Yearbook of Obstetrics and Gynaecology, Volume 5. RCOG Press, London, pp 233–245

Besinger RE, Moniak CN, Paskiewicz LS et al 1995 The effect of tocolytic use in the management of symptomatic placenta praevia. American Journal of Obstetrics and Gynecology 172:1770–1778

Caspi E, Lotan Y, Schreyer P 1983 Prolapse of the cord: reduction of perinatal mortality by bladder instillation and caesarean section. Israel Journal of Medical Sciences 19:541–545

Chetty RM, Moodley J 1980 Umbilical cord prolapse. South African Medical Journal 57:128–129

Cortis BS, Gensini GG 1977 Can the risks of myocardial infarction in pregnancy be reduced? Cardiovascular Diseases 4:49

Driscoll JA, Sadan O, Van Gelderen CJ et al 1987 Cord prolapse: can we save more babies? Case reports. British Journal of Obstetrics and Gynaecology 94:594–595

Duley L, Henderson-Smart D 2001 Drugs for treatment of very high blood pressure during pregnancy. In: The Cochrane Library, Issue 2, Update software, Oxford

Hankin GDU, Wendel GD Jr, Leveno KJ et al 1985 Myocardial infarction during pregnancy: A review. Obstetrics and Gynecology 65:139–146

Ladner HE, Danielsen B, Gilbert WM 2005 Acute myocardial infarction in pregnancy and the puerperium: a population based study. Obstetrics and Gynecology 105:480–484

Leerentveld RA, Gilberts EC, Arnold MJ et al 1990 Accuracy and safety of transvaginal sonographic placental localisation. Obstetrics and Gynecology 76:759–762, 1990

Johanson RJ, Cox C, Grady K et al 2003 Managing Obstetric Emergencies and Trauma: The MOET Course Manual. RCOG Press, London

Royal College of Obstetricians and Gynaecologists 2001 Placenta praevia: Diagnosis and management. Guideline No 27. RCOG, London

Towers CV, Pircon RA, Heppard M 1999 Is tocolysis safe in the management of third trimester bleeding? American Journal of Obstetrics and Gynecology 180:1572–1578

Tucker D, Liu DTY, Ramoutar P 1996 Myocardial infarction at term: a case report to consider management options. British Journal of Obstetrics and Gynaecology 6:522–524

Vago T 1970 Prolapse of the umbilical cord. A method of management. American Journal of Obstetrics and Gynecology 107: 967–969

Chapter **7**

Normal labour and delivery

David T Y Liu, Pamela M Thwaites

CHAPTER CONTENTS

Myometrial activity: pregnancy   45
Myometrial activity: labour   46
   Uterine work   46
      Intrauterine pressure   46
      General comments   47
   Effect of uterine activity on the cervix   47
      Before labour   47
      In labour   48
   Effect of uterine activity on the fetus   48
   Management of the delivery   48
      Position   48
      Aseptic conditions   48
      Medical attendant   48
      Delivery of the head   49
      Delivery of the shoulders   49
      Umbilical cord   49
      Management of the third stage   51
      Delivery of the placenta   51
   Effect of uterine activity on the mother   52
      Management guidelines   52

MYOMETRIAL ACTIVITY: PREGNANCY

During pregnancy the uterus is usually in a quiescent state. In the third trimester women experience low amplitude, poorly synchronised Braxton Hicks or practice contractions. Substances which contribute to the inhibition of myometrial activity include progesterone from placental syncytiotrophoblast and chorion; myometrial parathyroid hormone-related peptide; and nitric oxide and relaxin from the myometrium, decidua, chorion and amnion in addition to prostacyclins. The process of myometrial contraction requires activation of calmodulin, a calcium-binding protein with calcium ions which then in turn activates the enzyme myosin light chain kinase to produce adenosine triphosphate to power actin and myosin filaments to slide over each other to produce shortening. Inhibitors of myometrial activity act by increasing intracellular levels of cyclic nucleotides to prevent release of calcium ions from intracellular stores or by reducing myosin light chain kinase activity.

Towards term a number of processes occur which predispose to activation or preparation of the myometrium for onset of labour. Formation of gap junctions by increases in contraction-associated proteins such as connexin-43 enhance cell to cell coupling. Receptors for oxytocin and stimulatory prostaglandins are also increased. These changes are associated with myometrial stretch when the uterus enlarges and with the higher levels of oestrogens derived partly from placental conversion of fetal dehydroepiandrosterone (DHEAS) where they also exert a local oestrogen effect. In addition to increased DHEAS production, activation of the fetal hypothalamic–pituitary–adrenal axis in late pregnancy results in more fetal cortisol biosynthesis. Fetal cortisol competes to reduce the local progesterone effect and stimulate synthesis of corticotrophin-releasing hormone from placenta and fetal membranes for production of prostaglandins by the latter structures.

MYOMETRIAL ACTIVITY: LABOUR

Initiation of labour remains unclear, but prostaglandins have been implicated in myometrial contraction. Isoforms of phospholipase A_2 or C, activated by varying requirements for calcium ions, liberate arachidonic acids from membrane phospholipids. Prostaglandin synthase in amnion and chorion convert arachidonic acids to primary prostaglandins. For prostaglandin E_2 (PGE_2) there are four main receptor subtypes labelled from EP-1 to EP-4. These receptors are distributed in the myometrium in varying concentrations. Stimulation of EP-1 and EP-3 results in contractions whereas stimulation of the other two receptors leads to relaxation. These together with corticotrophin-releasing hormone-related cyclic AMP in the lower uterine segment contribute to fundal dominance.

Onset of labour is associated with a substantial increased myometrial sensitivity to oxytocin stimulation and a three- to five-fold increase in oxytocin production by chorio-decidual tissue. Oxytocin raises concentrations of free calcium in the myocytes to promote myometrial contraction.

Fetal membranes covering the internal cervical os exhibit a decreased production of the 15-hydroxyprostaglandin dehydrogenase enzyme which metabolises prostaglandins. More local prostaglandin production is available for cervical effacement and dilatation. This effect is supplemented by release of collagenase through increased cytokine activity.

Onset of labour is most likely between midnight and 0500 hours when maternal secretion of oxytocin peaks and the myometrium is most sensitive to oxytocin and prostaglandin. These changes in steroid and protein concentrations return to non-pregnant levels 48–72 hours post partum.

Uterine work

Myometrial contraction exerts a pull in circular and longitudinal directions (Figure 7.1)

The term fundal dominance is used to describe travel of myometrial contractions from the fundus of the uterus towards the cervix. The starting point or pacemaker for myometrial activity is situated near the point of insertion of the fallopian tubes into the uterus. The spread of myoelectrical activity through the uterus requires 1 minute. Approximately another minute is needed for adequate relaxation. Blood

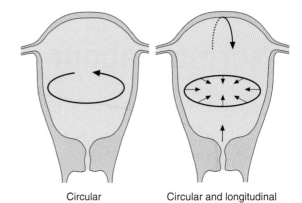

Circular   Circular and longitudinal

Figure 7.1 Myometrial contraction exerts pull in circular and longitudinal directions.

vessels must traverse the myometrium to reach the placenta. Contractions occurring more than once every 2 minutes contribute to poor myometrial relaxation and reduce blood and hence oxygen supply to the fetus. When two contractions are noted every 10 minutes for an hour consider possible onset of labour. In established labour the rate of contractions ranges between 3 and 5 per 10 minutes.

In early labour the uterus is not working at maximum capacity. This may be because the number of myometrial cells contracting is limited or contraction is poorly synchronised or of short duration. As labour progresses contractions becomes more efficient and uterine work increases. Capacity for work cannot, however, increase indefinitely. A stable phase for ability to work results once maximal work output is achieved for the individual mother. When the stable phase is achieved (Figure 7.2a) additional stimulation by oxytocics is of little value and can be harmful. Uterine work has been expressed as:

- Classically in Montevideo units which are intensity (mmHg) times number of contractions per 10 minutes. The intensity is taken as the height reached by the recorded contraction from the resting tone (Figure 7.2b).

- Kilopascals per 15 minutes. Included as a display in contemporary models of fetal monitors when intrauterine transducers are used. The range for normal labour is 700–1500 kPa per 15 minutes.

Intrauterine pressure

The viscoelastic myometrium always exerts pressure on the amniotic fluid. The resting pressure or tone is usually 6–12 mmHg. Amniotic fluid is not compressible.

Measurement is achieved by:

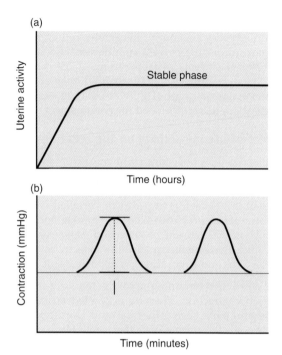

(a)

(b)

Figure 7.2 (a) Graph of uterine activity with stable phase (plateau) for individual woman. (b) Montevideo unit = intensity (amplitude of recorded contraction) × contractions per 10 minutes. The Alexandra unit, a refinement, takes into consideration duration of the contraction.

- Insertion of a fluid-filled polythene tube into the uterine cavity. This tube is connected to a transducer capable of measuring changes in hydrostatic pressure.
- Insertion of a catheter-tipped pressure transducer into the uterine cavity (Figure 7.3). This is a more costly but simpler system.
- Palpation and external (tocometers) assessment do not indicate intrauterine pressure.

Intensity of uterine contractions increases throughout pregnancy. Towards term pressures up to 30 mmHg may be recorded. During labour intrauterine pressure increases to levels of 60–80 mmHg. Contractions of this intensity are still detectable for 48 hours post partum but the frequency diminishes after 12 hours.

General comments
- Normal efficient uterine activity is associated with fundal dominance and regular synchronised contractions of good (more than 40 mmHg) intensity.
- Contractions should last between 40 and 60 seconds with an adequate interval in between when intrauterine pressure can return to resting tone.

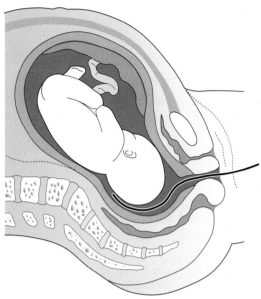

Figure 7.3 Intrauterine pressure measured by a catheter-tipped pressure transducer placed above presenting part is less affected by movement.

- Uterine contractions are more efficient when women lie on their side.
- Primiparous labour is generally associated with contractions of greater intensity than those in multiparae.
- Early amniotomy shortens labour with no detrimental effect on fetal outcome nor an increase in assisted delivery. In uncomplicated labours, the woman's preference must be considered. The increased uterine activity of labour exerts additional pressure on the amniotic fluid. Measurement of this intrauterine hydrostatic pressure (IUP) indicates the strength of the contraction.
- Epidural lengthens both first and second stage of labour, increased incidence of fetal malposition and vaginal instrumental delivery (incidence reduced by routine oxytocin).

Effect of uterine activity on the cervix

Before labour
In the weeks before labour that portion of the uterus between the internal os and the reflection of the uterovesical fold of the peritoneum is attenuated by stretch and Braxton Hicks contractions to form the lower segment. This allows the presenting part of the fetus, particularly in primiparous women, to settle or engage into the pelvis.

In labour

Labour is traditionally divided into two stages:

- First stage – onset of labour to full cervical dilatation. This includes the latent and active phase of labour.

- Second stage – full dilatation to delivery of the baby. The duration approximates 60 minutes in primiparas and 30 minutes in multiparas. Management/intervention should not be based solely on these suggested times. A little more time can be allocated to avoid unwelcome interference if both the fetus and the mother are well. On the other hand with complications or fetal distress, elective assisted delivery or a shortened second stage is advised.

Effacement precedes cervical dilatation. Initially uterine activity is expanded to achieve effacement. This period, the latent phase of labour, takes on average 9 ± 6 hours in the primiparas and 5 ± 4 hours in multiparas. The cervix is usually up to 2 cm dilated when labour begins. At the end of the latent phase cervical dilatation is usually between 3 cm and 4 cm. Once effaced further uterine activity produces rapid cervical dilatation of at least 1 cm per hour in both parous and nulliparous women. This, the active phase of labour takes on average 6 hours to reach full cervical dilatation (Figure 7.4). Multiparous women approach labour with more cervical effacement hence a shorter latent phase and thus a shorter labour.

It is common practice to plot the rate of cervical dilatation to indicate the progress of labour. This is usually charted on a single sheet of paper designed for recording labour events over a 24-hour period. Provision is also made for registering fetal heart rate (every 30 minutes), uterine contractions (every 30 minutes), rate of head descent and medication.

Cervical dilatation detected by vaginal examination is recorded every 2–4 hours. This graphic representation of parturition (partogram) summarises and depicts, visually, the events in labour (Figure 7.5). Cervical dilatation lagging 2–3 hours behind that expected from the normal graph (Figure 7.6), should suggest to medical attendants the need for reassessment.

Effect of uterine activity on the fetus

- Blood vessels traversing the myometrium to supply the placenta and fetus are compressed during uterine contractions. Delivery of nutrients and, particularly, oxygen is impeded or curtailed once the intrauterine pressure exceeds 40 mmHg. Increased myometrial tension or tone and rapid recurring contractions further reduce the capacity to supply the fetus and hence threaten hypoxic insult.

- Compaction or curling up of the fetus occurs with each contraction. Pressure is exerted on the presenting parts, such as the fetal head. During passage through the birth canal, the whole fetus is compressed and this can evoke vagal stimuli.

- The substantial increase in fetal catecholamine production helps switch off fetal lung liquid production.

- The fetus is gradually expelled into the vagina in the process of birth.

- The mechanism of labour is illustrated in Box 7.1.

Management of the delivery

Position

The squatting posture is well suited to delivery. A woman adopting the lithotomy position propped up with pillows and her legs drawn back essentially achieves this posture but has the added advantage of allowing attendant access to assist delivery.

Aseptic conditions

Gloves and gown are mandatory for the attendant conducting the delivery. Women should be draped and the vulval area cleansed. Deliver onto sterile towels.

Medical attendant

The medical attendant is usually stationed on the woman's right. Place the left hand on the fetal head as it 'crowns' (passage of the biparietal eminences through the vulva) to maintain flexion and prevent expulsive delivery.

The right hand is used to guard the perineum and cover the anus with a sanitary pad. If necessary assist

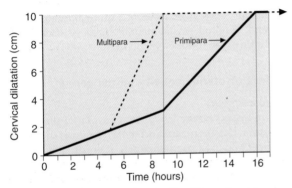

Figure 7.4 Partogram. Primipara and multipara showing latent phase and steep active phase to full cervical dilatation.

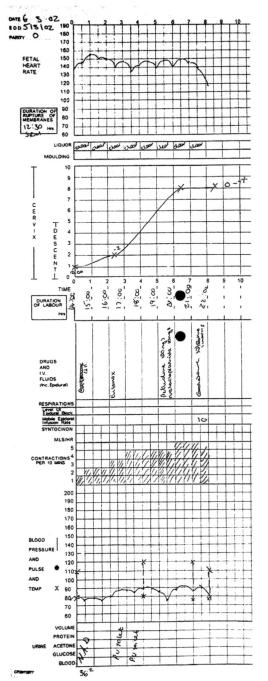

Figure 7.5   Example of a partogram in use showing a concise summary of events in labour.

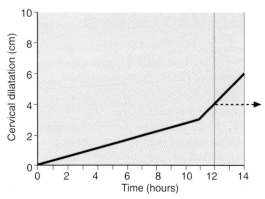

Figure 7.6   Partogram showing deviation (−) from the expected course.

extension of the fetal head by lifting the chin. Consider if an episiotomy is needed.

Delivery of the head
Instruct the woman to pant once the head is crowned. This prevents forceful pushing, and repeated gentle increase in intra-abdominal pressure created by panting nudges the head out. Aspirate the mouth and then the nose of the baby at the first opportunity. Give 0.5–1 ml of Syntometrine (a combination of the synthetic oxytocic Syntocinon 5 units/ml and ergometrine maleate, 0.5 mg/ml) intramuscularly to the mother. The oxytocic effect is evident in 2.5 minutes (Syntocinon) to 7 minutes (ergometrine). It assists uterine contraction and placental separation and thereby controls blood loss. For mothers at risk of haemorrhage, give ergometrine intravenously (oxytocic effect in 1 minute).

Delivery of the shoulders
Once external rotation is completed, direct the head gently downwards to assist delivery of the shoulders. When the anterior shoulder appears beneath the symphysis insert a finger into the anterior axilla and lift the body upwards watching the perineum at the same time to avoid extension of the episiotomy or tearing of the perineum.

Umbilical cord
Cut the cord within 1 minute of birth. This interval allows additional transfusion of more than a third of the fetal blood volume. Do not wait for cessation of pulsation as the placenta may be separated and fetal exsanguination can result. Free any loose cord around the neck over the head or shoulders and proceed with the delivery. If the cord is tight around the neck or

Box 7.1   Mechanism of labour

Flexion and entry

Uterine contractions cause further flexion and entry of the fetal head into the pelvis, usually in the occipito-transverse (Figure 7.7).

Descent and internal rotation

Descent occurs to the level of the ischial spines when levator ani muscles assist internal rotation to align the sagittal sutures for delivery through the widest anteroposterior diameter of the outlet.

Extension and delivery of the head

Distension of the lower part of the vagina evokes reflexes which stimulate the urge to push. Pushing is achieved by the Valsalva response and contraction of diaphragmatic and abdominal muscles. The head stretches the vagina and vulva as it delivers. Extension occurs once the head passes beneath the symphysis pubis. Fetal membranes usually rupture before this stage (shown in sequence in Figure 7.8).

Restitution, external rotation and delivery of the shoulders

The head rotates to occipitolateral or restitutes to align naturally perpendicular to the shoulders. The shoulders, having entered the pelvis in the oblique diameter, rotate so the bisacromial diameter of the shoulder delivers in the anteroposterior diameter of the pelvic outlet. Further rotation of the head laterally accompanies rotation of the shoulders (Figure 7.9).

Delivery of the body

The shoulders deliver assisted by lateral flexion of the body. Once this is achieved the rest of the fetus delivers readily as the uterus contracts down (Figure 7.10).

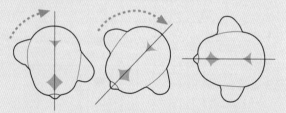

Figure 7.9   Restitution showing the relation of the sagittal axis of the fetal head to allow delivery of shoulders in the anteroposterior diameter of the pelvic outlet.

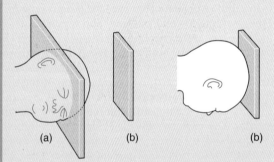

(a)   (b)   (b)

Figure 7.7   The widest part of the inlet (a) (transverse diameter) and outlet (b) (anteroposterior diameter) is represented geometrically. The fetal head enters in the occipito-transverse then rotates to address anteroposterior diameter of outlet.

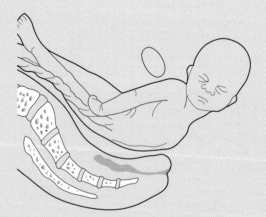

Figure 7.10   Delivery of the body by lateral flexion.

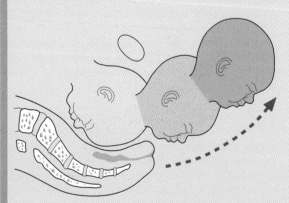

Figure 7.8   Delivery of the head by extension.

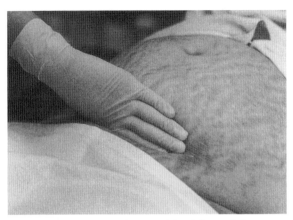

Figure 7.11 Placement of the hand for delivery of the placenta.

fetal resuscitation is anticipated clamp, cut the cord at once and deliver the baby.

Management of the third stage
The third stage is the internal between delivery of the fetus and delivery of the placenta. Placental separation is shown by:

- a lengthening of the cut cord
- a show of blood
- elevation of the fundus as the uterus contracts following separation of the placenta.

Delivery of the placenta
The placenta usually separates within 3 minutes and is delivered within 5 minutes after birth.

- Stand on the mother's right side. The uterus should be contracted.

- The left hand is placed suprapubically. Straddle the uterus with the thumb on one side and the rest of the fingers on the other for better control (Figure 7.11). Press backwards towards the mother to align the uterus with the vaginal axis. Figure 7.12 shows straightening of the uterus.

- Grasp the cord with the right hand and apply gentle traction in line with the pelvic axis (approximately 45° to the horizontal). If the cord springs back once pressure is removed, placental separation is not complete. Wait. If the placenta is separated, controlled traction will deliver the placenta (Figure 7.13).

- Rotate the placenta to wind the membranes into a cord to assist their complete delivery.

- Inspect the placenta (Box 7.2), the membranes and the cord for abnormalities and completeness.

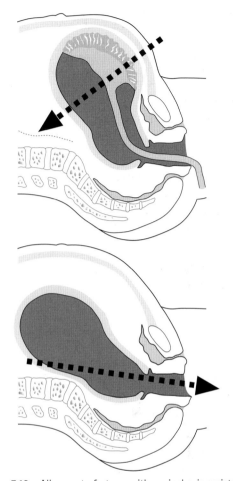

Figure 7.12 Alignment of uterus with vaginal axis assists the delivery of placenta.

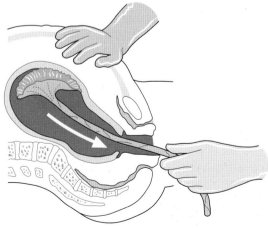

Figure 7.13 Controlled cord traction facilitates delivery of the separated placenta.

Effect of uterine activity on the mother

Management guidelines

- Labour evokes feelings of anxiety and anticipation particularly in the primipara, where labour is lengthy and when complications are present. Emphasise teachings from antenatal classes and offer support.

Box 7.2   Placental inspection

- Inspect and document all macroscopic features. Request histological examination for obstetric complications, e.g. growth restriction, stillbirth to determine possible aetiology. In twin pregnancy, confirmation of chorionicity is important.

- Karyotyping and genetic examination assist with diagnosis of fetal abnormalities, unexpected outcome and growth below the third centile.

- Take swabs from the chorion when infection is suspected.

- Pain threshold varies among individuals. Ensure comfort (Box 7.3) and avoid distress.

- Nurse the woman on her side or in a semi-reclining position (semi-Fowler) to assist labour and avoid compression of the inferior vena cava. Flexibility in attitude of the attendants is needed to accommodate individual preferences (check birth plans).

- Maintain energy requirements and electrolyte balance.

- Record the pulse, blood pressure and temperature at regular intervals.

- Special precautions are required if there is pre-existing maternal medical disease or complications (for example, supplementary hydrocortisone to cover stress of labour).

- Good communication and documentation is essential particularly when there is digression from standard practice.

Box 7.3   Administration of entonox

- Check that gas cylinders are not empty and that they have been stored at room temperature. The two gases may separate if stored at low temperatures ($-7\,°C$).

- Ensure the mask fits over the nose and mouth with no air leaks from the slides of the mask.

- Analgesia begins in 20 seconds and is maximum at 45 seconds. The interval between onset of uterine contractions and sensation of pain is 20–30 seconds in the latent phase and 10–15 seconds in the active phase of labour. Use the mask at the beginning of contractions for the maximum analgesic effect at the height of the contraction.

- Instruct the mother to inhale deeply through the mouth and exhale rapidly to make the machine click.

The gas mixture is only released from the demand valve in the machine when the mother inhales deeply.

- If the mother is particularly sensitive to nitrous oxide use the mask only when contractions become uncomfortable.

- For analgesia in the second stage, time contractions and breath 30 seconds before each contraction. Instruct women to take two to three quick deep breaths on the mask during a contraction prior to her pushing efforts.

- Women must be instructed to hold the mask themselves. Should they become anaesthetised the mask will fall away from the face and allow recovery.

Bibliography

Fox H 1997 Pathology of the Placenta. WB Saunders, London

Grammatopoulos DK, Hillhouse EW 1999 Role of corticotrophin-releasing hormone in onset of labour. Lancet 354:1546–1549

Howell CJ, Kidd C, Roberts W et al 2001 A randomised controlled trial of epidural compared with non-epidural analgesia in labour. British Journal of Obstetrics and Gynaecology 108:27–33

Lye SJ, Ou CW, Teoh TG 1998 The molecular basis of labour and tocolysis. Feto-Maternal Medical Review 10:121–136

Patel FA, Clifton VL, Chawalisz K et al 1999 Steroidal regulation of prostaglandin dehydrogenase activity and expression in human term placenta and chorio decidua in relation to labour. Journal of Clinical Endocrinology and Metabolism 84:291–299

Petraglia F, Florio P, Nappi C et al 1996 Peptide signalling in human placenta and membranes: autocrine, paracrine, and endocrine mechanisms. Endocrine Reviews 17:156–186

Sangha RK, Walton JC, Ensor CM et al 1994 Immunohistochemical localisation, mRNA abundance, and activity of 15-hydroxyprostaglandin dehydrogenase in placenta and fetal membranes during term and preterm labour. Journal of Clinical Endocrinology and Metabolism 78:982–989

Sparey C, Robson SC, Bailey J et al 1999. The differential expression of myometrial connexin-43, cyclooxygenase-1 and -2 and Gsα proteins in the upper and lower segments of the human uterus during pregnancy and labour. Journal of Clinical Endocrinology and Metabolism 84: 1705–1710

Steer PJ, Carter MC, Gordon AJ et al 1978 The use of catheter-tip pressure transducers for the measurement of intrauterine pressure in labour. British Journal of Obstetrics and Gynaecology 85:561

UK Amniotomy Group 1994 A multi-centre randomised trial comparing routine versus delayed amniotomy in spontaneous first labour at term. British Journal of Obstetrics and Gynaecology 101:307–309

Wu YW 2002 Systematic review of chorio-amnionitis and cerebral palsy. Mental retardation and Developmental Disabilities Research Reviews 8:25–29

Chapter **8**

Intrapartum nutrition and electrolytes

Paul Tomlinson, David T Y Liu

CHAPTER CONTENTS

Changes in labour   55
Nutrition in labour   56
  Controversy   56
  Management guidelines   56
    Uncomplicated/spontaneous labour   56
    Complicated labour: when fetal compromise/
      operative delivery more likely   56
Key points   56

Pregnant women approach labour with a mild degree of respiratory alkalosis and metabolic acidosis. Their capacity to use glucose is reduced. Defects in energy requirements are often met by increased lipolysis. This causes a small rise in plasma ketone levels throughout pregnancy. Ketonuria, however, is not observed unless plasma ketone concentration rises above 6–8 mmol/l. Gluconeogenesis does occur in the fetal liver and kidneys, but the main glucose supply is from the mother. This is provided by diffusion, across the placenta, down a concentration gradient. Fetal blood glucose levels are one-third to one-half that of the mother. As a result, fetal glucose rises and falls with changes in maternal nutritional state, and maternal starvation will reduce fetal plasma glucose. In labour, the fetal glucose requirement is 7–10 mg/kg per minute. Water diffuses freely across the placenta. Sodium and chloride concentrations are similar in maternal and fetal plasma, but potassium levels are higher in fetal than maternal blood, 6.4 mmol/l and 4.6 mmol/l, respectively. The likely mechanism of this is an active transport system.

CHANGES IN LABOUR

Labour further affects maternal metabolism and plasma electrolytes. Also, certain modern therapeutic measures employed in the management of specific problems in labour produce additional changes. The basic factors involved are:

- The energy of labour is provided predominantly by glucose, and most women enter labour with little reserve for sustained aerobic metabolism. Moderate accumulation of lactate causes a fall in maternal plasma pH to 7.34 and a fall in $PaCO_2$ to 4–4.5 kPa.

- Oral intake of food and water is often discouraged to reduce the risk of regurgitation of stomach contents and aspiration pneumonia (Mendelson's syndrome). This can occur in association with general anaesthesia, and abrupt changes in levels of consciousness produced by acute major pathology in labour or use of heavy sedation.

- Exertion, stress, and prolonged or high dose use of intravenous oxytocics (>16 mU/min Syntocinon) enhance antidiuretic hormone (ADH) production. This produces water retention and hyponatraemia.

- In a bid to avoid sodium retention, electrolyte-free dextrose solutions are commonly used to maintain hydration and to temporarily expand the vascular compartment when epidural analgesia is commenced. This practice can however cause hyponatraemia in the fetus and the mother. Rapid falls of plasma sodium to <128 mmol/l may produce cerebral oedema, confusion, convulsions, coma and even death.

- β-Sympathomimetics, such as salbutamol, are often used intravenously for reducing the risk of preterm labour. These drugs encourage migration of potassium into cells, producing hypokalaemia. There is an additional ADH effect and possible hyperglycaemia due to their sympathetic activity.

- Vomiting due to pain, stress or opioids and altered renal function due to complications such as preeclampsia (PET) can further contribute to water and electrolyte imbalance.

NUTRITION IN LABOUR

Controversy

Some obstetricians and midwives now believe that in the absence of risk factors that could lead to operative delivery of the baby (perhaps with the aid of general anaesthesia) or serious intrapartum morbidity (e.g. PET), strict limitations of oral intake in labour to small amounts of water could be relaxed (Michael et al 1991). Frye (1994) even claims that eating in labour allows women to feel normal and healthy. Their main argument, however, is that ingestion of adequate quantities of calories and water orally prevents significant acidosis and electrolyte disorders. Most protagonists of oral feeding in labour cite studies demonstrating that administration of clear fluids up to 2 hours before elective surgery does not increase gastric volume or acidity in non-pregnant patients, providing that they do not consume solid food (Kallar and Everett 1993). Applying the results

of such studies to women in labour may be ill-advised because:

- the interval between the last full meal and the onset of labour varies a great deal among women. Ultrasound examination will often demonstrate that two-thirds of pregnant women have solid gastric contents regardless of the time elapsed since their last meal (Kallar and Everett 1993).

- systemic administration of opioids to women in labour dramatically delays gastric emptying (Nimmo et al 1975). Epidural or spinal local anaesthetic/opioid mixtures may produce similar effects though not all studies agree on this.

- women in labour may require caesarean section or other life-saving interventions at any time. The interval between last oral intake and induction of anaesthesia could be substantially within 2 hours.

It is appropriate therefore to continue the practice of restricting oral intake in labour, probably to 60 ml/h water or other non-particulate fluid in uncomplicated pregnancies.

Management guidelines

Uncomplicated/spontaneous labour
- Assess condition after admission.
- Restrict oral intake to clear fluid.
- Prescribe opioids and antiemetics.
- Monitor fluid balance.

Complicated labour: when fetal compromise/ operative delivery more likely
- Assess condition after admission.
- Restrict oral intake to <60 ml/h water.
- Set up intravenous infusion: this should include 69 g glucose/m^2 per 24 hours to avoid ketonuria.
- Strict fluid balance chart.
- Regular urine checks for ketones.
- Regular plasma electrolyte checks.

KEY POINTS

- Nutrition in labour, especially in presence of complications, is important but requires much regular attention to detail.
- Opioid administration by any route may cause significant delays in gastric emptying.
- Women in labour who have not received appreciable quantities of parenteral opioid may be allowed up to 60 ml/h clear fluid to drink.

References

Frye A 1994 Nourishing the mother. Midwifery Today 31:25–26

Kallar SK, Everett LL 1993 Potential risks and preventative measures for pulmonary aspiration: new concepts in preoperative fasting guidelines. Anesthesia and Analgesia 77:171–182

Michael S, Reilly CS, Caunt JA 1991 Policies for oral intake during labour: a survey of maternity units in England and Wales. Anaesthesia 46:1071–1073

Nimmo WS, Wilson J, Prescott LF 1975 Narcotic analgesics and delayed gastric emptying during labour. Lancet i:890–893

Bibliography

Champion P, McCormick C 2001 Eating and Drinking in Labour. Books for Midwives, London

Royal College of Midwives 2005 Practice Guideline. Evidence Based Guidelines for Midwifery-led Care in Labour. RCM, London

Scrutton M, Metcalfe G, Lowy C et al 1999 Eating in labour: a randomised controlled trial assessing the risks and benefits. Anaesthesia 54:329–334

Chapter 9

Analgesia and anaesthesia

David M Levy

CHAPTER CONTENTS

Analgesia for labour   59
  Inhalational analgesia   59
  Parenteral opioids   60
  Transcutaneous electrical nerve stimulation   60
  Regional analgesia for labour   60
    Complications of regional analgesia   63
    Establishing regional analgesia – practical
      points   63
    Initial management of dural tap   64
    Epidural blood patch   65
    Pudendal block   65
Anaesthesia for caesarean section   65
  Pre-operative preparation   65
    Non-elective cases   65
  Spinal anaesthesia   66
    Establishing spinal anaesthesia – practical
      points   66
  Epidural anaesthesia   66
    Establishing epidural anaesthesia – practical
      points   67
  Combined spinal-epidural anaesthesia   67
  General anaesthesia   67
  Tocolysis and oxytocics   68
Postoperative analgesia   68
Placenta praevia   69
Pre-assessment   69
Pre-eclampsia   69
Eclampsia   69
  Practical points   70

Obstetric *analgesia* is the relief of pain in labour; *anaesthesia* is the abolition of sufficient sensation to allow operative delivery.

The experience of pain represents a complex combination of physiological, psychological, emotional and conditioned responses. Modern regional blocks can relieve pain in labour while preserving some sensation of uterine contractions and the ability to push. If instrumental delivery or caesarean section become necessary, it is possible to produce surgical anaesthesia rapidly by extension of the block. In the vast majority of cases general anaesthesia can be avoided.

General anaesthesia is nowadays reserved largely for those cases where a regional block is either contraindicated or has failed.

ANALGESIA FOR LABOUR

Inhalational analgesia

In the UK, 60–70% of labouring women seek to achieve analgesia by inhalation of a 50:50 mixture of nitrous oxide and oxygen (N_2O/O_2). Marketed as Entonox and Equanox, the gas mixture is supplied in cylinders with blue body and blue/white shoulders and is piped to delivery rooms in many hospitals.

The gas is self-administered by inspiration through a facemask or mouthpiece, which opens a demand valve. Diffusion from alveoli to pulmonary capillaries and delivery to the brain by the cardiac output is not instantaneous – inhalation should start as soon as a contraction begins so maximum effect is achieved at its peak (see Chapter 7, Box 7.3).

The drug is non-cumulative, and does not affect the fetus. N_2O/O_2 causes a variable degree of sedation. Some women appear to be dreaming or drunk; others become somnolent or even briefly unarousable.

Hyperventilation with N_2O/O_2 can be followed by a short period of apnoea, therefore the woman should hold the mouthpiece or mask herself. If she loses consciousness, she will let go. A few breaths of air eliminate the N_2O and consciousness will invariably be regained soon. A number of studies have questioned the analgesic effect of N_2O/O_2. Pain is still perceived under the influence of the drug – it is merely rendered more bearable by the intoxicated state.

The risk of cross-contamination between women sharing breathing systems dictates that mouthpieces and masks should be disposable or sterilised between users. Either a new disposable breathing system should be used for each woman, or a disposable breathing system filter interposed between the tubing and mouthpiece/mask.

Parenteral opioids

Clinical studies of pain scores have cast doubt on the analgesic efficacy of opioids in labour. The drugs are certainly sedative, inducing a feeling of disorientation and thereby making pain more tolerable. All opioids can induce maternal and neonatal respiratory depression (decreased Apgar and neurobehavioural scores). Gastric emptying is inhibited, and the incidence of nausea and vomiting increased.

Midwives can prescribe and administer controlled drugs in accordance with locally agreed policies and procedures. In the UK, pethidine is the most widely used intramuscular opioid. A usual dose of 100 mg lasts around 3 hours. Plasma pethidine concentrations are maximal in the neonate when the mother has received the drug about 3 hours before delivery. It is therefore illogical to withhold the drug if delivery is imminent, for fear of causing neonatal respiratory depression.

Naloxone is a specific opioid antagonist. The neonatal dose is $10\,\mu g/kg$ intramuscularly, repeated if necessary.

Comparisons of pethidine 100 mg with diamorphine 5 mg, meptazinol 100 mg and tramadol 100 mg have failed to demonstrate any convincing benefits. An antiemetic (e.g. cyclizine 50 mg or prochlorperazine 12.5 mg) should be given intramuscularly along with whatever the chosen opioid. Because of the additive risk of respiratory depression, intramuscular opioids should never be given in the event of inadequate regional analgesia without prior reassessment of the woman by an anaesthetist.

Transcutaneous electrical nerve stimulation

Electrical impulses applied to the skin via flexible carbon electrodes from a battery-powered stimulator

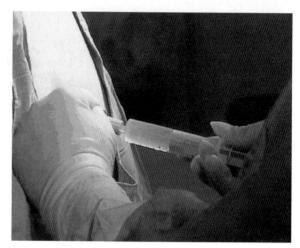

Figure 9.1 Advancement of Tuohy needle with loss of resistance to syringe plunger.

modulate the transmission of pain by closing a 'gate' in the dorsal horn of the spinal cord. The effect is similar to massage of the lower back by a birthing partner.

Transcutaneous electrical nerve stimulation (TENS) is used in about 1 in 20 labours in the UK. The technique is completely free from adverse effects, and can diminish the need for other analgesic interventions.

A study comparing TENS and 'sham' TENS' (TENS devices which appeared to be working but had been disabled) failed to demonstrate reduced pain scores in labour. After delivery, however, those women who had had working TENS retrospectively rated their analgesia more highly. More of these women stated they would choose TENS again in a future labour.

Regional analgesia for labour

Regional analgesia is the provision of pain relief by blockade of sensory nerves as they enter the spinal cord. Local anaesthetic can be introduced into the epidural or subarachnoid (intrathecal) space, or both.

The epidural space is identified by the loss of resistance to depression of a syringe plunger as a Tuohy needle is advanced (Figure 9.1) through the ligamentum flavum. A catheter is then threaded through the Tuohy needle (Figure 9.2) to facilitate top-ups or continuous infusion. The subarachnoid space (containing cerebrospinal fluid (CSF)) is a few millimetres deeper, inside the meninges. Needles used for spinal injection are much finer than Tuohy needles (Figure 9.3). A significant advance has been the development of 'pencil point' tips (Figure 9.4). Compared with standard cutting bevel or Quincke needle tips, the leak of

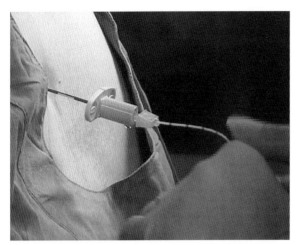

Figure 9.2 Tuohy needle advanced through the ligamentum flavum, with a catheter in the epidural space.

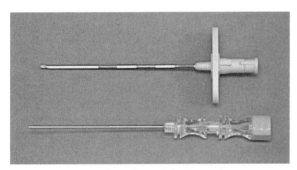

Figure 9.3 Epidural Tuohy (above) and spinal needles.

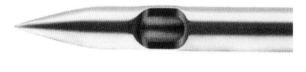

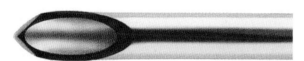

Figure 9.4 Pencil point (above) and cutting bevel tip spinal needles (courtesy of SIMS Portex Ltd).

CSF and likelihood of consequent headache are vastly reduced.

A trained anaesthetist *must* always be immediately available whenever regional analgesia is provided. Regional techniques improperly administered can be as hazardous as any general anaesthetic. Resources

Box 9.1   Resources for treatment of complications during the provision of regional analgesia

- Laryngoscope and blades
- Tracheal tubes and stylettes
- Oxygen source
- Suction source with tubing and catheters
- Self-inflating bag and mask for positive pressure ventilation
- Drugs – vasoconstrictor (e.g. phenylephrine, ephedrine), anaesthetic induction agent (e.g. thiopental), neuromuscular blocking drug (e.g. succinylcholine)

that should be available on every labour ward in the event of complications (see below) which might arise during the provision of regional analgesia are listed in Box 9.1.

Compared with every other analgesic technique, pain relief from regional blockade is undoubtedly superior. In the UK, 90% of consultant obstetric units provide a 24-hour epidural service; the average epidural rate is 24%.

Blockade of motor fibres causes relaxation of pelvic floor muscles and impairs expulsive efforts, therefore provision of adequate maternal analgesia with as little motor block as possible has emerged as a goal common to all regimens. Intermittent epidural boluses, continuous epidural infusions, and patient-controlled epidural analgesia all provide comparable pain relief and maternal satisfaction.

Unlike local anaesthetics, which prevent conduction of nerve impulses, opioids act on specific receptors in the spinal cord. Synergistic mixtures of local anaesthetic and opioids (usually fentanyl) have permitted significant reductions in the amount of local anaesthetic used. Side effects specific to the use of opioids are respiratory depression (in the most unlikely event that opioid spreads cephalad to reach the brainstem) and pruritus.

Combined spinal-epidural analgesia entails an initial subarachnoid injection of fentanyl mixed with a tiny amount of local anaesthetic. The resulting motor block is sufficiently minimal for women to retain sufficient muscle power to walk in labour. However, proprioception (information from joint receptors to maintain balance) can be impaired. In the absence of any proved advantage to mother or baby of walking in labour, some argue that it is hard to justify the risk of falling.

Table 9.1 Contraindications to regional analgesia, with associated risks

Contraindication	Risk
Uncorrected anticoagulation or coagulopathy	Vertebral canal haematoma
Local or systemic sepsis (pyrexia >38 °C not treated with antibiotics)	Vertebral canal abscess
Hypovolaemia or active haemorrhage	Cardiovascular collapse secondary to sympathetic blockade
Maternal refusal	Legal action
Lack of sufficient trained midwives for continuous care and monitoring of mother and fetus for the duration of the regional block	Maternal collapse, convulsion, respiratory arrest; fetal compromise

Signed consent is not necessary for regional analgesia in labour. Verbal consent is sufficient, and a brief record should be made in the notes of the risks/benefits that have been discussed.

Table 9.1 outlines the contraindications to regional analgesia, together with the associated risks.

A full blood count (FBC) is not required unless antepartum bleeding has occurred, anaemia is suspected, or there is evidence of pre-eclampsia. If the platelet count is normal, a coagulation screen is not necessary. If a pre-eclamptic woman's overall condition is deteriorating an FBC should have been processed no more than 2 hours before a regional block is undertaken. If platelet count is $70{-}100 \times 10^9$/l or if the trend is steadily downwards, a coagulation screen must be normal if spinal/epidural block is to be undertaken. Petechiae or platelet count $<70 \times 10^9$/l are indications for platelet transfusion. Aspirin therapy alone is not a contraindication to regional analgesia.

Low molecular weight heparins (LMWHs) pose the risk of vertebral canal haematoma and consequent spinal cord or nerve root compression. This risk has to be weighed against the risk of emergency general anaesthesia in a woman denied regional blockade. As far as possible, institution of regional blocks – and removal of epidural catheters – should be undertaken when anti-factor Xa activity is least. After delivery, continued vigilance for signs of haematoma is essential. If symptoms of leg weakness or numbness, back pain, or bowel/bladder dysfunction develop (onset can be delayed beyond 24 hours) neurological/neurosurgical advice should be sought without delay.

Although a vertebral canal haematoma or abscess is exceedingly rare, transient neuropathy has an incidence of about 1 in 2000. Women can be reassured that epidural analgesia does *not* cause new, long-term backache.

All women should be warned about the possibility of dural tap – the inadvertent tearing of the meninges by the Tuohy needle or epidural catheter, which should have an incidence of <1%. This complication can pre-

---

Box 9.2 Counselling before regional block

Before starting a regional block in labour inform women about:

- potential failure to site catheter or achieve perfect analgesia
- necessity to re-site catheter in 5–15% of cases
- localised backache for about 48 hours due to bruising
- maternal pyrexia (>38°)

Epidural analgesia is *associated* with the following:

- longer first and second stages of labour
- increased incidence of fetal malposition
- increased use of oxytocin
- increased incidence of instrumental vaginal deliveries

---

dispose to two potentially serious sequelae: total spinal anaesthesia, and post-dural puncture headache (PDPH). The vast majority of pregnant women who develop PDPH will require an epidural 'blood patch'. Other points worthy of explanation before performing a regional block in labour are listed in Box 9.2.

The rate of cervical dilatation, duration of second stage and the instrumental delivery rate are similar when epidural analgesia is established before or after 4 cm cervical dilatation. Regional analgesia does not result in an increase in the overall caesarean section rate or the rates specific for dystocia or fetal distress. However, a significant proportion of those women who undergo caesarean section for dystocia will have had epidural analgesia for labour. *Risk factors for dystocia produce painful labour and a desire for epidural analgesia.*

It is well worth explaining in advance to women with risk factors for operative delivery that *analgesia*

Table 9.2 Symptoms and signs of local anaesthetic toxicity

Symptoms	Signs
Numbness of tongue or lips	Slurring of speech
Tinnitus	Drowsiness
Light-headedness	Convulsions
Anxiety	Cardiorespiratory arrest

Box 9.3 Collapse in the obstetric patient

- Call for **help**.
- Clear the **airway**.
- Administer high-flow oxygen (10 l/min) by facemask.
- If apnoeic, ventilate with bag and mask. Apply cricoid pressure to occlude the oesophagus. Intubate the trachea as soon as is feasible.
- Relieve aorto-caval compression by manual displacement of the uterus or wedging the right hip with pillows.
- If pulseless, start external cardiac compressions.
- *Delivery by caesarean section is indicated if there is no response to advanced life support within 5 minutes.*

for labour can be converted to effective *anaesthesia* to facilitate forceps or caesarean delivery. Some women need time to consider the notion of being awake for a caesarean section.

Complications of regional analgesia

The two principal potential complications of epidural injection of local anaesthetic are *local anaesthetic toxicity* and *total spinal anaesthesia*. Aspirating the catheter to exclude intravenous or subarachnoid placement can prevent both. The delivery of local anaesthetic to the brain and heart by the bloodstream causes the symptoms and signs of toxicity (Table 9.2).

Epidural venous engorgement in the obstetric patient predisposes to blood vessel puncture in up to 1 in 5 epidurals. If blood is aspirated, flush with saline and withdraw the catheter by another 1 cm. If blood is still present, re-site at another interspace. Local anaesthetic toxicity is not an issue with spinals because the mass of drug injected is so much smaller.

Total spinal anaesthesia is the effect of excessive local anaesthetic within the subarachnoid space. If a dose intended for the epidural space is inadvertently delivered to the subarachnoid space, cephalad spread can cause respiratory arrest by blocking innervation of the diaphragm (C3–C5), and profound hypotension secondary to extensive sympathetic blockade.

A 'total spinal' can occur even when no CSF has been apparent on aspiration, and remains a possibility hours after initiation of an epidural block and following several top-ups. The risk of inadvertent subarachnoid block is not eliminated by epidural catheterisation at another interspace after the dura has been punctured, because the dural tear might still allow passage of local anaesthetic to the CSF.

In addition to local anaesthetic toxicity and total spinal anaesthesia, maternal collapse can occur as a result of:

- massive haemorrhage (which might be intrauterine or intraperitoneal)
- amniotic fluid embolism (anaphylactoid syndrome of pregnancy)
- pulmonary thromboembolism

- eclampsia
- intracranial haemorrhage
- myocardial infarction.

The management of collapse in the obstetric patient is detailed in Box 9.3.

All those working on a delivery suite should make sure they know where the resuscitation equipment and emergency drugs are kept, and keep up to date with the latest international algorithms.

Establishing regional analgesia – practical points

- The woman's cooperation must be secured to maximise the chances of success. Consider fentanyl 50 µg intravenously for the woman unable to keep still on account of intense pain. Particularly in multiparous women, it is worth checking that sudden escalation of pain is not indicative of imminent delivery or uterine rupture.

- Secure intravenous access (14 G or 16 G cannula) must be established using local anaesthesia. An intravenous crystalloid infusion must be started, although a fluid bolus is not required unless the woman is clinically dehydrated.

- Meticulous aseptic precautions are essential, with gown, gloves, hat and mask.

- Loss of resistance to saline is associated with a lower incidence of dural tap and patchy block compared with air. In the event of dubiety as to the origin of fluid appearing at the hub of a Tuohy needle, CSF and saline can be distinguished on the criteria detailed in Table 9.3.

- The epidural drug regimen used in two Nottingham teaching hospitals is given in Box 9.4.

Table 9.3   Distinction between CSF and saline

	CSF	Saline
Temperature	Warm	Cold
Protein	Present	Absent
Glucose	At least a trace	Absent
pH	7.5	<7.5

Box 9.4   Drug regimen for epidural analgesia

Either bupivacaine or levobupivacaine can be used.

Initial dose
Fentanyl 50 µg + (levo)bupivacaine 0.25% 10 ml given in two divided doses 5 minutes apart.

Subsequent infusion
Fentanyl 150 µg + (levo)bupivacaine 0.5% 10 ml + 0.9% saline to a total volume of 60 ml. Infuse at 5–15 ml/hour.

'Escape' top-up for inadequate analgesia
(Levo)bupivacaine 0.25% 5 ml, maximum of two doses per hour.

Levobupivacaine is equipotent with bupivacaine, but has less cardiac toxicity in the event of accidental intravenous administration. '(Levo)bupivacaine' means either drug is appropriate.

- A bilateral block to the sensation of cold (ice or ethyl chloride spray) to T10 (Figure 9.5) should relieve the pain of uterine contractions. If a block rises above T6 (Figure 9.5) the infusion should be stopped, and restarted at a lower rate when the block height has regressed to T10.

- If maternal systolic blood pressure falls below 75% of baseline (e.g. from 120 to 90 mmHg), administer O_2, turn on side, raise legs and give 500 ml fluid rapidly. If blood pressure remains low, phenylephrine 50 µg or ephedrine 3 mg intravenous increments should be given in preference to more fluid.

- Light diet is acceptable for women without obstetric risk factors.

- Any neurological deficit persisting >6 hours after the last top-up or discontinuation of an infusion should be referred for a neurological opinion.

Initial management of dural tap
- Either Tuohy needle or catheter can breach the meninges.

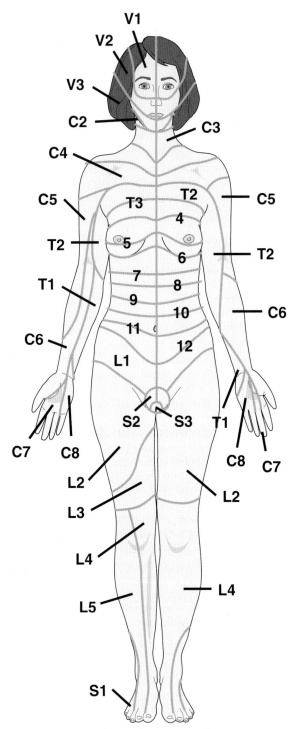

Figure 9.5   Map of (anterior) dermatomes (artwork by Rachel Ellaway © 2000 University of Edniburgh, with permission).

- If CSF flows from the hub of the needle, thread the catheter into the subarachnoid space. If CSF is aspirated from the catheter, leave the catheter in subarachnoid space. Alternatively, re-site the catheter at another interspace.

- If a catheter is used in the subarachnoid space, make sure that the filter is clearly labelled as *spinal*. Boluses of bupivacaine (or levobupivacaine) 0.25% 1–2 ml will provide excellent analgesia for labour. For caesarean section anaesthesia, titrate 0.5 ml increments of 0.5% hyperbaric bupivacaine.

- Only if headache develops during labour need elective instrumental delivery be advised at full dilatation. Caesarean section might be indicated in the rare instance of headache confining a woman to lying flat.

- There is no evidence that enforced postpartum recumbence will prevent development of PDPH. Ensure prescription of regular analgesia and a laxative such as ispaghula husk to prevent straining.

Epidural blood patch
- Indicated if *postural* headache or neckache persists beyond 24 hours. Note that the site of a headache is variable; the diagnostic feature is that it is worse after sitting up.

- In theatre, with full aseptic precautions, the epidural space is identified at or below the original puncture site, and unless limited by back or leg pain (due to arachnoid irritation), up to 20 ml of the patient's freshly aspirated blood is slowly injected.

- After lying flat for 1–2 hours, the woman can mobilise cautiously. About 1 in 5 women require a subsequent procedure.

- If headache is of insufficient severity to necessitate blood patch and the mother is discharged, arrangements must be made for review in the community. If her symptoms are not resolving within the next week, she should be readmitted. Chronic CSF leakage is not a benign condition – intracranial subdural haematoma is a rare complication of the reduced CSF pressure.

Pudendal block
This somatic nerve block provides anaesthesia for episiotomy/perineal repair and low forceps delivery. Both pudendal nerves are blocked as they pass under and slightly posterior to the ischial spines (see Chapter 11). Use of lidocaine 0.5% allows injection of a generous total volume (up to 40 ml). If epidural analgesia has been established during labour, pudendal block will be unnecessary. A top-up of (levo)bupivacaine 0.5% with the woman sitting (in order that the local anaesthetic might bathe the sacral nerve roots) will provide excellent anaesthesia.

ANAESTHESIA FOR CAESAREAN SECTION

Pre-operative preparation
Protracted deprivation of food and oral fluid should be avoided. Elective cases should no longer be instructed to be 'nil by mouth' from midnight. An appropriate fasting policy is:

- Last solid food **6 hours** pre-theatre
- Last cup of squash or tea/coffee (with semi-skimmed not full-fat milk) **2 hours** pre-theatre
- Unrestricted *sips* of *water* until operation.

Women scheduled for elective caesarean section should receive the following antacid prophylaxis because of the tiny risk of pulmonary aspiration of gastric contents in the course of general anaesthesia after failed regional block (and the remote possibility of high spinal anaesthesia causing inability to protect the airway):

- Two oral doses of ranitidine 150 mg, approximately 8 hours apart, and 30 ml 0.3 M sodium citrate immediately before transfer to theatre.
- Women in labour with significant risk factors for caesarean section should have oral ranitidine 150 mg 8 hourly.

Results of a recent FBC and blood group/antibody screen should be available. A haemoglobin concentration of 80–100 g/l (8–10 g/dl) should not usually be an indication for pre-operative transfusion, but a check should be made that serum has been saved by the laboratory in case a cross-match becomes necessary. Urea and electrolytes are requested only if specifically indicated.

Non-elective cases
- *Only about 10% of emergency caesarean sections are totally unpredictable.* Anaesthetists, obstetricians and midwives should discuss those women whose babies have prior evidence of compromise (e.g. intrauterine growth restriction, or poor biophysical profiles/umbilical artery Doppler studies).

- Unless a senior obstetrician is certain that vacuum extraction/outlet forceps delivery will succeed, regional blockade should be sufficient to facilitate immediate caesarean section, should it prove necessary.

> **Box 9.5 Maternal mortality attributable to anaesthesia**
>
> - Failed tracheal intubation (and reintubation)
> - Pulmonary aspiration of gastric contents
> - Anaphylaxis to induction/neuromuscular blocking drugs
> - Airway obstruction from neck haematoma after central line insertion
> - Regional block without intravenous access
> - Total spinal anaesthesia (complicating combined spinal-epidural anaesthesia)
> - Inadequate antagonism of neuromuscular block

- When a decision to proceed to caesarean section is made for a woman labouring with an epidural, it is important to be clear how long the obstetrician is prepared to wait for surgical anaesthesia. Placental abruption, uterine scar dehiscence, prolonged fetal bradycardia and cord prolapse are indications for *immediate* caesarean section (not necessarily under general anaesthesia in all cases). Dystocia ('failure to progress') should allow plenty time for topping up an epidural.

- Emergency patients should be transferred in left lateral position, with Syntocinon discontinued. All women should be positioned on the table with 15° left lateral tilt.

- Monitoring of electrocardiogram, noninvasive blood pressure and pulse oximeter is essential for all cases. For general anaesthesia, capnography (CO_2 monitoring) is vital to confirm tracheal intubation. Inhalational agent monitoring will aid prevention of awareness. Suction must be working and close to hand.

Causes of maternal mortality directly attributed to anaesthesia are listed in Box 9.5.

Spinal anaesthesia

Spinal anaesthesia has become the most common technique for elective caesarean section, on account of its speed and efficacy compared with epidural anaesthesia. Placental blood flow is maintained provided that hypotension is avoided. The possibility of having to resort to general anaesthesia should always be mentioned, and the airway evaluated pre-operatively.

Only rarely should pressure of time preclude institution of a spinal block for a woman who has been labouring without epidural analgesia.

Establishing spinal anaesthesia – practical points

- Avoid aortocaval compression at all times.

- Atropine (0.6 mg) and phenylephrine (1 mg, diluted to 100 µg/ml) and ephedrine (30 mg, diluted to 3 mg/ml) should be drawn up, with drugs for general anaesthesia readily available.

- Establish intravenous infusion (14 or 16 G cannula).

- All drugs for subarachnoid injection must be drawn up through a particulate filter.

- **Hyperbaric** (heavy) **bupivacaine 0.5% 2.5 ml** is appropriate for most patients. Pre-term women (28–35 weeks) have a requirement for more local anaesthetic compared with those at term (>38 weeks), probably because of reduced caval compression and displacement of the dura by engorged epidural veins.

- Preservative-free **morphine 0.1 mg** or **diamorphine 0.25 mg** mixed with the local anaesthetic will provide prolonged postoperative analgesia in conjunction with regular paracetamol and nonsteroidal anti-inflammatory drug (NSAID) unless contraindicated (see Box 9.6 below).

- Infuse a litre of Hartmann's or 0.9% saline rapidly. Maintain systolic arterial pressure above 100 mmHg by administration of intravenous boluses of phenylephrine 50 µg or ephedrine 3 mg.

- Hypotension with tachycardia (heart rate >100 beats per minute) is best treated with 50–100 µg increments of phenylephrine, which tends to increase blood pressure with concomitant decrease in heart rate. There is less fetal acidosis after maternal administration of phenylephrine as opposed to ephedrine.

- *Anaesthesia* (inability to appreciate light touch) should extend from S5 to T4 (Figure 9.5) at the time of delivery. A block to cold from S4 to T4 should be confirmed and documented before surgery starts. Because spinal anaesthesia virtually guarantees complete sensory loss below the most cephalad level, the lower dermatomes do not need to be tested.

- In the event of an inadequate block, a second intrathecal injection should not be administered, because it is difficult to estimate an appropriate safe dose. If time permits, site an epidural catheter and top up cautiously with (levo)bupivacaine 0.5%. If delivery is urgent, general anaesthesia will be indicated.

Epidural anaesthesia

This is most often used when epidural *analgesia* has been established during labour. There are *very* few occasions when a woman with a working epidural in labour should need general anaesthesia for caesarean section on the grounds of lack of available time to establish surgical anaesthesia.

Epidural anaesthesia is indicated in certain clinical conditions (e.g. congenital heart disease) when a regional technique is preferable to general anaesthesia but spinal anaesthesia is relatively contraindicated because of its potential for sudden sympathetic blockade.

Epidural anaesthesia might be favoured when provision of optimal postoperative analgesia by infusion of (levo)bupivacaine/fentanyl in a high-dependency area is warranted, e.g. severe pre-eclampsia.

Establishing epidural anaesthesia – practical points

- The top-up to achieve surgical anaesthesia should be administered in theatre with full monitoring attached, rather than in the delivery room.

- (Levo)bupivacaine 0.5% (plain) 15–20 ml works as fast and as reliably as any other solution for transformation of low-dose epidural analgesia into surgical anaesthesia. Note that about 7 times as much local anaesthetic is required for an equivalent effect from drug administered into the epidural as opposed to subarachnoid spaces.

- Opioids both improve the quality of the block during surgery (e.g. when the uterus is exteriorised) and provide postoperative analgesia in conjunction with an NSAID. Epidural fentanyl in labour does not preclude a further perioperative dose of up to 100 µg (e.g. 50 µg during establishment of the block and a further 50 µg after delivery). The subsequent epidural administration of diamorphine 2.5 mg will provide excellent postoperative analgesia.

- Epidural anaesthesia may leave normal sensation in the most caudal (sacral) dermatomes. Block of the sacral roots is important to prevent pain during traction and pressure on the vagina. All dermatomes from S5 to T4 (Figure 9.5) should be tested to cold on both sides, and the upper and lower limits of the block (and any missed segments) documented.

- Intraoperative pain is more likely with epidurals than spinals. Intravenous alfentanil in 0.5 mg increments can be used to control breakthrough pain, and should not be withheld for fear of neonatal respiratory depression. Isoflurane 0.25% in 50% oxygen/50% nitrous oxide administered by anaesthetic breathing system is also effective. Unrelieved, persistent pain must be managed with general anaesthesia.

Combined spinal–epidural anaesthesia

- The initial subarachnoid injection can be deliberately conservative, to reduce the risk of a dangerously high block (e.g. in the morbidly obese, or patients with difficult airways). In addition, the haemodynamic consequences of spinal anaesthesia will be minimised.

- The subarachnoid block can be augmented by subsequent epidural top-ups (particularly useful if protracted surgery is anticipated).

- The epidural catheter can be used in the postoperative period (e.g. severe pre-eclampsia).

General anaesthesia

- With good antenatal education and pre-operative explanation of the benefits of regional anaesthesia, few women should insist on general anaesthesia.

- Women should be fully assessed wherever possible before transfer to theatre. Pre-oxygenation and cricoid pressure should be explained, and the airway assessed.

- The anaesthetic machine and equipment for management of the difficult airway, e.g. McCoy laryngoscope, gum elastic bougie, laryngeal mask airway (LMA), Combitube, and cricothyrotomy device must be checked. *Never reach for an unfamiliar device for the first time in a crisis*!

- A dedicated trained assistant must be available to apply pressure on the cricoid cartilage to occlude the oesophagus.

- Site a 14 G or 16 G cannula in the hand or wrist with Hartmann's solution or 0.9% saline running. Ensure establishment of left-lateral tilt.

- Optimise head and neck position for intubation. In addition to left lateral tilt, a slight head-up position should offer some protection against gastro-oesophageal reflux.

- Pre-oxygenate via a close-fitting facemask for 3 minutes or until the end-tidal oxygen concentration approaches 90%.

- Administer a precalculated bolus of thiopental 5 mg/kg or etomidate 0.3 mg/kg. Give succinylcholine 100 mg or rocuronium 0.6 mg/kg and instruct assistant to apply cricoid pressure.

- In the event of failure to intubate the trachea, maintain cricoid pressure and attempt to ventilate the lungs with 100% oxygen via facemask. If ventilation proves impossible, release cricoid pressure (which might be causing airway obstruction).

Regurgitation and pulmonary aspiration of gastric contents is neither inevitable nor necessarily fatal.

- An LMA can restore airway patency by displacing the tongue, epiglottis, or larynx from the posterior pharyngeal wall. Again, any increased risk of regurgitation compared with a tracheal tube is of secondary importance to establishing oxygenation. If recovery from succinylcholine has occurred, surgery can proceed with spontaneous respiration of vapour in 100% O_2.

- Mechanical ventilation should be instituted after successful tracheal intubation or placement of an LMA when a non-depolarising neuromuscular blocker has been used. Check for continued pulmonary inflation and adjust minute volume to maintain end-tidal CO_2 at around 4.0 kPa.

- With the airway secured and recovery from succinylcholine block confirmed, give increments of a non-depolarising relaxant, e.g. atracurium 25 mg or rocuronium 30 mg, guided by the response to peripheral nerve stimulation. *Smaller doses will be required in the presence of therapeutic serum magnesium concentrations.*

- Adjust fresh gas mixture to 33–50% O_2 in N_2O plus approximately 0.75 MAC (end-tidal) of volatile agent (isoflurane or sevoflurane).

- Concerns about the effects of anaesthetic agents on the newborn baby and uterine tone have been over-emphasised in the past. Excessively light general anaesthesia risks awareness and has a detrimental effect on utero-placental blood flow.

- After the cord is clamped, give intravenous morphine 10–20 mg. Do not discontinue inhalational anaesthesia until surgery has been completed.

- Reverse neuromuscular block using a peripheral nerve stimulator to confirm full recovery.

Tocolysis and oxytocics

On occasions, uterine relaxation might be requested to facilitate procedures such as delivery of a second twin.

- Intravenous increments of glyceryl trinitrate (GTN) **50 μg** are effective. Hypotension does not seem to occur in women already venodilated by a regional block. GTN can alternatively be given by metered dose (400 μg) sublingual spray.

- Syntocinon 5 units should be given by slow intravenous bolus at every caesarean section as soon as the cord has been clamped (the last cord if multiple pregnancy). This dose can be repeated. Syntocinon can cause transient vasodilatation, hypotension

---

Box 9.6   Contraindications to diclofenac

- Hypovolaemia or continuing bleeding (risk of renal hypoperfusion).
- Pre-existing renal impairment (including poor urine output in pre-eclampsia). If diclofenac is withheld, reconsider prescription once oliguria has resolved.
- Asthma with history of sensitivity to NSAIDs (OK to prescribe if patient has previously taken other NSAIDs without adverse effects).
- Peptic ulceration.
- Coagulopathy.
- Hypersensitivity to NSAIDs.

---

and tachycardia, that are effectively treated with intravenous increments of phenylephrine 50 μg.

- The requirement for a Syntocinon infusion (40 units over 6 hours) can be anticipated in certain cases. Women with a large uterine cavity after multiple pregnancy or macrosomic baby, and those who have had a prolonged labour, antepartum haemorrhage or placenta praevia are at risk of postpartum haemorrhage.

- Avoid the large unnecessary fluid load of successive 500 ml bags containing Syntocinon (with its antidiuretic effect) by using small diluent volumes administered by syringe pump.

POSTOPERATIVE ANALGESIA

- Unless contraindicated, **diclofenac** 100 mg + **paracetamol** 1 g suppositories should be administered at end of surgery. Prescribe *regular* diclofenac, 50 mg 8 hourly + **paracetamol** 1 g 4–6 hourly, maximum 4 g/24 h both oral or PR. **Dihydrocodeine** 30–60 mg orally, 4 hourly (maximum 240 mg/24 h) is prescribed 'as required'.

- Contraindications to diclofenac (and other NSAIDs) are listed in Box 9.6.

- Because of the risk of respiratory depression, it makes sense to restrict *parenteral* administration of opioids by midwives for at least 6 hours after spinal or epidural fentanyl and 12 hours after morphine or diamorphine. Following general anaesthesia, titrate morphine intravenously. For the postnatal ward, prescribe morphine 10–15 mg intramuscularly 3 hourly 'as required' *or* 1 mg boluses (5 min lockout) via patient-controlled analgesia system (PCAS).

- Ensure a LMWH has been prescribed (pulmonary embolism is the leading cause of 'direct' maternal death in the UK).

Discharge to the ward only when cardiovascular and respiratory variables are acceptable and stable. Women must not be left alone in single rooms. Monitoring of respiratory rate, sedation, pulse and blood pressure must be charted in accordance with the unit's protocol.

PLACENTA PRAEVIA

The anaesthetist should engage in discussion with the obstetrician regarding the placental site and how much bleeding is anticipated. The risk of major haemorrhage is significantly increased if a previous section has been performed and the placenta is adherent to the myometrium (placenta accreta).

- Regional anaesthesia is not necessarily contraindicated. However, the woman should be made aware that significant blood loss might ensue, and that being awake while large quantities of blood are rapidly infused might not be a pleasant experience. In the event of serious difficulty securing haemostasis, general anaesthesia might become desirable.

- Ensure that at least 4 units of red cells are available. Two intravenous lines (14 G or 16 G cannulae) should be established with rapid fluid infusion devices primed. *Senior obstetricians and anaesthetists should be present in theatre.*

- Cell salvage has gained acceptance in obstetric practice, although blood recovery should not take place during removal of the amniotic fluid.

- Because the lower segment does not contract as effectively as the upper segment, there is a risk of postpartum haemorrhage after caesarean section for placenta praevia. Close postoperative monitoring and a Syntocinon infusion for at least 6 hours are essential.

PRE-ASSESSMENT

All units should have a referral system between obstetricians and obstetric anaesthetists. Trainees providing out-of-hours cover should never be presented with complex cases 'out of the blue'. Consider anaesthetic referral for any woman referred to a specialist physician's clinic (e.g. cardiology).

Anaesthetists' principal concerns are:

- the feasibility of epidural/spinal block, which depends on flexion of the lumbar spine and normal blood coagulation
- whether tracheal intubation at emergency caesarean section might be hazardous, e.g. because of limited neck flexion/mouth opening

- the influence of medical conditions and their treatment on the safe conduct of regional or general anaesthesia.

Criteria for referral are listed in Box 9.7.

PRE-ECLAMPSIA

Anaesthetists' contributions include provision of analgesia, blood pressure control, intravenous fluid/blood product administration and physiological monitoring. Regional analgesia is strongly indicated to eliminate the pain and stress of labour and thus prevent further rises in blood pressure and improve uteroplacental blood flow. A regional block should not be regarded as a first-line treatment for hypertension – specific antihypertensive therapy should be administered first.

Spinal anaesthesia does not cause excessive hypotension (the hypertension of pre-eclampsia is mediated humorally, not neurally by the sympathetic nervous system). Standard IV boluses of phenylephrine or ephedrine do not cause an exaggerated hypertensive response.

General anaesthesia is indicated if there is a coagulopathy or symptoms (especially piercing headache) of impending eclampsia. Specific problems include laryngeal oedema, which might necessitate a smaller tracheal tube. Prior communication with the neonatal paediatrician is essential so that preparation can be made for antagonism of opioid or provision of ventilatory support.

The induction regimen should protect the cerebral circulation from hypertensive surges. Have a low threshold for direct arterial pressure monitoring. Attenuate the pressor response to intubation with alfentanil 10 µg/kg or remifentanil 2 µ/kg prior to rapid sequence induction.

In the presence of therapeutic serum concentrations of magnesium sulphate, use reduced doses of non-depolarising drugs for maintenance of neuromuscular block (e.g. mivacurium 0.15 mg/kg). A peripheral nerve stimulator is *essential* to monitor the degree of block.

Before extubation, consider specific therapy (e.g. labetalol in 10–20 mg increments) to avert a dangerous pressor response. If a swollen larynx was evident at laryngoscopy or intubation was traumatic, be extremely wary of post-extubation stridor.

ECLAMPSIA

Seizures occurring in late pregnancy and labour should be regarded as eclamptic unless proved otherwise. Alternative diagnoses include epilepsy,

---

Box 9.7 Criteria for antenatal anaesthetic referral

Cardiovascular problems
- Congenital heart disease
- Valvular heart disease
- Arrhythmias
- Cardiomyopathy
- Poorly controlled hypertension

Respiratory problems
- Severe asthma (requiring steroids or hospital admission)
- Breathlessness which limits daily activity
- Cystic fibrosis, or any other chronic chest disease

Neurological/Musculoskeletal problems
- Any back surgery, e.g. laminectomy, surgery for scoliosis (rods may have been inserted)
- Congenital conditions, e.g. spina bifida
- Muscular dystrophy, myotonia
- Myasthenia gravis
- Demyelinating disease (multiple sclerosis)
- Spinal cord injury
- Rheumatoid arthritis or any condition affecting neck/jaw
- Cerebrovascular disease, e.g. aneurysm, arteriovenous malformation

Haematological problems
- Anticoagulation
- Blood clotting/platelet disorders

- Patients who have been treated for malignancy, e.g. lymphoma, leukaemia

Airway problems
- Previous difficulty with intubation
- Inability to open mouth or move jaw or head normally

Drug-related problems
- Cholinesterase abnormalities – succinylcholine (Scoline) apnoea
- Allergy or adverse reaction to anaesthetic drugs
- Malignant hyperthermia
- Drug misuse

Other problems
- Morbid obesity – body mass index (weight ÷ height squared) >40 kg/m^2
- Needle phobia
- Panic attacks
- Any obscure eponymous syndrome that no one seems to have heard of, which may pose problems if emergency anaesthesia is needed
- Any women with concerns regarding analgesia or anaesthesia, e.g. previous problems with inadequate epidural for labour, or pain/awareness during caesarean section

---

amniotic fluid embolism (anaphylactoid syndrome of pregnancy), intracranial pathology (tumours, vascular malformations, haemorrhage), water intoxication, and local anaesthetic toxicity.

Practical points

- Maintain airway patency and give 100% oxygen. If a clear airway cannot be achieved with facemask and Guedel airway, summon skilled anaesthetic assistance and intubate the trachea. Use a generous dose of thiopental or propofol ideally with alfentanil to help obtund the pressor response. Avoid aortocaval compression, and attempt to prevent trauma to the mother and fetus.

- Most initial fits will be self-limiting. After the convulsion has terminated, examine the mother for signs of pulmonary aspiration (tachypnoea, crackles/wheeze), and institute SpO$_2$ monitoring. Ensure that the fetal heart rate is determined without

delay. Signs of fetal compromise secondary to maternal hypoxaemia or placental abruption will signal the need for emergency caesarean section.

- Depending on the conditions of mother and fetus, a regional anaesthetic *may* be appropriate (a single fit is not a contraindication to a regional block).

- Postoperatively, all eclamptic women who have an emergency caesarean section under general anaesthesia should be transferred to an intensive care unit for a period of sedation and ventilation. Ideally, brain imaging should be performed *en route* in order to exclude intracranial haemorrhage and ascertain whether there is evidence of cerebral ischaemia.

- Treat as for a non-pregnant patient with brain injury/cerebral ischaemia. If neuromuscular block is used, arrange neurophysiological monitoring (e.g. cerebral function analysing monitor) so that further seizure activity might be identified.

Bibliography

Burnstein R, Buckland R, Pickett JA 1999 A survey of epidural analgesia for labour in the United Kingdom. Anaesthesia 54:634–640

Carroll D, Tramèr M, McQuay H, Nye B, Moore A 1997 Transcutaneous electrical nerve stimulation in labour pain: a systematic review. British Journal of Obstetrics and Gynaecology 104:169–175

Elbourne D, Wiseman RA 2005 Types of intra-muscular opioids for maternal pain relief in labour. Cochrane Database of Systematic Reviews 2005 Issue 2. John Wiley & Sons, Chichester

Shibli KU, Russell IF 2000 A survey of anaesthetic techniques used for caesarean section in the UK in 1997. International Journal of Obstetric Anesthesia 9:160–167

Why mothers die 2000–2002. Report on confidential enquiries into maternal deaths in the United Kingdom. London: Royal College of Obstetricians and Gynaecologists, 2004. http://www.cemach.org.uk

Chapter 10

Intrapartum fetal surveillance

David T Y Liu
Mentors: Rosemary Buckley, Toby Fay

CHAPTER CONTENTS

Physiology and pathophysiology   73
Fetal heart rate: background   74
　Further points   74
Fetal heart rate: types   75
　Baseline FHR   75
　Transient changes in heart rate   76
　　Transient acceleration   76
　　Early decelerations   76
　　Combined patterns – variable
　　　decelerations   76
　　Late decelerations   77
Improving fetal heart rate recording   77
　Requirements for electronic heart rate
　　monitoring   77
　Fetal heart rate pattern changes   78
　　Incomplete progress of patterns   78
　　Palisade patterns   78
　Display of uterine contractions   78

Measurements of uterine contractions   79
　Tocometer   79
　Catheter-transducer system   80
　Pressure-tipped catheter   80
Fetal acid–base balance   80
　Fetal pH   80
　Fetal blood sampling   81
　　Procedure   81
　Management of the abnormal fetal heart rate
　　trace   82
　　Further points   82
Fetal acidaemia, Apgar scores and neurological
　outcome   82
Meconium and meconium aspiration   82
　Management of meconium in amniotic fluid   83
Other considerations   83
　Severe moulding   83
　Fetal movements   83

Most babies deliver without problems. In complicated pregnancies, however, birth can be a hazardous process for the fetus. Intrapartum surveillance by manually assessing contractions and listening (60 seconds) at intervals (15 minutes in first stage, 5 minutes in second stage) to check the fetal heart rate is a well-established obstetric practice for uncomplicated pregnancies. Electronic instrumentation has been introduced to facilitate continuous intrapartum fetal monitoring (when auscultation suggests abnormality, when there is evidence of or potential fetal compromise). The fetus signals potential compromise by:

- alterations in heart rate
- the development of acidosis
- the passage of meconium
- the presence of excessive moulding
- excessive movements.

PHYSIOLOGY AND PATHOPHYSIOLOGY

The fetal cardiac output is controlled mainly by the heart rate rather than stroke volume. Cardiac output also varies with gestation. About half (50%) of the fetal cardiac output is directed to the low resistance placental circulation for oxygenation and nutrients. Flow rate in the umbilical vein is approximately 100 ml/kg per minute. The following statements are relevant to understanding intrapartum fetal surveillance:

- Normal fetal heart rate (FHR) is between 110 and 160 beats per minute. Vagal response slows the rate, for example during fetal head or cord compression, whereas in a healthy fetus sympathetic response or catecholamine release following anaemia, hyperthermia, sepsis or hypoxia will produce tachycardia up to a maximum of 220 beats per minute.

- A fetus with an intact brain and myocardium exhibits FHR accelerations of 15 beats per minute for more than 15 seconds above baseline recordings in response to fetal movements, tactile or auditory stimulation.

- The healthy fetus exhibits an intrinsic baseline FHR variability of 5–25 beats per minute. A 'flat' or 'silent' pattern with fewer than 5 beats per minute variability for 40 or less minutes can indicate fetal inactivity or fetal 'sleep'.

- The fetus can improve myocardial oxygenation through a reflex compensatory mechanism or 'diving reflex' by slowing the heart rate during uterine diastolic. This mechanism can produce transient changes described as variable or late decelerations which in about 50% may signal the likely presence of metabolic acidaemia (normal umbilical artery pH 7.26 ± 0.08). Fetal blood sampling is required to differentiate between physiological or pathological heart rate responses.

- Umbilical vein compression causes a reflex vagal parasympathetic response and produces transient variable decelerations. Like late decelerations, persistent appearance of these patterns correlate with possible presence of fetal acidaemia.

FETAL HEART RATE: BACKGROUND

FHR can be recorded intermittently by auscultation with a Pinard stethoscope or electronically by a Doppler instrument. Doppler recordings rely on ultrasound registration of the Doppler shift to signal FHR. Continuous electronic FHR monitoring (Figure 10.1) was introduced to provide uninterrupted intrapartum recordings. A fetal scalp electrode and intrauterine pressure recordings were used to provide the described classic patterns of transient FHR changes. Intrapartum pressure recording of uterine activity, however, is now usually replaced by use of external transducers to register sequential changes in uterine contraction. Correct placement of this external contraction device is important. Idiosyncrasies between the intrauterine and external methods for recording uterine contraction must be appreciated. The universal principle of need to understand the workings of tools used must

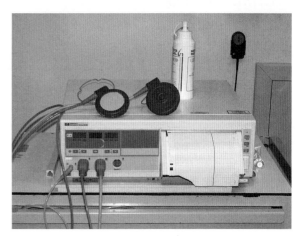

Figure 10.1   A machine used for continuous fetal heart rate monitoring.

apply since FHR change is read against the peak of the displayed uterine contraction.

Continuous electronic FHR monitoring is a screening adjunct for intrapartum fetal surveillance. Interpretation remains problematical and emphasises the need for constant education since failure to appreciate and react to signals of fetal insult is consistently identified as an avoidable factor in intrapartum fetal hypoxic damage or demise. Contemporary recommendation is that there should be an ongoing programme of education for interpretation of FHR changes for all involved in intrapartum care (Willis 2005).

Screening fetal welfare by recording FHR changes (cardiotocograms (CTGs)) should:

- interpret changes against a set of accepted definitions (for example, National Institute for Health and Clinical Excellence (NICE) 2001).
- interpret against the clinical presentation and background.

Further points

- Drugs, e.g. pethidine can blunt FHR responses whereas procedures such as insertion of an epidural block, vomiting, catheterisation and toileting can be followed by changes reflecting placental blood flow or vagal responses. Over 40% of fetuses in labour may show non-reassuring or abnormal traces. Discrepancy between fetal outcome, FHR and pH emphasises that non-reassuring FHR changes should be interpreted as a need for review and/or check fetal pH where appropriate. At best only 60–70% pathological changes are indicative of fetal acidaemia.

- There is intra- and inter-observer variation in interpretation. Attempts to standardise interpretation is thwarted by the lack of an internationally accepted guideline for interpretation and consensus for terminology or definition.

- A tocodynamometer essentially indicates only presence of a contraction. The peak of uterine contraction registered by an external tocometer need not equate with recordings from an intrauterine catheter. The peak of the contraction using an external tocodynamometer (photo) varies with the site of placement on the mother's abdomen.

- There is no clear understanding of the relation between FHR changes and fetal myocardial or cerebral oxygenation.

- A normal CTG pattern reassures that only 2% of babies will have a pH of <7.25 at birth.

- A well-grown healthy fetus should withstand 90 minutes of hypoxic stress before the pH falls. Fetal reserve is less in a compromised fetus. The preterm fetus is more susceptible to hypoxia, in particular, damage of the type II pneumocytes. There is, however, no means to indicate how much hypoxic insult a healthy fetus can withstand.

- In 90% of cases of cerebral palsy the causative event occurs before onset of labour. In the remaining 10% intrapartum signs of hypoxia may reflect the presence of pregnancy compromise such as intrauterine growth restriction, fetal damage or infection.

- Usually hypoxaemia and metabolic acidaemia are progressive processes and timing of onset is difficult. Signs of fetal compromise are often insensitive and not specific to any particular cause.

- The fetus may be able to compensate until attendant effects of uterine contractions or strength of contractions produce added insult and threat of irreversible neurological damage.

- Fetal acidaemia may indicate ability of the fetus to respond appropriately to hypoxia. Metabolic acidaemia at birth is common (2%) and most of these babies do not develop neurological damage. Pathological acidaemia associated with increased risk of neurological damage is a pH <7.00 and a base deficit of >12 mmol/l. Existing fetal compromise must be kept in mind.

- The fetus is unlikely to be acidaemic if the FHR baseline is between 110 and 160 beats per minute, variability is within 5 and 25 beats per minute and there is no deceleration. Acidaemia is likely if there is bradycardia, no variability and persistent late or variable decelerations. In acute hypoxia the pH drops by 0.1 units/min.

- Fetal metabolic acidosis (pH <7.00 and base deficit of 12 mmol/l or more) is associated with increased risk of subsequent neurological deficit such as spastic quadriplegia.

- After 32 weeks the FHR patterns can be interpreted as for term babies. Before this gestation there are fewer accelerations and less than 20 second decelerations can occur spontaneously.

- Fetal sepsis is not usually associated with a low pH (pH <7.20) until the late stage of labour.

- A scalp electrode should not be used in women with the human immunodeficiency virus (HIV) or herpes simplex virus. Do not attach the clip to a fetus with a bleeding disorder, e.g. haemophilia.

FETAL HEART RATE: TYPES

During labour the FHR is described in terms of baseline rates (readings between contractions) and transient changes (readings during contractions). Four features – baseline rate, variability, presence of acceleration and deceleration – are used to assess fetal welfare.

Baseline FHR

- Normal – accepted as between 110 to 160 beats per minute recorded over 5 or 10 minutes (NICE 2001).

- Tachycardia – above 160 beats per minute. Sympathetic or catecholamine response. It is severe if above 180 beats per minute. Causes include maternal diseases such as infection and thyrotoxicosis; administered drugs, for example atropine, β-sympathomimetics and hydralazine; fetal infection and hypoxia. A rate of between 161 and 180 beats per minute is non-reassuring.

- Bradycardia – below 110 beats per minute. Progressive or sudden slowing to less than 100 beats per minute suggests fetal decompensation. Known contribution by administered drugs such as opioids and local anaesthetics; fetal cardiac abnormalities, for example heart block and fetal hypoxia. A rate between 100 and 109 beats per minute is non-reassuring.

- Baseline variability – as a consequence of a fixed stroke volume, the FHR speeds and slows to maintain a stable blood pressure and cardiac output. Normally this variability is more than 5 beats per minute (distance between two faint horizontal score lines on recording paper) to 25 beats per

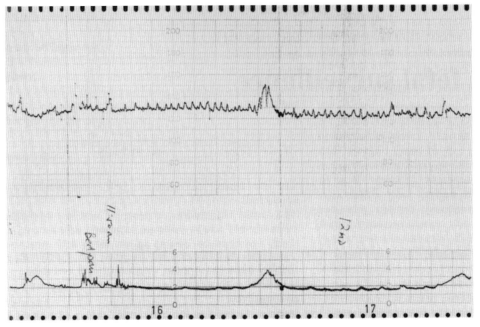

Figure 10.2 Example of transient acceleration in the heart rate.

minute. The term 'flat trace' or the electronic term 'silent trace' is used to describe variability of less than 5 beats per minute. The controlling centre for cardio-acceleration and deceleration is in the medulla. Variability is affected by:

- hypoxia – flat trace, sinusoidal patterns (smooth, sinewave pattern of 5–15 beats per minute recurring 3 to 5 times per minute lasting more than 10 minutes)
- depressant drugs, for example opioids, diazepam (flat trace)
- anaemia (sinusoidal patterns)
- machinery averaging techniques (display trace with less variability)
- neural tube abnormalities affecting control centre, e.g. anencephaly (flat trace)
- Doppler technique for FHR (produces a 'noisy' or irregular trace masking true variability).

- A flat trace for less than 20 minutes is non-reassuring or suspicious and is abnormal if the duration is longer than 20 minutes. Note fetal sleep pattern (up to 40 min). Interpret by considering all aspects, e.g. the trace of associated deceleration patterns.

Transient changes in heart rate

The fetus is subjected to compression and transient hypoxic stress during uterine contractions. Contrac-

tions above 4–6 kPa interrupt placental intervillous blood flow. The healthy fetus tolerates these impositions without much change in heart rate. With fetal compromise and/or non-physiological uterine contractions, patterns of transient FHR changes are observed reflecting the degree of fetal response. It takes 60–90 seconds for reoxygenation of the intervillous blood hence contraction intervals should not be less than 120 seconds.

Transient acceleration
An increase in heart rate (15 beats per minute or more and lasting 15 or more seconds) throughout contraction is an early response to sympathetic stimuli (Figure 10.2) and reflects a fetus in good condition.

Early decelerations
An early deceleration is indicated by a decrease in heart rate (15 beats per minute or more and lasting 15 seconds or more) with the onset of contractions and a return to baseline rate at the end of the contraction (Figure 10.3). Vagal stimulation, the oxygen conserving diving reflex and response to hypoxia all contribute to this pattern of heart rate change.

Combined patterns – variable decelerations
Between early and late decelerations are patterns in which there is a mixture of accelerations and decelerations to suggest varying severity of stress

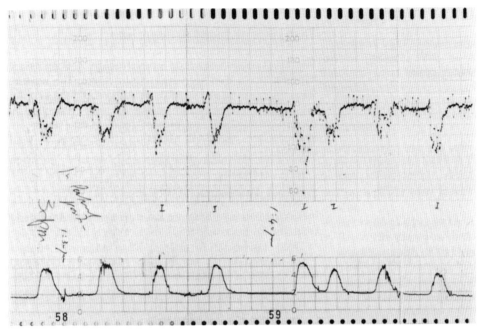

Figure 10.3 Example of a flat trace, early deceleration and combined patterns of acceleration/deceleration in the heart rate.

intermediate between the pure patterns. These patterns are considered to be associated with umbilical vein compression. Patterns in which acceleration precedes deceleration indicate possible less fetal compromise than decelerations with rebound accelerations. Patterns with slow return to baseline, biphasic deceleration and lost of variability are atypical and suggest abnormality. There is also variable timing of deceleration against uterine contraction (Figure 10.3).

Late decelerations

Fetal hypoxic insult is suggested by decelerations commencing after mid to end of contraction and nadir more than 20 seconds after peak of contraction. Decelerations may be shallow or deep. A long lag time or delay before decelerations, a prolonged nadir (more than 3 minutes) or slow return to baseline signifies more severe compromise (Figure 10.4). Evidence from studies and international consensus advise significance only if the patterns recur and persist.

IMPROVING FETAL HEART RATE RECORDING

Doppler ultrasound techniques (via abdominally placed transducers) may produce poor quality recordings. Application of a fetal scalp clip (Box 10.1) gives more satisfactory and more easily interpretable

records. These clips may also be applied to the fetal buttocks when the fetus presents by the breech.

Contemporary interpretation of FHR tracing advises assessment of fetal welfare based on the baseline rate, baseline variability and presence or absence of accelerations and decelerations (early, late and variable).

- Reassuring trace is one where the baseline rate is between 110 and 160 beats per minute, variability is between 5 and 25 beats per minute, with accelerations and no decelerations.

- Non-reassuring or suspicious trace displays the above described non-reassuring features in rate and variability. Early and variable decelerations are present but no accelerations.

- An abnormal or pathological trace displays a rate below 100 or above 180 beats per minute. Variability is less than 5 beats per minute for more than 90 minutes or there are sinusoidal patterns (over 10 minutes) and the presence of late or atypical variable decelerations.

Requirements for electronic heart rate monitoring

- Ensure compromised or at risk fetuses are offered the benefit of electronic FHR monitoring. The

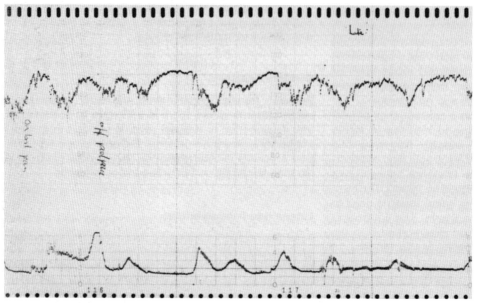

Figure 10.4 Example of a flat trace tachycardia and late deceleration

Clinical Negligence Scheme for Trusts (CNST) standards require guidelines for use and interpretation of antenatal and intrapartum electronic FHR monitoring.

- Check that the CTG machines are regularly serviced and standardised, for example the running paper speed should be 1 cm/min.
- All medical staff engaged in the use of electronic FHR monitoring must receive training and regular updating to maintain competency. Training includes drills every 6 months to respond appropriately when non-reassuring or pathological patterns are detected (Willis 2005).
- The FHR trace is a medical record. Events, timing and medical staff involved must be carefully documented on the trace.
- It is a requirement that these FHR traces are kept for a minimum of 25 years.

Fetal heart rate pattern changes

Labour is associated with progressively stronger and more frequent uterine contractions, hence increasing fetal stress. When fetal compromise is present this increase in neurological and hypoxic stimuli initiates a progression of FHR pattern changes displaying the range from no response, transient acceleration, early decelerations, variable decelerations and late decelerations. In certain circumstances such as excessive oxytocic usage or immediately after placement of an epidural block simple measures such as reduction in oxytocic administration, placing the woman on her side and/or giving oxygen through a facemask for a short time can revert these changes. Many sequences of pattern changes and recovery throughout labour forewarn of the need for a short second stage.

Incomplete progress of patterns

The recognised sequence of FHR changes to and from innocuous to non-reassuring and pathological patterns in response to circumstantial situations, for example women using bedpan or positional postural hypotension, contributes to the acknowledged difficulty in interpretation of FHR traces.

Palisade patterns

The combination of hypoxia and vagal stimuli at the second stage of labour often produces deep decelerations with usually rapid recovery after each contraction. Deep (fewer than 100 beats per minute) heart rate decelerations and tall amplitudes of contraction combine to give the appearance of a fence, hence the term palisade patterns. When these patterns occur assess cervical dilatation. As there is a hypoxic component, these patterns must not be allowed to continue for too long.

Display of uterine contractions

An external tocometer only indicates the presence of a contraction. The amplitude of the trace displayed on

Box 10.1   Application of scalp clip

- The mother can be in either the dorsal semi-Fowler or the lateral position for application.
- Aseptic precautions are essential.
- Select the appropriate available clip (Figure 10.5).
- Perform a vaginal examination to determine cervical dilatation, confirm the rupture of membranes and establish presentation of the fetus.
- Direct the clip to a safe area of the scalp or gluteal surface (away from the face, the fontanelles or the fetal perineum).
- Check correct application by examining display of the FHR on the monitor.

- Anchor the extravaginal part of the clip to the mother's thigh making sure allowance is made for some slack to accommodate movement (Figure 10.6).
- Note: Do not apply clips if there is a fetal bleeding disorder or if the mother is carrying HIV or herpes simplex virus.

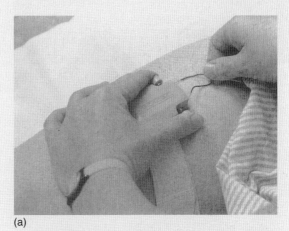

(a)

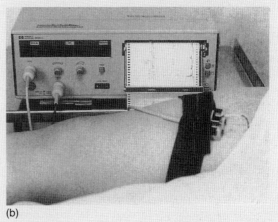

(b)

Figure 10.6   (a,b) Anchorage of a clip to the thigh.

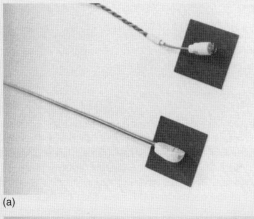

(a)

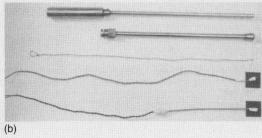

(b)

Figure 10.5   (a) Scalp 'clips' used for direct FHR monitoring. (b) With applicator.

the recording chart is not representative of intrauterine pressure. Compared with excursions recorded simultaneously from an intrauterine recording system, excursions registered by an external tocometer can precede or follow those derived from an intrauterine system. Classically, early and late decelerations refer to the situation where an intrauterine measuring system is used. Decelerations cannot be timed with accuracy when external tocometers are used because correct placement is often difficult. This statement is

particularly important for correct interpretation of FHR recordings.

Measurements of uterine contractions

Tocometer

An external tocometer (Figure 10.7) has a button or disc which is depressed when the uterus hardens during a contraction (Figure 10.8). The tocometer is placed on the most convex area of the uterus during

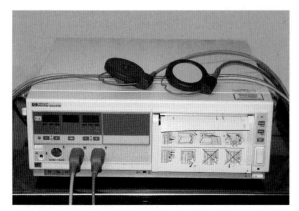

Figure 10.7   Example of an external tocometer.

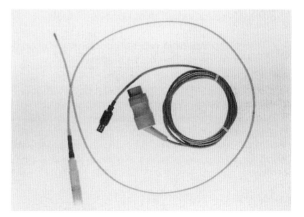

Figure 10.9   Pressure-tipped catheter

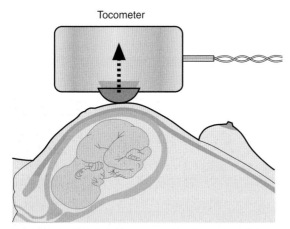

Figure 10.8   The signal is generated by depression of the button by the mother's abdomen.

contraction to obtain a good display on the recording chart. The amplitude of the contraction displayed is less obvious in overweight women. Frequent alteration of the recording site throughout labour is necessary to obtain good displays. External tocometers have the advantage that they can be used when membranes are not ruptured.

Catheter-transducer system

A saline-filled polythene catheter is placed through the cervix into the amniotic cavity to record the hydrostatic pressure during contractions. This hydrostatic pressure is measured by a transducer with a strain gauge. It requires constant attention (flushing to avoid blockage). There is a risk of infection. When amniotic fluid is reduced towards the end of labour, the amplitude of the displayed excursions becomes less representative of true intrauterine pressure. This system is

used to produce the classic descriptions for FHR recordings. It has been largely superseded by pressure-tipped catheter systems.

Pressure-tipped catheter

A closed system is placed at the tip of a catheter to register increased intrauterine pressure. Increased hydrostatic pressure alters the electrical frequency response of the transducer system which is displayed to reflect the intensity of uterine contractions. It is convenient, less affected by alterations between the level of the uterus and the recording transducer, and is more acceptable to women and attendant staff (Figure 10.9). Avoid entrapment of catheter tip (the tip should be free in the amniotic cavity).

FETAL ACID–BASE BALANCE

Fetal pH

Fetal hypoxia promotes anaerobic metabolism and the production of lactic acid which accumulates to lower fetal pH (pH = the logarithm of the reciprocal of hydrogen ion concentration; it expresses presence or absence of acidaemia). The pH at the onset of labour in a normal fetus is about 7.33 (range 7.20–7.50). There is a slight drop to 7.27 at the time of delivery. This is due to accumulation of lactic acid generated during transient hypoxia associated with contractions. Fetal acidaemia correlates poorly with the Apgar score of the newborn. Acidaemia is evident in 2% of uncomplicated births and most of these babies do not develop cerebral palsy.

The measurement of base excess in fetal capillary blood gives further insight into the acid–base status of the fetus. Base excess in mEq/l or mmol/l is the amount of acid or base needed to titrate the blood

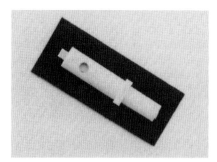

Figure 10.10   A guarded blade used to induce capillary ooze.

sample to a pH of 7.40 at a pCO_2 of 40 mmHg and a temperature of 37°C. Metabolic acidosis means that the available buffer base is used up and a state of base insufficiency or base deficit exists. The prefix minus (−) denotes a negative balance of buffer bases. Normal umbilical artery base excess is in the range of 6.7 mEq/l. In acute anoxia the pH falls by 0.1 unit/min. Negative base excess or base deficit of more than −12 mmol/l suggests the presence of acidaemia.

Fetal blood sampling

The pH of capillary blood from the fetal scalp or the gluteal area should be checked whenever fetal compromise is suspected.

Procedure
* Place the woman in the lithotomy position with 15° lateral tilt or preferably in a left lateral position.
* Aseptic precautions include gowns, gloves, cleansing of the vulval area and sterile drapes.
* Check that the cervical dilatation is 3 cm or more with easy access to the fetus.
* Select an amnioscope of the appropriate size and digitally guide it through the cervix onto the fetal skin. Remove the obturator and attach a light source. Alternatively, the speculum or an endoscope can be guided through the cervix under direct vision with a fibreoptic light attached.
* Apply the endoscope firmly to the fetal skin to exclude seepage of amniotic fluid.
* Rub the fetal skin with a swab to clean it and use ethyl chloride spray to produce reactive hyperaemia.
* Coat the skin surface with silicone gel so the blood will form a globule. For a hairy surface, part or remove the hair to prevent smudging of the blood trickle.
* Press the prepared skin firmly once or twice with a 2 mm guarded blade to make an incision (Figure 10.10).

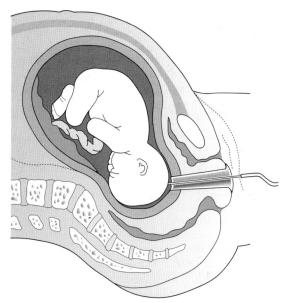

Figure 10.11   Fetal blood sampling.

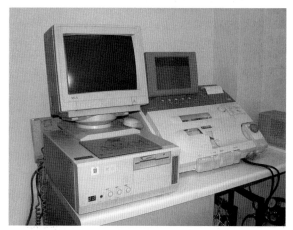

Figure 10.12   A blood gas analyser for measuring fetal pH and base excess.

* Collect the blood into heparinised capillary tubes by gravitation (Figure 10.11). Suction through a tube is not advised because of potential risk of infection.
* Collect sufficient blood for three consecutive readings. Tubes are sealed after a small segment of iron filing ('flea') is inserted. This filing is moved up and down the tube with a magnet to mix the blood.
* Apply pressure or silicone wax to the incision to secure haemostasis.
* Process samples immediately (Figure 10.12). Prolonged exposure to air will raise pH.

- In the breech presentation, blood from the buttocks is interpreted in the same way as for cephalic presentation.
- Fetal blood sampling is contraindicated in the presence of maternal infection, e.g. HIV, herpex simplex, and fetal bleeding disorders, e.g. haemophilia or prematurity of less than 34 weeks.

Management of the abnormal fetal heart rate trace

General principles and care paths are as follows:

- Try to determine cause.
- Check maternal pulse, blood pressure and medication. Is the woman in pain, anxious or febrile?
- Turn the woman on her side. Select side away from placental bed (usually turn to left side away from inferior vena cava).
- Adjust or switch off intravenous oxytocin. Give a tocolytic, e.g. subcutaneous terbutaline 0.25 mg if hypercontractility persists.
- Assess cervical dilatation. Exclude cord prolapse.
- If appropriate give the woman oxygen by using a face mask. Avoid prolonged use of oxygen as can be harmful to the fetus.
- Expedite delivery if the cervix is fully dilated and there are no contraindications.
- Sample fetal blood if cervix is not fully dilated.
- Assess the total clinical situation. Caesarean section and early delivery can be more appropriate than fetal blood sampling, e.g. deceleration of more than 3 minutes.
- Notify paediatrician/neonatologist.
- Check pH and base excess of cord blood (arterial and venous) at delivery when there is evidence of intrapartum fetal compromise, need for assisted delivery or if baby is delivered in poor condition.

Further points

- Use your common sense. When FHR changes indicate severe compromise in an at-risk fetus, immediate delivery rather than fetal blood sampling is appropriate. Consider delivery rather than repeat sampling if there is fetal compromise and the fetal pH is borderline (7.21–7.25).
- With complete anoxia pH falls at a rate of 0.1 pH units per minute. The interval between repeat sampling must be flexible and should be guided by close observation of the FHR.
- Acidaemia is accepted as being present when the fetal pH is less than 7.20. With pH of 7.21 to 7.25 repeat in 15–30 minutes or consider delivery if non-reassuring FHR abnormalities persist. Consider base deficit results.

- Maternal lactic acidaemia aggravated by hyperventilation can add to fetal acidosis as there is free transplacental interchange of acid metabolites. The fetal scalp pH is 0.1 pH units below that of the maternal venous blood. A fetal pH of more than 0.2 pH units below that of the maternal venous blood means that fetal acidosis is independent of any maternal influence.

- A fetal scalp caput, uterine contractions and the occasional bubble in the collecting tube should not influence pH readings.

FETAL ACIDAEMIA, APGAR SCORES AND NEUROLOGICAL OUTCOME

It is accepted that there is disconcordance between FHR, fetal acidaemia subsequent Apgar scores and eventual neurological sequelae. The fetal acid base status should be checked when the FHR patterns show persistence of a non-reassuring or pathological trace.

When there is disconcordance between the FHR trace and fetal pH check the acid–base status within 30 minutes. In the presence of continuing pathological patterns the fetus should be delivered. Cord blood pH and base deficit status should be checked after delivery.

MECONIUM AND MECONIUM ASPIRATION

- Meconium (Greek word for opium poppy) is present in fetal gut from 10 weeks' gestation. Passage into the amniotic fluid is uncommon before 34 weeks but is detected in 14–30% of pregnancies by 40 weeks (up to 50% at 42 weeks) and reflects gastrointestinal maturity.

- Meconium in amniotic fluid is also more likely if a fetus is more than 4000 g and mothers are of African origin (1.5 times more compared with white mothers).

- Parasympathetic activity mediated by the hypothalamus, local peristaltic reflexes and the intestinal hormone motilin all contribute to passage of meconium.

- Infection will produce fetal enteritis, which initiates passage of meconium even in the preterm fetus.

- Hypoxia per se does not lead to passage of meconium. In the presence of normal FHR patterns fetal outcome is similar with or without meconium in the amniotic fluid.

- It is difficult to determine the exact time when meconium is passed.

- Meconium aspiration is defined as presence of meconium below the vocal chords and occurs in 35% when amniotic fluid is meconium stained.

- Most meconium aspiration occurring in utero is associated with fetal gasping (response to hypoxaemia) but not with irregular deep breathing, which increases with fetal maturity. The fetus inhales 200 ml/kg per 24 hours of amniotic fluid.

- Meconium aspiration is more likely when meconium concentration is described as thick (usually reflecting the presence of oligohydramnios) and if the pH is <7.20.

- Aspirated meconium damages the fetal lungs by its biochemical properties, and furthermore it predisposes to infective pneumonitis.

- In the absence of hypoxia aspiration is asymptomatic in 90% or is only associated with mild disease. Meconium aspiration is usually (95%) associated with thick meconium, and when severe and compounded by hypoxia it is predictive of a high risk of neonatal death (up to 40%).

Management of meconium in amniotic fluid

- Check and record presence of meconium after membrane rupture.
- Fetal blood sampling is not indicated if FHR pattern is normal.
- The presence of non-reassuring FHR patterns indicates that risk of fetal acidaemia is increased. Check fetal pH.
- Amnio-infusion cannot prevent passage or inhalation of meconium but only dilutes its concentration. Its value awaits confirmation.
- Pharyngeal aspiration if performed must be gentle to avoid trauma and expedient to prevent further risk of hypoxia.

- When meconium-stained amniotic fluid is evident continuous, FHR monitoring is advised. By the same token avoid maternal hypotension, maternal hypoxia, excessive uterine contractions or situations which may precipitate fetal hypoxia.
- Aspirate the oropharynx, then the nose as soon as the fetal head is delivered.
- A paediatrician/neonatologist should attend the delivery (especially when there is thick particulate meconium).

OTHER CONSIDERATIONS

Severe moulding

Fetal skull bones are not fused thus permitting a certain amount of movement (separation or overlap) when the fetal head adjusts during its passage through the maternal pelvis. This adjusting or moulding is noticed first at the occipital-parietal sutures. The next suture involved is the parietal-frontal suture and lastly the parietal-parietal suture. Moulding is described as of minor degree when the bones just approximate. Overlapping of bones, which can be readily separated digitally, is observed with further moulding. Severe moulding is evident when the overlapping bones cannot be separated. Severe moulding is associated with FHR decelerations, lower pH value and poor Apgar scores hence is considered a sign which signals fetal compromise. Where there is overlapping the situation must be reviewed and delivery considered if it is not safe to continue labour.

Fetal movements

Excessive or turbulent fetal movements are sometimes observed during labour and should be viewed with concern as indicative of fetal compromise. Steps should be taken to check the FHR pattern and if necessary the fetal pH.

References

National Institute for Clinical Excellence 2001 Clinical Guidelines. The Use of Electronic Fetal Monitoring. London, RCOG

Willis 2005 CNST Maternity Clinical Risk Management Standards. NHSLA, London

Bibliography

Alexander GR, Hulsey TC, Robillard PY et al 1994 Determinants of meconium stained amniotic fluid in term pregnancies. Journal of Perinatology 14:259–263

Baker PN, Kilby MD, Murray H 1992 An assessment of the use of meconium alone as an indication for fetal blood sampling. Obstetrics and Gynecology 80:792–796

Beard RW, Morris ED, Clayton SG 1967 pH of fetal capillary blood as an indicator of the condition of the fetus. Journal of Obstetrics and Gynecology of the British Commonwealth 74:812–822

Beard RW, Filshie GM, Knight CA et al 1971 The significance of the changes in the continuous fetal heart rate in the first stage of labour. Journal of Obstetrics and Gynecology of the British Commonwealth 78:865–880

Becker RF, Windle WF, Barth EE et al 1940 Fetal swallowing, gastro-intestinal activity and defaecation in amnio. Surgery Gynaecology Obstetrics 70:603–614

Brotanek V, Hendricks CH, Yoshida T 1969 Changes in uterine blood flow during uterine contractions. American Journal of Obstetrics and Gynecology 103:1108–1116

Cree JE, Meyer J, Hailey DM 1973 Diazepam in labour: its metabolism and effect on the clinical condition and thermal genesis of the newborn. BMJ 4:251–255

Duenholter JH, Pritchard JA 1976 Fetal respiration: quantitative measurements of amniotic fluid inspired near term by human and rhesus fetuses. American Journal of Obstetrics and Gynecology 125:306–309

Duenholter JH, Pritchard JA 1977 Fetal respiration: a review. American Journal of Obstetrics and Gynecology 129:326–338

Falciglia HS 1988 Failure to prevent meconium aspiration syndrome. Obstetrics and Gynecology 71:349–353

Fleischer A, Schulman H, Jagani N et al 1982 The development of fetal acidosis in the presence of an abnormal fetal heart rate tracing. American Journal of Obstetrics and Gynecology 144:55–60

Guyton AC 1991 Behavioural and motivational mechanisms of the brain, the limbic system and the hypothalamus. In: Guyton AC, ed. Textbook of Physiology, 8th edn. WB Saunders, Philadelphia, pp 651–656

Hobbel CJ, Hyvarinen MA, Oh W 1972 Abnormal fetal heart rate patterns and fetal acid base balance in low birthweight infants in relation to the respiratory distress syndrome. Obstetrics and Gynecology 39:83–88

Liu DTY, Thomas G, Blackwell RJ 1975 Progression in response patterns of fetal heart rate throughout labour. British Journal of Obstetrics and Gynaecology 82: 943

Low JA 1997 Intrapartum fetal asphyxia: definition, diagnosis and classification. American Journal of Obstetrics and Gynecology 176:957–959

Low JA, Cox MJ, Karchmar EJ et al 1981 The prediction of intrapartum fetal metabolic acidosis by fetal heart rate monitoring. American Journal of Obstetrics and Gynecology 139:299–235

MacLennan A 2000 A template for defining a causal relationship between acute intrapartum events and cerebral palsy. International Consensus Statement. Australian New Zealand Journal Obstetrics and Gynaecology 40:13–21

Mohmoud EL, Benirschke K, Vaucher YE et al 1988 Motilin levels in term neonates who have passed meconium prior to birth. Journal of Paediatric Gastro-enterology and Nutrition 7:95–99

Moss D, Holm BA, Spitale P et al 1991 Inhibition of pulmonary surfactant function by meconium. American Journal of Obstetrics and Gynecology 164:477–481

Naeye RL, Peters EC, Bartholomew M et al 1989 Origins of cerebral palsy. American Journal of Diseases of Children 143:1154–1161

Romero R, Hanaoka S, Manzor M et al 1991 Meconium stained amniotic fluid: a risk factor for microbial invasion of the amniotic cavity. American Journal of Obstetrics and Gynecology 164:859–862

Rossi EM, Philipson EH, Williams TG et al 1989 Meconium aspiration syndrome: intrapartum and neonatal attributes. American Journal of Obstetrics and Gynecology 161:1106–1110

Schulze M 1925 The significance of the passage of meconium during labour. American Journal of Obstetrics and Gynecology 10:83–88

Steer PJ, Eigbe F, Lissauer TJ et al 1989 Inter-relationships among abnormal cardiotocograms in labour, meconium staining of the amniotic fluid, arterial cord blood pH and Apgar scores. Obstetrics and Gynecology 74:715–721

Stewart KS, Philpott RH 1981 Fetal response to cephalo-pelvic disproportion. British Journal of Obstetrics and Gynaecology 87:641–649

Sykes G, Molloy PM, Johnson P et al 1982 Do Apgar scores indicate asphyxia? Lancet i:494–495

Umstad MP, Permeezel M, Pepperell RJ 1994 Intrapartum cardiotocography and the expert witness 34:20–23

Winkler CL, Hauth JC, Tucker JM et al 1991 Neonatal complications at term as related to the degree of umbilical artery acidaemia. American Journal of Obstetrics and Gynecology 164:637–641

Yeomans ER, Gilstrap LC, Lebeno KJ et al 1989 Meconium in the amniotic fluid and fetal acid base status. Obstetrics and Gynecology 73:175–178

Chapter 11

Episiotomy and tears

David T Y Liu

CHAPTER CONTENTS

Types of incision   85
   Medial incision   85
   Mediolateral Incision   85
   J-shaped incision   85
Technique   86
Timing   86
Do   87
Do not   87
Repair of an episiotomy   88
Resuturing episiotomies   88
Tears in the perineum   89
Consequences of perineal trauma for women   90

Episiotomy is the term used for an incision in the perineum. Not all women require an episiotomy for delivery but considerable experience is necessary to determine when it is not needed. This incision is made:

- when a perineal tear is imminent, thus avoiding uncontrolled damage
- to relieve pressure on the soft preterm fetal head
- to expedite delivery when birth is delayed by an unyielding perineum
- to provide adequate room for assisted delivery.

TYPES OF INCISION

Medial incision

Medial incisions are made in the anatomical plane and are comfortable. There is less bleeding, and they are easy to repair. However, access is limited and the incision carries the risk of extension into the rectum, hence it is only used by someone experienced (Figure 11.1a).

Mediolateral Incision

This incision is safe, easy to perform, and thus the most commonly used. It is associated with least risk of anal sphincter damage. The cut must begin at the mid-point of the fourchette and is directed towards the ischial tuberosity into the ischiorectal pad of fat (Figure 11.1b).

J-shaped incision

This type of incision has the advantage of the medial incision and provides better access than the mediolateral approach. The lateral incision is made tangential

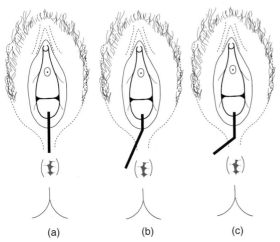

Figure 11.1 (a) Medial incision, (b) mediolateral and (c) J-shaped incision.

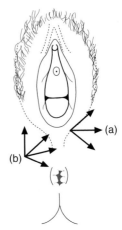

Figure 11.3 Infiltration of local anaesthetic in fan formation starting either at (a) the middle of the fourchette, or (b) near the ischial tuberosity to cover the area of the incision.

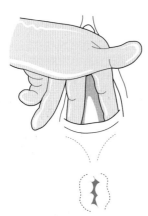

Figure 11.2 Using the fingers the fourchette is drawn away from the presenting part of the fetus before infiltration.

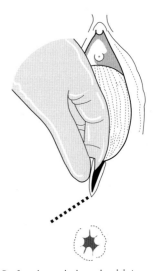

Figure 11.4 Performing a J-shaped episiotomy.

to the brown of the anus (Figure 11.1c). It is excellent for the experienced surgeon.

TECHNIQUE

- An existing epidural can provide adequate anaesthesia; if not infiltrate with a local anaesthetic. The fingers are placed inside the introitus to protect the presenting parts of the fetus (Figures 11.2 and 11.3).

- The index and middle fingers are placed in the introitus along the direction of intended cut. The thumb is apposed to stabilise the perineum. A single cut 3 cm long starting from the mid-point of the fourchette is made with scissors.

- In the J-shaped incision, the thumb, middle and index fingers are apposed in the midline of the

fourchette. The tip of the thumb is placed 0.5–1 cm above the brown of the anus. A midline incision to the tip of the thumb is made. The thumb and fingers are kept firmly apposed. The scissors are then rotated to align transgentially to the brown perianal area and another incision is then made (Figure 11.4).

TIMING

Episiotomy should be performed:

- when tearing of the vagina becomes obvious. This is indicated by a show of fresh blood when the presenting part of the fetus distends the perineum as the mother pushes

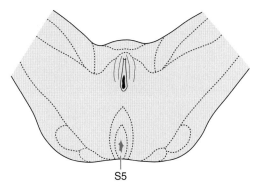

Figure 11.5   Dermatomes of the perineum. Perianal area is supplied by S5.

- when the overstretched perineum may be seen to tear
- electively with a thick unyielding perineum
- electively before traction on the forceps or before proceeding to breech delivery (when a breech is on the perineum).

DO

- Place women in the lithotomy position.

- Unless in an emergency, ensure there is adequate anaesthesia. Epidural anaesthesia may not be sufficient. Pudendal block anaesthetises only S2–S4 hence perineal infiltration with additional local anaesthetic is required to cover S5 of the perianal area (Figure 11.5).

- Remember the total amount of local anaesthetic used should not exceed 200 mg of lidocaine. This is especially important in women who have been given an epidural block.

- The pudendal nerve enters the pudendal canal approximately 1 cm below and 1 cm cephalad to the ischial spine when the woman is supine. The pudendal vessels are beside the nerves (Figure 11.6), therefore aspirate back before infiltration to prevent intravascular injection.

- Perform episiotomy with one or two strokes and not with multiple bites.

- In repeat episiotomy follow the previous properly made incisions.

- If an episiotomy must be made before the perineum is fully stretched by the presenting part of the fetus, simulate that situation by applying gentle traction on the perineum before making the incision. This will reduce the bulk of tissue incised, hence minimising bleeding and trauma.

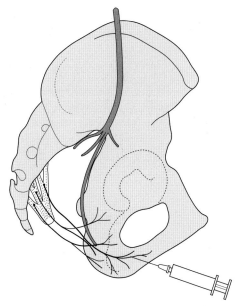

Figure 11.6   The pudendal nerve crosses the ischial spine medial to the pudendal artery.

- Tie off or place a clip on any spurting vessels to reduce blood loss. For the same reason repair episiotomies as soon as possible.

- Ensure the apex of the incision is identified before repair. If there is extension into the fornices a general anaesthetic or epidural block will aid proper exploration of damage and subsequent repair.

- Check the vaginal incision for any gaps in the suturing. Finally examine the rectal aspect of the incision. Any stitch through into the rectum should be cut to prevent infection and fistula formation. Ensure haemostasis is achieved.

- Consider subcutaneous sutures for the skin.

DO NOT

- Perform an episiotomy as a routine.
- Perform the episiotomy too early because vaginal delivery may not be possible, and blood loss and discomfort are increased when women receive both a perineal and an abdominal incision.
- Incise beyond an obstruction to ready delivery due to a thick or unyielding posterior fourchette (Figure 11.7).
- Incise beyond the bony ischial tuberosities. Outlet obstruction due to bony structures is not relieved by an episiotomy. A generous episiotomy is not generous for the woman.

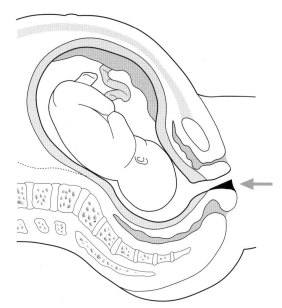

Figure 11.7 Obstruction caused by unyielding posterior fourchette (shaded) area

- Make an episiotomy before rotation with Kjelland's forceps. Vaginal delivery may not be achieved and rotation can extend the episiotomy.
- Leave any vaginal pack behind.
- Pull stitches too tight. This only increases discomfort and oedema.

REPAIR OF AN EPISIOTOMY

- The mother should be in the lithotomy position. Cleanse the surgical field, drape and maintain aseptic technique. Commence suturing from above the apex and appose the vaginal mucosa with continuous loose locking stitches placed 1 cm apart and 1 cm from the edge of the wound. Tie off at the vaginal mucocutaneous junction of the fourchette (Figure 11.8). Ensure anatomical apposition especially at hymenal remnants and mucocutaneous junction.

- This is followed by interrupted sutures placed perpendicular to the skin (Figure 11.8b). These sutures occlude any dead space and appose the subcutaneous tissue and the levator ani and perineal muscles. Avoid putting sutures through the rectal mucosa.

- The subcutaneous sutures are placed 1 cm deep and 1 cm apart to close the cutaneous wound. Polyglactin 910 sutures, which produce less tissue reaction and less pain during suture removal are recommended (Figure 11.8c, d).

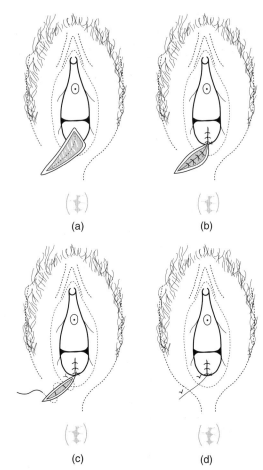

(a) (b) (c) (d)

Figure 11.8 Repair of an episiotomy: (a) episiotomy, (b) continuous locking vaginal stitches and interrupted sutures, (c) subcutaneous sutures and (d) repair complete. Steps (c) and (d) can be replaced by interrupted sutures.

- Check the vagina to ensure no gaps are present in the suture line and haemostasis is achieved. Perform a rectal examination to exclude any stitch which may have come through the rectal mucosa or the presence of a haematoma. Any rectal stitch must be cut. A haematoma must be evacuated.

RESUTURING EPISIOTOMIES

Breakdown of an episiotomy often follows infection of a haematoma. The following procedure should be adopted:

- Take swabs from the infected wound and vagina for bacterial culture.
- Epidural or general anaesthesia facilitates proper repair.

- The old episiotomy must be opened up in total, any haematoma if present evacuated, the wound edges freshened and the repair effected by interrupted sutures to allow drainage.
- Superficial dehiscence of the wound edges need not be resutured. Keeping the wound clean by regular bathing will promote rapid healing by secondary intention.
- Prescribe approximate broad-spectrum antibiotics.

TEARS IN THE PERINEUM

Eighty-five per cent of vaginal deliveries are associated with some perineal trauma. These are graded as:

- First degree – superficial lacerations, skin only, underlying muscles not damaged.

- Second degree – lacerations involving tearing of perineal muscles.

- Third degree – damage involving partial or complete disruption of the anal sphincter. These have an incidence of 2%, and are subdivided into:
  - less than 50% external sphincter injured
  - more than 50% external sphincter affected
  - torn internal anal sphincter.

- Fourth degree – there is complete disruption of the external and internal sphincters and the rectal mucosa.

Tearing is associated with:

- the woman's tissue type, ethnicity, age and health
- primiparous delivery
- prolonged second stage of labour
- narrow suprapubic arch
- poorly flexed head and occipitoposterior position
- precipitate labour
- big baby (more than 4000 g)
- shoulder dystocia
- assisted vaginal delivery (e.g. forceps, but much less with ventouse extractions).

Superficial grazes and tears, if they are not bleeding, can be left. Second degree tears are repaired as for episiotomies. Skin edges, because they are ragged, may need interrupted rather than subcutaneous sutures.

Third and fourth degree tears are associated with 4% of vaginal deliveries with mediolateral episiotomy. Severe tears are more common in the nullipara (4%) birthweight over 4 kg (2%), occipitoposterior position (3%), long second stage (4%) and forceps delivery (7%).

Repair of a third degree tear requires:

- Epidural or general anaesthesia (allow anal sphincter to relax and facilitate adequate repair).

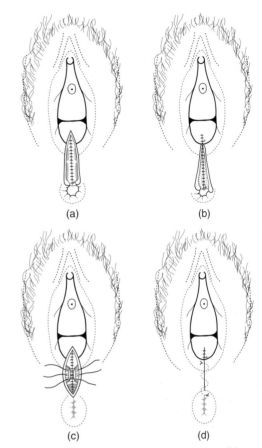

(a)   (b)

(c)   (d)

Figure 11.9 Repair of third-degree tear. Repair of (a) rectal mucosa, (b) vaginal mucosa and (c) rectal sphincter. (d) Subcuticular sutures.

- Continuous suture to repair the rectal mucosa. Commence above the apex of the tear; the mucosa is everted into the rectum. Tie-off at the mucocutaneous junction (Figure 11.9a). Use monofilament suture if available, e.g. polyglactin 910.

- The vaginal mucosa is repaired as for an episiotomy (Figure 11.9b).

- The severed ends of the rectal sphincter, which usually retract, are identified and apposed by interrupted sutures (Figure 11.9c). End-to-end repair of the sphincter may result in poorer subsequent function if the ends retract. Overlapping the ends of the sphincter provides more perineal bulk and better function. The anus should accommodate a finger after the sphincter muscles are approximated. The skin is apposed by subcutaneous and interrupted sutures (Figure 11.9d). Ensure that the vaginal introitus accepts two fingers at the end of the repair.

- Avoid constipation. A low-fibre diet and faecal softeners are advised, e.g. lactulose and Fybogel for 10 days. Do not use oil-based aperients. They inhibit healing of wound edges and encourage rectovaginal fistula formation.

- Prophylactic antibiotics reduce infection and wound dehiscence. Use metronidazole and broad-spectrum antibiotics.

- Prescribe adequate postoperative analgesia.

- Advise elective caesarean section for subsequent births since further vaginal delivery increases risk of anal incontinence.

- Clear documentation of findings and management is essential.

- Ensure follow-up and review.

CONSEQUENCES OF PERINEAL TRAUMA FOR WOMEN

- In 10% pain and discomfort will last 3–18 months after delivery.
- 20% will experience superficial dyspareunia for about 3 months.
- 3–10% report faecal incontinence (30% flatus incontinence).
- 20% experience urinary incontinence.

> **Box 11.1 Third degree tears: faecal incontinence**
>
> - About 13% of women experience a degree of incontinence, usually flatus, or rectal urgency after vaginal delivery.
> - Faecal incontinence is due to nerve and external and internal anal sphincter injury. Both nerve and muscle are damaged when injury is severe.
> - Mediolateral episiotomy may not prevent third degree tears. Two-thirds of third degree tears occur in women with an episiotomy.
> - Poor repair will result in subsequent sphincter defect with 50% of women having a degree of incontinence (flatus, faecal).
> - About 10% of women may experience wound disruption necessitating further surgery.
> - All women with third degree tears should be reviewed 3 months after surgery.

- Occult anal sphincter damage occurs in 36% after vaginal delivery and is evident in 70% (range 54–88%) despite repair of third and fourth degree tears.

Review women with severe tears 6 months or a year after delivery. Box 11.1 gives further information on third degree tears.

Bibliography

Bek KM, Laurberg S 1992 Risk of anal incontinence from subsequent vaginal delivery after a complete obstetric and sphincter tear. British Journal of Obstetrics and Gynaecology 99:724–726

Browning GG, Motson RW 1983 Results of Parks operation for faecal incontinence after anal sphincter injury. BMJ (Clinical Research Edition) 286:1873–1875

De Leeuw JW, Struijk PC, Vierhout ME et al 2001 Risk factors for third degree perineal ruptures during delivery. British Journal of Obstetrics and Gynaecology 108:383–387

Glazener CMA, Abdalla M, Stroud P et al 1995 Postnatal maternal morbidity: extent, causes, prevention and treatment. British Journal of Obstetrics and Gynaecology 102:286–287

Mackrodt C, Gordon B, Fern E et al 1988 The Ipswich Childbirth Study: 2 A randomised comparison of suture materials and suturing techniques for repair of perineal trauma. British Journal of Obstetrics and Gynaecology 105:441–445

Royal College of Obstetricians and Gynaecologists 2004 Guideline No. 23. Methods and Materials used in Perineal Repair. RCOG, London

Sultan AH, Kamm MA, Hudson CN et al 1993 Anal sphincter disruption during vaginal delivery. New England Journal of Medicine 329:1905–1911

Sultan AH, Kamm MA, Hudson CN et al 1994 Third degree obstetric anal sphincter tears and risk factors and oucome of primary repair. BMJ 308:887–891

Venkatesh KS, Ramanujam PS, Larson DM et al 1989 Anorectal complications of vaginal delivery. Diseases of colon rectum 32:1039–1416

Wood J, Amos L, Rieger N 1998 Third degree anal sphincter tears: risk factors and outcomes. Australian and New Zealand Journal of Obstetrics and Gynaecology 38:414–417

Chapter 12

The newborn

David A Curnock

CHAPTER CONTENTS

Physiological considerations   92
  Acid–base   92
  Cardiovascular system   92
  Lung liquid   92
  Body temperature   92
Resuscitation at birth   92
  Preparation   92
  Procedure at delivery   92
Special situations   93
  Meconium in the amniotic fluid   93
  Low birthweight infants   94
  Hypovolaemic shock (asphyxia pallida)   94
  Drug depression   94
Emergencies due to congenital abnormalities   95
  Choanal atresia   95
    Presentation   95
    Treatment   97
  Upper airway obstruction at vocal cord
    level   97
    Presentation   97
    Treatment   97
  Diaphragmatic hernia   97
    Presentation   97
    Treatment   97
  Tracheo-oesophageal fistula   97
    Presentation   97
    Treatment   97
  Pulmonary haemorrhage   97
    Presentation   97
    Treatment   97
  Pneumothorax   97
    Prevention   97
    Treatment   99
Birth trauma   99

Next to the risks encountered during labour, the transition from intrauterine to independent extrauterine existence is the second most critical period of the newborn's life. Mismanagement or failure to anticipate difficulties result in unnecessary damage to or death of the newborn. At every delivery a person should be present who has been trained in neonatal resuscitation. In addition, a paediatrician or a nurse practitioner with advanced resuscitation skills should be called to attend the delivery when there is:

- severe intrauterine growth retardation
- multiple births
- preterm delivery at less than 34 weeks' gestation
- vaginal breech delivery
- intrapartum fetal distress, e.g. pathological cardiotocograph, pH on fetal blood sample <7.2
- rotational forceps (e.g. Kjelland's) delivery
- urgent or emergency caesarean section
- elective caesarean section under general anaesthesia for placenta praevia or multiple births
- meconium staining of the liquor
- maternal insulin-dependent diabetes
- maternal myasthenia gravis
- known serious fetal abnormality, e.g. diaphragmatic hernia, hydrops fetalis
- severe rhesus disease.

Aftercare is most effective if:

- All labour ward personnel understand neonatal physiology and are familiar with resuscitative procedures.
- The neonatal condition is assessed accurately and the correct resuscitation measures are promptly undertaken. There is no place for deliberation or a 'wait and see' policy when a baby fails to establish regular respiration.

- Well-drilled teamwork is ensured.
- Equipment for resuscitation is well maintained.

PHYSIOLOGICAL CONSIDERATIONS

Acid–base

Before labour the normal fetus has a pH around 7.3, pCO_2 about 35 mmHg and pO_2 between 35 and 40 mmHg. At the end of labour repeated episodes of hypoxia associated with uterine contractions result in the normal newborn having a pH of 7.22–7.26, pCO_2 of 50 mmHg, pO_2 of 20 mmHg and a base excess of −5 to −8. This change equates with subjecting a normal fetus to 2 minutes of total anoxia. After 8–10 minutes of total anoxia, permanent brain damage would result.

Cardiovascular system

The fetal lungs in utero receive only 10% of the fetal right ventricular output. At birth the newborn's first breath expands the lungs and reduces pulmonary vascular resistance, thus allowing increased pulmonary flow. At the same time systemic vascular resistance rises when the umbilical cord is clamped. These changes and rising pO_2 result in closure of the shunts, foramen ovale and ductus arteriosus, establishing the pulmonary and systemic circulation. Hypoxia, acidosis and pulmonary atelectasis increase pulmonary vascular resistance and hence prevent closure of the shunts, thus limiting oxygenation of the blood. Prompt resuscitation will:

- encourage expansion of the lungs
- allow ventilation to reduce pCO_2 and increase pO_2
- reduce acidosis.

Breathing is stimulated by exposure to the extra-uterine environment and by the increasing fetal plasma carbon dioxide (pCO_2). Air is drawn in during the first breath. However, this air is expelled again through a partly closed glottis to effect the cry we hear from a healthy baby. During the first few minutes, breathing may be irregular or even intermittent but this is followed by more regular breathing at 40–60 breaths a minute. Regular breathing lowers pCO_2 and raises pO_2.

Normal acid–base status is only achieved at the end of 1 or 2 hours. Any complication which depresses the newborn prolongs this recovery period.

Lung liquid

In utero the fetus secretes fluid continuously from its lungs. Compression of the thorax during labour helps to expel this lung fluid. It is thought that raised fetal plasma adrenaline following the stress of labour is important in switching off the mechanism for lung fluid production and thus preparing the fetus for extrauterine existence. The residual lung liquid at birth is usually rapidly absorbed into the capillaries or lymphatics. Infants delivered electively by caesarean section have less opportunity for removing this lung fluid and therefore may develop some respiratory distress (transient tachypnoea) due to retention of lung liquid. Spontaneous resolution is expected and, while an increased oxygen concentration may be needed for a time, artificial ventilation is seldom necessary.

Body temperature

Keeping the baby warm is essential. The newborn's large surface area to body volume ratio, especially if preterm or of low birthweight, allows rapid cooling. A rapid drop in body temperature increases the need for oxygenation and exacerbates metabolic acidosis. Maintenance of body temperature is therefore particularly important in depressed infants. Failure to maintain adequate body temperature in preterm neonates is a major contributory factor to mortality due to respiratory distress syndrome. All neonates should be dried quickly, wrapped in a prewarmed towel and placed in a warm environment. Most resuscitation trolleys now incorporate an overhead radiant heater which should be switched on well in advance (Figure 12.1).

RESUSCITATION AT BIRTH

Preparation

Whenever there is time before the baby is born, obtain the obstetric history and check the resuscitation trolley and the equipment. Switch on the overhead heater. Request additional help if appropriate, e.g. for babies of less than 34 weeks' gestation or for multiple births. Introduce yourself to the parents.

Procedure at delivery

At the moment of birth start the clock, and dry and cover the baby in the warm towel. Assessment at birth is commonly by the Apgar score which documents five criteria (Table 12.1). Each criterion is scored from 0 to 2 to describe the spectrum from poor to good. The maximum score is 10 points. The infant is examined at 1 minute and again at 5 minutes after birth, scores being allocated at these two intervals. The score does not predict the outcome for the baby, and it is not useful in the management of individual babies, but it can be repeated again at regular intervals to document the response to resuscitation.

Decide on the baby's need for resuscitation by assessing four of the Apgar score signs – breathing, colour, heart rate and tone. The baby will then be in one of four groups and the appropriate management is followed (Table 12.2) proceeding in the order **ABCD**:

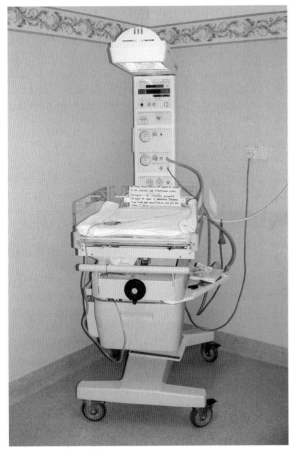

Figure 12.1   A resuscitation trolley.

- Airway – open the airway.
- Breathing – inflate the lungs and breath for the baby.
- Circulation – ensure an effective circulation, with chest compressions if necessary.
- Drugs – consider drugs to achieve this if initially unsuccessful.

Boxes 12.1–12.3 describe the resuscitation procedures and Figure 12.2 illustrates the use of mask ventilation.

In addition to the Apgar score, the biochemical indices of pH and base excess from combined venous and arterial cord blood can provide useful information about the duration of stress suffered. Mean cord pH in babies with normal Apgar scores is 7.3. Babies with birth asphyxia usually have cord pH <7.0 but the majority who develop hypoxic ischaemic encephalopathy have pH <6.8.

SPECIAL SITUATIONS

Meconium in the amniotic fluid

If the meconium is thick or particulate and the baby is not breathing or has a low heart rate:

- Place the baby on the resuscitation trolley and visualise glottis with laryngoscope. If meconium is present around glottis, suck under direct vision or, if skilled at intubation, it is appropriate to intubate immediately and apply direct suction to the tube.

- Maintain suction as the tube is withdrawn. A core of meconium will accompany the tube. Repeat this procedure until the tube comes out clear of meconium. An experienced operator can achieve three of four intubations within the first minute.

- Ventilate with oxygen only when the tube is clear.

If no meconium is seen around the glottis, clear the airways and treat as a normal baby.

Table 12.1 The Apgar score			
Physical sign	Score value		
	0	1	2
Heart rate	Absent	Below 100/minute	Over 100/minute
Respiratory effort	Absent	Slow, irregular gasping	Good, crying
Muscle tone	Limp/flaccid	Some flexion	Normal with movement
Response to stimulation	No response	Facial grimace	Good response with cry
Colour of trunk	White	Blue	Pink

Table 12.2   Resuscitation at birth

Condition at birth	Management
1. Breathing/crying Pink Heart rate >100 Good tone	Deliver the baby directly onto the mother's abdomen, and dry with a towel. This enhances bonding and maintains temperature by direct skin to skin contact
2. Apnoeic/gasping Blue Heart rate >100 Reasonable tone	Stimulate the baby by rubbing the back with a towel or gently tapping the feet. Open the airway (head in neutral position) and clear by performing gentle oral, followed by nasal suction. Give facial oxygen. If no response is shown by 1 minute of age, i.e. the heart rate is falling or the baby remains blue, then bag and mask ventilation should be commenced (see Box 12.1). Check for chest movement. If there is no improvement by 2 minutes of age, i.e. the heart rate has not increased, consider intubating the baby
3. Apnoeic Blue/pale Heart rate <100 Some tone	Bag and mask ventilation should be commenced immediately (see Box 12.1). Check for chest movement. If there is no response within 2 minutes, then intubate the baby
4. Apnoeic White Heart rate <60 Flaccid	Full cardiopulmonary resuscitation is required Intubate immediately (see Box 12.2) and commence intermittent positive pressure ventilation (IPPV). If no-one experienced at intubation is immediately available, or it is technically difficult, then bag and mask ventilation should be given until help arrives. After 30 seconds reassess heart rate by auscultation. If heart rate is <60 commence chest compressions (see Box 12.3) Note: The commonest reason for failure of the heart rate to improve is ineffective lung inflation. Check that there are good chest movements *before* commencing chest compressions. If there is no/poor chest movement, reposition the airway (head in neutral position, and a second operator applies jaw thrust) If there is no response to IPPV and chest compressions an umbilical venous catheter should be inserted and adrenaline and sodium bicarbonate given (see Box 12.3)

Low birthweight infants

Whether due to prematurity or poor intrauterine growth, these infants are susceptible to rapid heat loss and require expert resuscitation.

Hypovolaemic shock (asphyxia pallida)

This follows bleeding from the feto-placental vessels (abruptio placentae, placental shunting in twins, intrapartum bleeding and fetal trauma). A poor Apgar score, low circulatory blood volume and metabolic acidosis are characteristic. Proceed as follows:

1. Resuscitate as for an infant in group 4 (Table 12.2).
2. Expand the blood volume; uncross-matched O negative whole blood is given – 5–10 ml/kg bodyweight can be given over 2–3 minutes (normal neonatal blood volume is 70–90 ml/kg).

Shock produces vascular constriction. Following recovery with ventilation or replacement of blood volume, peripheral vessels will dilate and this can cause secondary hypotension and shock. The recovery phase therefore must be carefully monitored, as relapse after initial recovery may indicate the need for additional replacement.

Drug depression

Drugs used in obstetrics for sedation or analgesia will cross the placenta and affect the fetus, causing respiratory depression, poor thermal regulation and depressed reflexes.

- Opioids (pethidine, papaveretum) cause depression if administered to the mother within 3 hours before birth. The antidote, naloxone (Narcan), is a specific narcotic antagonist, given intramuscularly or intravenously. It must not be given to the baby of an opiate-dependent mother as it may cause acute withdrawal. The dose is 10 µg/kg. Narcan Neonatal contains 20 µg/ml. Naloxone is effective for 20 minutes after intravenous use, or 1–2 hours after being given intramuscularly. This is shorter than the action of the narcotics and therefore infants must be observed closely for a relapse when further doses of naloxone will be required.

- Diazepam (Valium) more than 30 mg given to the mother in 24 hours can produce apnoeic spells, carbon dioxide retention and a floppy newborn at birth. Keep the baby under close observation and give warmth and support for 24–48 hours. Phenothiazines may produce similar effects in the newborn.

Box 12.1 Bag and mask ventilation

- Airway-opening techniques

  The head should be tilted back gently to a neutral position and the chin lifted forward taking care not to compress the floor of the mouth.

  A folded towel placed under the neck and shoulders may help to maintain the neutral position.

  Use a 10 FG (black) suction catheter for a term baby or 8 FG (blue) catheter for a preterm baby to gently clear the mouth and pharynx.

- Use a soft silicon mask which is big enough to cover the face from the bridge of the nose to below the mouth. A good seal must be obtained around the infant's face (Figure 12.2).

- Use a T-piece or a bag with 500 ml capacity and a blow-off valve set at approximately 40 cm of water, and an oxygen flow rate of 5 l/min.

- Inflation breaths – the first five breaths ('inflation' breaths) should be given slowly to clear the lung fluid and establish a functional residual capacity, compressing the bag with the fingers for 2–3 seconds and achieving initial pressures of 30 cmH$_2$O.

- Following the first five breaths, ventilation should continue with 0.5 second inflation time and at a rate of 30–40 breaths per minute.

- Observe the chest wall for good movement. Listening with a stethoscope may be misleading because of transmitted upper airway sounds. If there is poor inflation check that the airway is not obstructed. Reposition the head, making sure the neck is not overextended and get a second operator to support the chin or to apply jaw thrust. If necessary perform gentle oral suction.

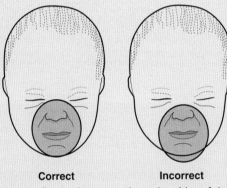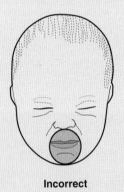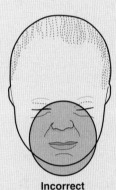

| Correct | Incorrect | Incorrect | Incorrect |

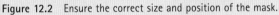

Figure 12.2 Ensure the correct size and position of the mask.

- Clomethiazole (Heminevrin) for sedation of pre-eclampsia/eclampsia can produce a sleepy baby. There is no specific antidote. Observe, support and keep the infant warm.

- Magnesium sulphate, prescribed for pre-eclampsia, can cause neonatal depression. The antidote, calcium gluconate 100 mg intravenously, is effective (30 mg/kg slowly).

- Local anaesthetic. Regional anaesthetic agents administered to the mother can reach the fetus in 30 minutes or less and cause hypotonia and depress myocardial activity. The half-life of these agents in the fetus varies from 3 to 9 hours. There is no antidote. Observe the infant closely.

- Gaseous anaesthetic agents can contribute to neonatal depression but these agents are cleared rapidly and therefore present less of a problem.

EMERGENCIES DUE TO CONGENITAL ABNORMALITIES

Certain abnormalities will limit the newborn's ability to establish respiration. Some have a subtle, gradual presentation whereas others are acute life-threatening conditions.

Choanal atresia

A bony or membranous septum is present across one or both posterior nasal air passages, obstructing breathing.

Presentation
The infant presents with respiratory distress from birth. Newborns are obligatory nose breathers and cannot breathe satisfactorily through the mouth. A catheter cannot pass up through the nostril.

Box 12.2   Endotracheal intubation and intermittent positive pressure ventilation (IPPV)

- Position baby on resuscitation platform and use airway-opening techniques and suction as for mask ventilation.
- Equipment: A 3 mm endotracheal (ET) tube should be used for a baby of ≥32 weeks' gestation, and a 2.5 mm ET tube for a baby <32 weeks' gestation, with a straight-bladed laryngoscope and a pressure manometer.
- Set the oxygen flow to 4–8 l/min via a bag and valve or via a T-piece attached to a pressure manometer.
- Pre-oxygenate the baby using mask ventilation.
- Hold the laryngoscope in the left hand and insert it into the right side of the baby's mouth so that the tip of the blade lies in the oesophagus.
- Use the laryngoscope blade to sweep the tongue across the midline to the left.
- Gently lift the laryngoscope forwards and upwards, withdrawing it very slightly from the oesophagus until the larynx and vocal cords come into view.
- Application of cricoid pressure either by an assistant or by using the little finger of the left hand may be helpful.
- Hold the ET tube with the right hand and gently insert it into the right side of the baby's mouth so that it does not obscure the view of the vocal cords.
- Advance the tip of the ET tube through the cords for 1–2 cm. The approximate length of the ET tube at the lips for infants of 1, 2, and 3 kg is 6.5, 7.5 and 9.0 cm, respectively.
- Remove the laryngoscope, and attach the ET tube to the bag and mask or to the T-piece and pressure manometer.
- The first five inflation breaths should be held for 2 seconds to establish the functional residual capacity.
- Then ventilate the baby at a rate of 30 breaths per minute, and adjust the peak inspiratory pressure so that it is sufficient to provide good chest movement.
- Observe chest movement, and auscultate over both axillae and over the stomach to asses the correct position of the tube.
- Fix the ET tube, and when the baby is stable check the tube position with a chest X-ray.

Note:

1. *Never* attach a baby's ET tube to the oxygen supply without a pressure limiting device within the circuit.
2. Do not spend longer than 30 seconds trying to intubate the infant before recommencing mask IPPV, for a minimum of 1 minute before attempting intubation again.

Box 12.3   Circulation and cardiac compressions

- External cardiac compressions must be started if the heart rate is <60/minute.
- The baby will already be receiving IPPV via an endotracheal tube, or, if this is not possible, by bag and mask.
- There are two techniques:
  1. The chest is encircled with both hands so that the fingers lie behind the baby and the thumbs are opposed over the sternum.
  2. Two fingers of the same hand are used to compress the sternum.
- The thumbs or fingers should be positioned over the middle third of the sternum, 1 cm below the inter-nipple line. The sternum should be compressed to a depth of 1.5–2 cm.
- The compressions should be at a rate of 120/min and a ratio of 3 compressions to 1 ventilation.
- External cardiac compressions should continue until the heart rate is >80 beats per minute and increasing.
- If there is no response to IPPV and cardiac compressions insert an umbilical venous catheter (UVC).
- Obtain a baseline blood gas, blood sugar, and haemoglobin sample.

- Give the following drugs via the UVC:
  - Adrenaline 10 μg/kg (i.e. 0.1 ml/kg of 1 in 10 000) followed by a 0.5–1.0 ml normal saline flush.

Continue ventilation and cardiac compressions. Reassess the heart rate and if there is no response after 1 minutes give:

- Sodium bicarbonate (4.2%) 1 mmol/kg (i.e. 2 ml/kg) followed by a saline flush, followed by further doses of adrenaline 10 μg/kg every 3–5 minutes if there is no response. An increased dose of 30 μg/kg can be considered in this situation.
- Glucose (10%). During prolonged resuscitation, hypoglycaemia (blood glucose <2.6 mmol/l) may occur and this may interfere with resuscitation. Give 10% glucose 2.5 ml/kg followed by a saline flush.

Note: All drugs should be checked before giving, and a record of drug administration kept. If there is no response to resuscitation by 20 minutes, then resuscitation should be discontinued, the decision being made by the registrar or consultant.

Treatment

Intubate and ensure the baby is comfortable. Replace the endotracheal tube with an oral airway. Resolve the obstruction surgically as a planned procedure.

Upper airway obstruction at vocal cord level

Presentation

The infant presents with respiratory distress and stridor.

Treatment

Ventilation and intubation may not be possible. Tracheostomy or, in less experienced hands, insertion of a wide-bore needle into the trachea below the level of the obstruction can allow ventilation until expert help arrives.

Diaphragmatic hernia

There is an incidence of 1/4000 live births. Usually the posterolateral part of the diaphragm fails to develop and almost always on the left side.

Presentation

The infant presents with cyanosis, severe respiratory distress, a scaphoid abdomen, poor breath sounds and the heart sound displaced to the right side of the chest. Often diagnosed before birth by routine scanning.

Treatment

Intubate, ventilate and stabilise before surgery.

Tracheo–oesophageal fistula

This is an additional problem in 90% of babies with oesophageal atresia. Fifty per cent of these infants have congenital heart disease and imperforate anus. The upper oesophageal pouch is usually blind. The distal oesophagus opens into the trachea above its bifurcation (Figure 12.3).

Presentation

Polyhydramnios is present during pregnancy. At birth the infant is 'mucusy' or 'bubbly', with gaseous abdominal distension. Diagnose before first feed to avoid aspiration pneumonia.

Treatment

Pass a wide-bore tube (FG 10 or 12), preferably double lumen with radio-opaque line, called a Replogle tube. Aspirate the contents from the upper pouch and take

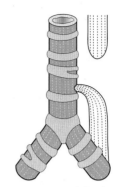

Figure 12.3   Tracheo-oesophageal fistula.

an X-ray to confirm the level of the blind end. Apply continuous suction on the tube and nurse the baby tilted head up to reduce reflux of gastric acid through the fistula until surgery is arranged.

Pulmonary haemorrhage

Bleeding into the alveoli can follow intrapartum pneumonia, severe rhesus disease, intracranial haemorrhage, congenital heart disease and growth retardation with severe intrapartum hypoxia.

Presentation

The infant presents with severe respiratory distress with fresh blood in the trachea. There may be evidence of disseminated intravascular coagulation.

Treatment

Intubate, ventilate using positive end expiratory pressure (PEEP), transfuse with whole blood and treat the cause.

Pneumothorax

This may present spontaneously at birth or occur in association with meconium aspiration or respiratory distress especially if resuscitation has been over-vigorous.

Prevention

The main danger is tension pneumothorax which rapidly causes respiratory distress and cyanosis. Reduced breath sounds on affected side and cardiac shift suggest pneumothorax but do not indicate the present or absence of tension. Transillumination with a light source is helpful. Confirm with a chest X-ray if there is no urgency.

Table 12.3 Types of birth trauma and their management at birth

Types of trauma	Description	Causes	Treatment
Minor superficial injuries	Bruises, abrasions, petechiae, subconjunctival haemorrhages, compression marks	Normal delivery, forceps, caesarean sections	Observe infant, reassure mother
Caput succedaneum (substitute head) (Figure 12.4)	Oedematous swelling over the vertex or occiput	Scalp lymphatics and venous stasis producing a serous collection separating aponeurosis and periosteum. Associated with labour. Degree reflects length and difficulty of labour	Observe. Spontaneous resolution within 24 hours
Cephalhaematoma (Figure 12.4)	Well-defined swelling over the parietal bone	Collection of blood beneath the periosteum, usually of the parietal bone and is limited by the suture lines. Associated with normal delivery, forceps, Ventouse extraction, fracture of skull bones	Observe, may increase in size. Resolves in 2–3 weeks. Can contribute to jaundice
Skull fractures	Linear hairline fracture or depressed fractures	Spontaneous deliveries, following trials of labour, assisted deliveries such as forceps or caesarean sections	No treatment unless there is cerebral bleeding, focal neurological irritation or paresis is observed
Subdural haemorrhage	Bulging fontanelle, cerebral irritation, retinal haemorrhage and low Apgar score	Excessive moulding, preterm delivery, difficult forceps, difficult rotation, breech extraction, ruptured veins in the subdural space	Subdural taps. Confirm diagnosis and relieve intracranial pressure
Intracranial haemorrhage	Shocked or stillborn with tear or tears in the tentorium cerebelli identified at post-mortem	Spontaneous rapid delivery or follows difficult labour, preterm delivery, breech extraction or assisted delivery	Condition tends to be fatal. If the infant survives lumbar puncture can confirm and ultrasound can be used to localise and determine the extend of bleeding to provide an idea of prognosis
Hypoxic ischaemic encephalopathy	Low Apgar score followed by irritability and high-pitched cry. A full fontanelle and tonic convulsions	All events which contribute to fetal hypoxia	Observe, sedate if irritable. Resolution of the condition may be complete or result in various degrees of handicap
Facial palsy	Paralysis of facial muscles, inability to close eye on affected side	Usually follows forceps delivery where the facial nerve is compressed just behind the stylomastoid foramen	Spontaneous recovery within a few days. Apply facial massage to maintain tone. Protect cornea of affected eye
Sternomastoid tumour	Haematoma of the sternomastoid	Rotational delivery, large babies with shoulder problems, breech deliveries after Lovset's manoeuvre	Check the neck of all difficult deliveries. If the condition is missed torticollis may result. Physiotherapy and muscle stretching three to four times daily is helpful

Table 12.3   *Continued*

Types of trauma	Description	Causes	Treatment
Brachial plexus palsy	Erb-Duchenne cervical 5, 6 nerve sheath is torn and nerves compressed by bleeding. Arm on affected side is limp with pronation of forearm and flexion at the wrist. Klumpke's cervical 7 and 8 nerve damage. Produces a wrist drop and paralysis of hand	Stretch injury following difficult delivery of the shoulders or difficult Lovset's manoeuvre	Support arm in position of relaxation. Arm is flexed and abducted for Erb's variety of damage. Physiotherapy three to four times daily, and consider referral for expert surgical decompression
Fractures	Greenstick fractures of limbs or clavicle. Pseudoparalysis or reluctant to move a limb should alert	Mainly with breech delivery or shoulder dystocia. Occasionally may follow normal delivery	Confirm by radiology. Splint to rest affected arm
Visceral damage	Large liver and spleen may be damaged	Breech delivery when the hands are placed too high for the Lovset's manoeuvre particularly in a small or preterm fetus. May also follow vigorous resuscitation	Deteriorating neonatal condition and suspicion of acute abdomen. Necessitates laparotomy

Treatment

Aspirate with a needle to reduce tension. This must be followed by a chest drain and an underwater seal.

BIRTH TRAUMA (Table 12.3)

Good obstetric practice and better judgement for the mode of delivery have reduced the incidence of birth trauma. It is important to appreciate that sometimes birth trauma can follow an easy spontaneous delivery.

Trauma is most likely in:

* prolonged labour
* trials of labour
* preterm delivery
* operative delivery, and this includes caesarean section.

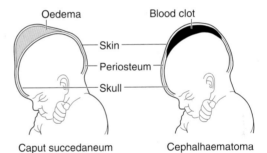

Figure 12.4 Comparison of the features of caput succedaneum and cephalhaematoma.

Bibliography

Nelson KB, Ellenberg JH 1981 Apgar scores as predictors of chronic neurologic disability. Pediatrics 68:36–44

Resuscitation Council (UK) 2001 Resuscitation at Birth – The Newborn Life Support Provider Course Manual. Resuscitation Council (UK), London

Roberton CMT, Finer NN, Grace MGA 1989 School performance in survivors of neonatal encephalopathy associated with birth asphyxia at term. Journal of Pediatrics 114:753–760

Chapter **13**

Preterm labour and preterm premature rupture of membranes

David T Y Liu
Mentor: Ronald Lamont

CHAPTER CONTENTS

Preterm labour 101
Preterm labour: general statements 101
Preterm labour at 23–26 completed weeks 102
Cervical cerclage 103
Preterm labour: antibiotics and infection 103
Preterm premature rupture of membranes 104
Preterm labour and tocolytics 105
Preterm delivery 106

PRETERM LABOUR

The World Health Organization (1992) defined preterm birth as delivery before 37 weeks of pregnancy. On the basis of this definition between 6% and 10% of births are preterm (5.6% in Oceania, 5.8% in Europe, 11–12% in America) but around 50% deliveries are more than 35 weeks' gestation with near 100% survival expected of babies born after 32 weeks of pregnancy. Intact survival exceeds 50% after 27 weeks and improves as gestation increases towards 32 weeks. In this group (27–32 weeks' fetus) every effort must be made to enhance survival and optimise quality of life.

The International Classification of Diseases uses 22 completed weeks as the beginning of the perinatal period when birthweight corresponds to 500 g. In practice the lower limit of fetal viability is influenced by available care and varies between 23 and 25 weeks of pregnancy. Delivery at these extreme preterm periods of gestation, 23 weeks to 26 weeks and 6 days, account for the majority of neonatal deaths and subsequent handicaps. At 24 weeks 50–80% of babies die. Half the survivors are disabled, 50% of them are severely disabled, only 13% survive intact.

PRETERM LABOUR: GENERAL STATEMENTS

When preterm labour presents the following considerations are important:

- Detailed pathophysiology of preterm labour is unknown hence the dilemma of effective therapy. Attempts to improve outcome for this obstetric complication (currently some 13 000 000 preterm deliveries worldwide) include efforts to predict or prevent its occurrence by risk scores, sonographic cervical assessment, uterine activity monitoring or

Table 13.1   Preterm labour: proposed guidelines for management

Cervical status	Cervical dilatation (cm)	Uterine contraction	Suggested management
Effaced	>3	Nil	Cerclage
Not effaced	3 or less (with scan showing funnelling or length <20 mm)	Two in 10 minutes lasting more than 40 seconds for 1 hour	Treat if present for more than 2 hours
Effaced	4 to 5	As above	Urgent therapy with loading dose regimen
Effaced	6 or more	Established labour	Preparation for delivery

tests for presence of fibronectin in cervico-vaginal secretions. Correct diagnosis of onset of labour is important (Table 13.1).

- Obstetric associations include congenital fetal abnormalities, preterm membrane rupture (30–40%), placental separation, intrauterine infection (10–15%) and fetal death. Perform ultrasound scan to exclude contraindications for therapy.

- Only infection and spontaneous onset of uterine activity are amenable to treatment. Past or current history of infection, presence of membrane rupture and stage of cervical dilatation must be considered.

- The most experienced obstetrician on duty should assess all suspected preterm labours. Accurate diagnosis and proper assessment is essential for correct management. Fetal age, numbers, weight and presentation are significant factors governing outcome. If in-house expertise or facilities are not available, consider transfer to a tertiary hospital.

- Obtain detailed obstetric and medical history from the patient. Identify conditions which contraindicate drug therapy or attempts to stop preterm labour or delivery.

- Management of preterm labour, particularly at the extremely preterm periods of gestation, can have significant psychosocial consequences for the parents. There is also clinical risk of mortality and morbidity for the woman from prolonged tocolysis, haemorrhage (more than 1000 ml) thrombosis and sepsis if surgery is performed. Some 6% uterine scars dehisce in future pregnancies after a classical caesarean section.

- Senior neonatologists and obstetricians must counsel parents fully (preferably at a joint meeting) about complications, likelihood of neonatal survival and eventual outcome. Parents must be made aware that expected outcome can change after delivery depending on the baby's condition at birth, presence of infection, sex of the baby and results of

neonatal care such as residue lung disease or intracranial lesions. Respect the parents' informed choice. They have to live with the consequences.

PRETERM LABOUR AT 23–26 COMPLETED WEEKS

Preterm labour and delivery at these extremely early gestations presents both ethical and clinical challenges. The following current evidence will help counselling:

- Between 23 and 24 weeks every extra day increases survival by 3%. From 24 to 26 weeks there is a 2% increase.

- Increase in birthweight especially between 600 g and 800 g enhances survival.

- Females and Afro-Caribbean babies have survival advantages compared with Caucasian babies.

- Pregnancy complications leading to delivery at these extremely early gestations do not influence survival before discharge.

- Singleton babies are more likely to survive compared with twins, especially among those between 700 g and 999 g.

- Overall prevalence of moderate or severe cerebral palsy is 1.5–2.5 per 1000 live births. Below 1500 g at birth the incidence is 50 per 1000. Table 13.2 gives examples of survival rates and incidence of major handicaps such as neurodevelopmental deficits with spastic diplegia, hemiplegia, quadriplegia or sensory and intellectual impairment after delivery at extremely early gestations.

- A poorly formed lower uterine segment necessitates use of classic caesarean section for delivery.

- Before 26 completed weeks of gestation there is no evidence to suggest benefit or danger for corticosteroid administration. A full course of corticosteroids (two doses of 12 mg dexamethasone 12 hours apart) for fetuses between 28 and 34 weeks' gestation reduce mortality, incidence of respiratory distress

Table 13.2 Percentage survival and survival with handicap between gestations 23–26 weeks and 6 days				
Gestation (weeks)	23	24	25	26 + 6 days
Survival (%)	15	40	50	60
Survivors with handicap (%)	65	35	30	25

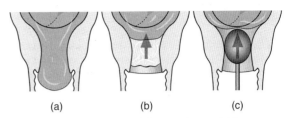

Figure 13.1   Reduction of bulging membranes (a) by gauze roll (b) or inflated balloon (c).

and intraventricular haemorrhage. Use of thyrotrophin releasing hormone is not recommended. Repeat courses of corticosteroids is also not recommended.

- β-Adrenergic agonists (e.g. ritodrine) are currently not indicated before 23 weeks' gestation. There is more risk than benefits associated with ritodrine use in twin or high multiple pregnancies between 23 and 26 weeks and 6 days. The Royal College of Obstetricians and Gynaecologists (2002) does not recommend use of these drugs.

- Neonatal outcome is not improved by prophylactic antibiotic therapy at this early gestation. However, appropriate antibiotics in early pregnancy for pathological colonisation reduce the incidence of preterm birth.

- Before 23 weeks in utero transfer is seldom indicated. Perform caesarean section when there is a maternal indication. Compassionate care only for the baby is acceptable.

- Between 23 and 26 weeks and 6 days, if clinically appropriate, transfer for delivery at a tertiary hospital. Perform caesarean section only after full discussion with the woman and her partner.

- Delay in cord clamping is likely to be beneficial because of reduced need for transfusion.

- An experienced neonatologist must attend the delivery. The parents' wishes must be considered regarding neonatal care immediately after delivery. The condition at delivery significantly affects outcome.

CERVICAL CERCLAGE

Emergency cerclage has been performed for gestations as late as 26 completed weeks with intact membranes and cervical dilatation between 3 cm and 10 cm. The reported rate of perinatal survival is 45–63%. When compared with conservative management with bed rest the incidence of infection, need for caesarean section and perinatal mortality appeared similar. A successful outcome is more likely before 20 weeks' gestation for cervical dilatations of less than 4 cm, when C-reactive protein is less than 4 mg/dl and

the white cell count is below 14 000. Cervical cerclage requires:

- Intact membranes and no uterine contractions.

- Counselling the woman about risks, e.g. infection, possible outcome of procedure, e.g. fetal membrane rupture, and potential for success.

- Commencing tocolytics 2 hours before surgery. These should be continued for 24 hours after surgery. Whether amnioreduction before cerclage improves success rates remains controversial.

- Placing the woman in a slightly head down position for surgery. General anaesthesia with halothane or tocolytics and spinal anaesthesia help relax the uterus.

- Placing sponge forceps at positions 3, 6, 9 and 12 of the cervix to provide countertraction. Bulging membranes are reduced by gentle traction on all four sponge forceps followed by gentle insertion of a lubricated gauze roll through the cervix. Alternatively, insert a Foley catheter and inflate the balloon (Figure 13.1).

- Once the membranes are reduced insert cervical sutures (usually in form of a tape) as high as is feasible. Note position of bladder and ureters. Take interrupted bites above placement of the sponge forceps and tie the knot at 3 or 9 o'clock for easy access. Do not tie beneath bladder as the knot will cause irritation.

- Bed rest following surgery for 24–48 hours. Ambulate when there is no uterine irritability.

There is a place for an abdominal approach for cervical cerclage. Before leaving hospital advise to watch for discharge, vaginal infection and onset of labour.

PRETERM LABOUR: ANTIBIOTICS AND INFECTION

Vaginal microorganisms such as bacterial vaginosis, group B streptococci, *Listeria monocytogenes* and *Gardnerella vaginalis* are associated with preterm labour and preterm premature rupture of membranes (PPROM). Current understanding is:

- Use of antibiotics showed significant advantage after PPROM in maternal (e.g. chorioamnionitis or endometritis) and neonatal outcome (respiratory distress syndrome, intraventricular haemorrhage, sepsis and cerebral palsy).

- Whether antibiotic treatment of vaginal microorganisms prevent preterm labour or PPROM remains controversial. There are, however, reports of infection as a cause in 40% of spontaneous preterm labour and administration of intravenous antibiotics have delayed delivery. Incidence of preterm birth is reduced when appropriate antibiotics for pathological infections are prescribed early in pregnancy.

- For PPROM, antibiotic therapy can prolong delivery for 1 week and reduce maternal and neonatal infection. Hence it should be used, especially between 23–26 completed weeks (see below).

- Around 10–15% of pregnant woman carry group B haemolytic streptococci. A history of fever and 'flu-like' illness may indicate *Listeria monocytogenes* infection. If infection is suspected prescribe ampicillin (2 g stat and 1 g 6 hourly intravenously for 10 days or until delivery). Add metronidazole (1 g per rectum three times a day) if chorioamnionitis is likely. If penicillin is contraindicated substitute ampicillin with a cephalosporin, for example cefotaxime (1 g intravenously 8 hourly). Note there is 5–10% cross-sensitivity with cephalosporins. Alternatively erythromycin 250 mg (drug of choice, see below) in divided doses can be used. Notify the neonatologist.

PRETERM PREMATURE RUPTURE OF MEMBRANES

The incidence of spontaneous rupture of fetal membranes before 37 weeks' gestation is around 3–6%. Contributory factors include infection (e.g. group B haemolytic streptococci, bacterial vaginosis, listeriosis and *Gardnerella* infection) polyhydramnios or collagen defect. Some 30–40% of preterm labour is preceded by membrane rupture. This complication is the most significant factor in the likelihood of preterm labour and delivery (Table 13.3). Once membranes rupture, 50% of woman will go into labour spontaneously in 24 hours and 80% will commence labour in 48 hours. When PPROM is suspected:

- Perform speculum examination with strict aseptic technique. A pool of liquor in the posterior fornix

Table 13.3 Impact of listed conditions on likelihood of preterm delivery following preterm labour

Factor	Calculated weight	Weighting given in preterm labour score
Membranes	1.45	1.5
'Show'	1.17	1
Dilatation	1.38	1.5
Contributory factors	1.05	1
Contractions	0.71	–

is a classic sign. Fetal fibronectin testing is expensive. A negative test suggests labour is unlikely but even if the test is positive some 80% need not deliver in the near future. Actim Partus (insulin-like growth factor binding protein-I is said to be more specific). If 'negative' labour is not likely, if 'positive' membranes are ruptured. If membranes are ruptured exclude cord prolapse.

- Take swabs for bacterial culture. Chorioamnionitis is often present, threatening wound infection and neonatal sepsis.

- Look out for signs of herpetic infection.

- Chorioamnionitis is associated with maternal tachycardia with or without fever (pyrexia may be absent in gram negative septicaemia). There is uterine tenderness on palpation and evidence of fetal tachycardia or ominous fetal heart rate changes. An offensive vaginal discharge may be evident. When infection is established consider delivery whatever the gestation. Some 10% of fetuses will be infected.

- For gestations of 32 or more weeks with confirmed membrane rupture, risk of cord prolapse and infection outweigh preterm delivery. Allow preterm labour to continue if there are no contraindications (for example footling breech which necessitates caesarean section). In the absence of uterine contractions and cervical conditions not favourable for induction of labour, adopt conservative management (hospitalisation, bed rest and antibiotics).

- Uterine infection, if not present, will occur after 4 hours of membrane rupture. Deliver by caesarean section if active herpetic lesions are evident and time since membrane rupture is less than 4 hours.

- Between gestations of 27 and 32 weeks, adopt conservative management if there is no uterine activity. Prescribe corticosteroids. With preterm labour and no contraindications, tocolytics and antibiotics can be used to gain an extra week to reduce maternal and fetal morbidity.

Box 13.1   Comments regarding use of β-sympathomimetics

- Can delay delivery for 48 hours.
- No effect on perinatal mortality or morbidity.
- Maternal heart rate must not exceed 130–140 beats per minute.
- The woman must be closely monitored. Hypotension can result.
- Monitor fluid balance. If pulmonary oedema is diagnosed stop treatment and prescribe diuretics.
- Do not prescribe β-sympathomimetics to woman with cardiac disease. The increased cardiac output can cause myocardial ischaemia.
- Woman with diabetes will need adjustment of blood sugar levels since carbohydrate metabolism is affected.

- β-sympathomimetics can cross the placenta to produce similar effects in the fetus as the mother (e.g. fetal tachycardia).
- About 14% of women stop treatment because of side effects such as tachycardia, dyspnoea, palpitation or chest pain. Use is not recommended by the Royal College of Obstetricians and Gynaecologists.
- An oxytocin antagonist is a safer alternative. It is 10 times less likely to cause cardiovascular side effects and 15 times less likely to result in discontinued therapy.

Box 13.2   Management of preterm labour and delivery

- Clinical assessment by the most experienced obstetrician on duty when a woman presents with possible preterm labour. Perform sterile speculum examination. Take swabs for microscopy and culture. Define cervical status. Address reasons for admission if diagnosis is not confirmed. Follow guidelines in Table 13.1.

- Check medical and obstetric history. If delivery is not imminent determine gestational age and clinical status. Perform ultrasound scan. Note contraindications to stop preterm delivery and exclude risk of medical treatment with tocolytics. Consider need for in utero transfer. Tocolysis is not likely to succeed if labour is established and the cervix is ≥5 cm dilated (Table 13.1).

- Between 27 and 34 weeks' gestation and no contraindications to stop labour, prescribe tocolytics and corticosteroids. Arrange transfer if indicated and safe. Discuss with the woman and her partner and neonatologists to obtain an agreed mode for delivery if tocolysis fails.

- For preterm labour at 23–26 weeks and 6 days' gestation note above discussed statements. Respect the parental wishes. An experienced neonatologist must attend delivery to determine if active resuscitation is appropriate. External cardiac massage and adrenaline may not improve survival. Request for neonatologist to attend delivery of babies less than 23 weeks' gestation is principally for supporting the parents.

- Monitor the fetal heart rate continuously by ultrasound throughout labour. Prompt response is required to prevent hypoxic damage of these susceptible fetuses.

- An epidural block provides the best form of analgesia and obviates need for opioids which aggravate neonatal respiratory problems.

- Do not use the ventouse. An episiotomy can facilitate delivery. Forceps are designed for a term baby. A small Wrigley forceps may be more appropriate for assisted vaginal delivery.

- Erythromycin 250 mg four times daily for 10 days can prolong pregnancies and benefit neonatal outcome. Co-amoxiclav is not recommended because of its association with increase in occurrence of neonatal necrotising enterocolitis. Add metronidazole if chorioamnionitis is suspected.

PRETERM LABOUR AND TOCOLYTICS

- β-Adrenergic agonists such as salbutamol, terbutaline and especially ritodrine were the most commonly used tocolytics. Magnesium sulphate, nifedipine and prostaglandin synthase antagonist are not licensed for use. Prostaglandin synthase antagonists cross the placenta and cause serious fetal vascular side effects such as closure of the ductus arteriosis (see Box 13.1).

- Exclude contraindications for stopping preterm labour and use of drugs (for example maternal heart disease).

- Before 26 weeks and 6 days use of β-agonists may confer more harm than benefit.

- Strict surveillance of β-agonist usage is essential. Careful fluid balance, avoidance of intravenous saline, monitoring with electrocardiography and frequent auscultation of lung basis to exclude pulmonary oedema are recommended.

- The aim is to prevent delivery for 24–48 hours to allow corticosteroid therapy to enhance fetal lung maturity. Significant fetal benefit has not been shown (perinatal mortality, morbidity and increase in birthweight). Corticosteroids are not used if there is chorioamnionitis, tuberculosis or porphyria.

- Potential better tocolytics such as selective cyclo-oxygenase-2 enzyme inhibitors and prodrug prostaglandin synthase inhibitors with predominantly maternal effects suggest potential. The oxytocin antagonist atosiban (Tractocile) is licensed for treatment of preterm labour. This competitive inhibitor of oxytocin is as effective as a β-agonist in delaying delivery for 48 hours and safer for the mother but neonatal outcome is the same (Box 13.1).

PRETERM DELIVERY

Preterm labour and delivery remain serious complications with significant sequelae for mothers and their newborns. The informed views of the women and their partners, neonatologists and obstetricians must be considered, preferably at a joint meeting, to determine an agreed best plan of management. Established preterm labour seldom responds to tocolytics for any length of time hence the main focus must be on the most competent place and most suitable mode of delivery for best results. Where necessary, appropriate and safe in utero transfer is preferred. There is a place for compassionate care for the extremely preterm baby especially if delivered in poor condition. General guidance for preterm labour and delivery management is presented in Box 13.2.

References

Royal College of Obstetricians and Gynaecologists 2002. Tocolytic drugs for women in preterm labour. Guidelines 1(b). London, RCOG

World Health Organization 1992

Bibliography

Anon 1995 Effect of corticosteroids for fetal maturation on perinatal outcomes. NIH Consensus Development Panel on the effect of corticosteroids for fetal maturation on the perinatal outcomes. JAMA 273:413–418

Banks BA, Caan A, Morgan MA et al 1999 Multiple courses of antenatal corticosteroids and outcome of premature neonates. North American Thyrotropin Releasing Hormone Study Group. American Journal of Obstetric and Gynecologists 181:709–717

Canadian Preterm Labour Investigators' Group. 1992 Treatment of pre-term labour with the beta-adrenergic agonists ritodrine. New England Journal of Medicine 327:308–312

Datospian Study Group, Goodwin TM, Palenzuela GJ, Silver H et al 1996 Dose ranging study of the oxytocin antagonists atosiban in the treatment of pre-term labour. Obstetrics and Gynecology 88:331–336

Gyetvai K, Hannah ME, Hodnett ED et al 1999 Tocolytics for preterm labour: a systematic review. Obstetrics and Gynecology 94:869–877

Finnstrom O, Olausson PO, Sedin G et al 1997 The Swedish National Prospective Study on extremely low birthweight (ELBW) infants. Incidence, mortality, morbidity and survival in relation to level of care. Acta Paediatrica 86:503–511

Kenyon SL, Taylor DJ, Tarnow-Mordi 2001 Broad spectrum antibiotics for spontaneous preterm labour: the ORACLE II randomised trial. Lancet 357:989–999

Lam PM, Yuen PM, Lau TK et al 2001 Relationship between birthweight and repeated courses of antenatal corticosteroids. Australian and New Zealand Journal of Obstetric and Gynaecology 41:281–284

Lamont RF 2003 The development and introduction of anti-oxytocic tocolytes. British Journal of Obstetrics and Gynaecology 110(Suppl 20):108–112

Lembet A, Eroglu E, Ergin T et al 2002 New rapid bed-side test to predict preterm delivery: phosphorylated insulin-like growth factor binding protein-I in cervical secretions. Acta Obstetrica et Gynecologica Scandinavica 81:706–712

Elder MG, Romero R, Lamont RF (eds) 1997 Preterm Labour. Churchill Livingstone, New York

Romero R, Sibai BM, Sanchez-Ramos et al 2000 An oxytocin receptor antagonist (atosiban) in the treatment of preterm labour: a randomised, double-blind placebo controlled trial with tocolytic reserve. American Journal of Obstetric and Gynaecology 182:1173–1183

2003 Strategies to prevent the morbidity and mortality of preterm labour. Proceedings of the First International Preterm Labour Congress, 27–30 June 2002, Montreux, Switzerland. British Journal of Obstetrics and Gynaecology 20:Supplement 20

The World Wide Atosiban A versus Beta agonists Study Group 2001 Effectiveness and safety of the oxytocin antagonists Atosiban versus beta adrenergic agonists in the treatment of pre-term labour. British Journal of Obstetrics and Gynaecology 108:133–142

Welsh A, Nicolaides K 2002 Cervical screening for preterm delivery. Current Opinion in Obstetrics and Gynaecology 14:195–202

Chapter 14

Abnormal labour

David T Y Liu
Mentor: Martin Whittle

CHAPTER CONTENTS

Abnormal uterine activity   109
  False labour (spurious labour)   109
    Management   109
  Precipitate labour and delivery   110
    Management   110
  Sudden cessation of labour   110
    Management   110
Prolonged labour   110
  Abnormal contractions (powers)   110
    Infrequent weak contractions (hypotonic
      uterine activity)   110
    Frequent strong contractions (hypertonic
      contractions)   110
    Incoordinate uterine activity   111
  Passenger   112
  Abnormal descent (passage)   112
    Management   113
  Deficient/delayed cervical dilatation
    (passage)   114
Consequences of prolonged labour   114
  Fetus   114
  Mother   114
  General management   114
Trial of labour   114
  Contraindications   114
  Requirements   115
  Failed trial of labour   115
Trial of scar or vaginal delivery   115
  Contraindications   115
  Requirements   115

Spontaneous onset of labour followed by efficient uterine activity and delivery around a time of 8 hours for multiparous and 12–14 hours for primiparous women is accepted as normal. Labour complicated by problems of uterine contractility or integrity (powers), adequacy of the pelvis (passage) and fetal complications (passenger) is considered abnormal.

ABNORMAL UTERINE ACTIVITY

False labour (spurious labour)

Braxton Hicks or practice contractions may be exceptionally uncomfortable or of longer duration, thus giving the impression that labour has started. Repeated episodes of false labour or spurious labour on the other hand can signify fetal compromise and the need for early delivery to avoid fetal death.

Management
- Assess the woman to establish whether or not she is in labour. Observe contraction strength and frequency; check cervix on admission and review 1–2 hours later. If the cervix is <4 cm and there is no dilatation over the observation period, she is either in the latent phase of labour or not in labour. Assess fetal wellbeing using a 20 minute cardiotocograph (CTG) (this is not a requirement of the National Institute of Health and Clinical Excellence). If deemed not in active labour and fetus is satisfactory, she may go to the ward to await events. If appropriate some women may even go home.

- The presence of risk factors, i.e. abnormalities in the pregnancy or a non-reassuring CTG, indicate the need for close surveillance with consideration to augment or induce labour.

- Women should be fully informed, contribute to plans for their care and be aware of the reasons for the steps taken.

Precipitate labour and delivery

Labour resulting in delivery less than 2 hours after onset of uterine contractions is accepted as rapid or precipitate. Dangers include delivery in an unsuitable or non-sterile environment with risk of fetal and maternal trauma. Precipitate labour and delivery are possible in the following conditions:

- When there is little resistance to delivery. With an effaced cervix 3 cm or more dilated and the presenting part engaged and well applied, little harm is likely if labour is properly conducted in an appropriate environment. Women with a history of precipitate labours should be admitted around 38 weeks for induction of labour to control the situation.

- Rapid labour may follow sensitivity to or excessive use of oxytocics. The fetus is pushed rapidly through the birth canal by strong frequent uterine contractions. Fetal hypoxia and trauma together with soft tissue damage of the birth canal are likely. This should not happen in well-conducted labours.

Management
- Anticipate the situation from the obstetric history. Women must be carefully selected for oxytocin stimulation. This is particularly important in grand multipara or in women with a history of short labours.
- Anticipate the condition if pelvic findings suggest the likelihood of rapid labour.
- The maternal and fetal conditions must be closely monitored. A midwife must be in attendance to supervise labour.
- Myometrial sensitivity to oxytocin (Syntocinon) is enhanced after prostaglandin usage.
- Following delivery, examine the soft tissue of the birth canal for possible damage.

Sudden cessation of labour

When labour stops suddenly suspect uterine rupture. Uterine rupture is usually, but not always, preceded by evidence of fetal distress and continuous lower abdominal pain.

Management
- Confirm the diagnosis.
- Assess maternal condition, treat if shocked.

- The globular outline of the uterus is lost, fetal parts may be readily palpable, the fetal heart sounds may be absent, lie may not be longitudinal.
- Cross-match blood, summon an experienced anaesthetist and senior obstetrician.
- Perform emergency laparotomy.
- If repair of the uterus is not possible proceed to hysterectomy. There is a place for subtotal hysterectomy in this situation.

Box 14.1 gives more information on uterine rupture.

PROLONGED LABOUR

Labour is prolonged if it lasts more than 24 hours. This concept is dangerous if it suggests the mistaken connotation that labour can continue for 24 hours before delay is diagnosed. Labour should be considered prolonged once it lags behind the normal partogram by 2–3 hours. This definition draws attention earlier to development of abnormality. Labour is prolonged because of:

- abnormal contractions (powers)
- abnormal descent of the presenting part of the fetus (passenger)
- deficient/delayed cervical dilatation (passage).

Abnormal contractions (powers)

Infrequent weak contractions (hypotonic uterine activity)
Most likely reason is misdiagnosis of labour. It has been said that the overstretched uterus does not labour well but evidence for this is thin.

Management
- Assess the woman's status, support her morale and correct ketoacidosis.
- If there are no contraindications (exclude disproportion and malpresentation), augment labour by amniotomy with or without intravenous oxytocics.
- Maintain close surveillance.

Frequent strong contractions (hypertonic contractions)
These can follow the inappropriate use of oxytocics. Prolonged labour associated with strong contractions is seen principally in multiparous mothers with disproportion. The practised uterus mounts an increased effort to overcome the obstruction. The resultant frequent strong contractions and increased uterine tone result in both maternal and fetal distress. If allowed

Box 14.1   Uterine rupture

Classification
Rupture may be incomplete (intact peritoneum) or complete (uterine cavity communicates directly with peritoneum cavity). This complication occurs in between 1 in 140 and 1 in 300 labours with a uterine scar.

Associations
- Previous uterine damage or surgery, e.g. myomectomy that encroached into the uterine cavity, hysterotomy and perforations.

- Caesarean sections, particularly classic sections (may rupture before onset of labour). Multiple sections or sections with inadvertent extension or need for an inverted T incision (Chapter 17). History of infection may mean poor healing and a weaker scar.

- Obstructed labour.

- Oxytocic usage. The very unfavourable cervix, previous lower segment caesarean section and oxytocic augmentation in multiparous women require careful assessment and close observation.

- Prostaglandin pessaries should be used with caution when priming a cervix in the presence of a previous caesarean scar.

- Instrumental delivery, e.g. rotation forceps.

- Intrauterine manipulations, e.g. internal podalic version for assisted breech delivery. This complication contributes to maternal and high perinatal mortality. Prevention by attention to the above is important.

Diagnosis
See Chapter 17.

Subsequent care
- Provide an opportunity for counselling to explain reasons for this traumatic incident.
- Elective caesarean section and close antenatal surveillance is mandatory if further pregnancies are allowed when the uterus is salvaged.

---

to continue tetanic uterine activity can occur. A retraction ring denoting the junction between the strong contracting upper uterine segment and the overstretched lower segment is observed as a late sign of imminent uterine rupture.

Management
- An abnormal fetal heart rate is often an early sign and should alert the attendant to the problem.

- Exclude overstimulation by oxytocics.

- Caesarean section is indicated for tetanic contractions and an overstretched lower segment. This should be considered even if the fetus is dead. Destructive operations for a dead fetus increase the risk of uterine rupture.

- If the situation is less acute, reassess presentation and position of the presenting part of the fetus. The mode of delivery will depend on the findings and include trial of forceps, rotation forceps or more usually caesarean section.

- Excessive uterine activity can sometimes be reduced using salbutamol (a tocolytic) by inhalation for immediate effect.

Incoordinate uterine activity
The pacemaker for myometrial activity is normally situated at the cornu of the uterus. When pacemaker activity develops at alternative sites and interrupts fundal dominance, irregular uterine contractions are produced and incoordinate uterine activity results. Incoordinate uterine activity produces poor uterine propulsive effort, increased uterine tone and intermittent painful strong uterine contractions (Figure 14.1). This is usually, but not exclusively a condition of primiparous women in whom an element of disproportion is present. This condition is more likely if the woman is frightened, distressed or anxious as in a first labour, particularly if she is over the age of 35 years.

Management
- Reassure, sedate if appropriate and prescribe analgesia. Epidural anaesthesia is particularly effective.
- More than 50% of these women may require assisted delivery. Group and save blood.
- Re-examine the woman to exclude absolute disproportion.
- If appropriate, rupture the membranes and apply direct fetal heart rate monitoring.
- Prescribe intravenous oxytocics if there is no contraindication to further labour. The use of oxytocics overrides pacemaker influence.
- Deliver by caesarean section if there is no progress after 2–4 hours of oxytocic therapy or if fetal distress develops.

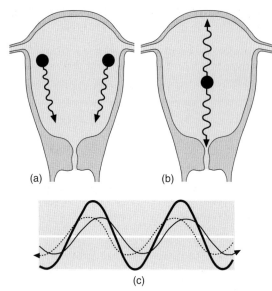

Figure 14.1 Fundal dominance with (a) normal pacemaker activity and (b) ectopic pacemaker and incoordinated uterine activity. (c) Schematic illustration of ectopic pacemaker activity resulting in high amplitude and attenuated contraction waves of incoordinated activity.

Passenger

Another cause for failure to progress is due to problems with the passenger (fetus/fetuses). There are four main factors:

1. malposition
2. fetus too big (macrosomia)
3. malpresentation
4. fetal abnormality.

It is essential to exclude these factors when poor progress presents. Malposition can sometimes be corrected by the use of oxytocin but its injudicious use in the other situations may result in uterine rupture.

The occipitoposterior position (see Chapter 16) is a common cause of slow progress, particularly in primigravid mothers. Frequently this malposition is associated with backache and early membrane rupture. Potential for deflection, hence a larger fetal head diameter, together with need to rotate from a posterior position to a more optimum occipitoanterior position contributes to prolonged labour. Adequate uterine activity is necessary to ensure rotation. In an android pelvis, failure to achieve rotation to occipito-anterior results in arrest at occipitotransverse. This will need assisted rotational delivery if the fetal head is low down and disproportion is excluded. At mid-pelvic level the correct approach is for delivery by caesarean section.

Fetal abnormality includes conjoined twins or tumours, for example, cystic hygromas. In contemporary practice most of these are identified antenatally on ultrasound scanning. In twin labour, consider 'locking' when there is failure of descent despite ideal conditions. Caesarean section is usually required. The risk is highest when the first twin is breech.

Fetal abnormality also includes growth restriction. See Box 14.2 for procedures in cases of intrauterine growth restriction.

Abnormal descent (passage)

Any condition, which hinders descent, will prolong labour. Obstruction to descent is due to the following:

- Obstruction by a mass or tumour outside the uterus, for example, an ovarian cyst. Malpresentation and malposition is usual. Obstruction can be at any level such as the pelvic brim or upper half of the pelvis. This complication should be identified before the onset of labour. Delivery is by caesarean section. An experienced obstetrician is required to conduct or supervise any additional surgery.

- Masses such as fibroids arising from the uterus or cervix can interfere with descent of the fetus. Occasionally after a lengthy labour when little residual liquor is present, the uterus may be wrapped tightly around the fetus preventing descent. Caesarean section is required. A possible exception is where forceps delivery is prevented by tonic uterine contraction. When this occurs the uterus can be relaxed by amyl nitrate, salbutamol inhalation or halothane administration to allow vaginal delivery.

- The presence of an unsuspected degree of placenta praevia.

- Disproportion. This term describes the situation where the proportions or diameters of the pelvis are inadequate for the passage of the fetus. This terminology describes inadequacy of the pelvis to accommodate the fetal head, which has the largest diameter and is least compressible. Cephalo-pelvic disproportion is a relative concept. A larger than normal baby can produce disproportion in a pelvis which is of normal size. This concept is particularly relevant in multiparous labours. The present fetus may be larger in size than a fetus in a previous pregnancy so previous spontaneous delivery should not encourage complacency. Alternatively, a small or preterm baby may deliver with ease through a small or contracted pelvis. Disproportion may arise at any stage of labour or at any site

---

Box 14.2   Intrauterine growth restriction

- Confirm diagnosis from obstetric history and ultrasound measurements. Umbilical artery Doppler waveform and CTG trace can indicate impaired fetal–placental perfusion. Late-onset growth restriction may be associated with normal umbilical artery Doppler findings despite fetal compromise because of compensatory mechanisms.

- Determine if the fetus is anatomical and chromosomally normal. Fetal weight less than 500 g, presence of reverse end diastolic flow velocity in umbilical arteries, umbilical vein pulsations and CTG fetal heart rate decelerations forewarn of poor prognosis.

- Review situation with the woman and her partner and a neonatologist. Offer counselling where appropriate.

- Determine mode of delivery. Consider past obstetric history, past labour patterns and presenting cervical conditions. Before 34 weeks of pregnancy presence of severe fetal compromise and anticipated viability justifies elective caesarean section. Use intravenous oxytocin to induce labour (starting at 2–4 mU/min). This is similar to performing a contraction stress test. Appearance of decelerations necessitates delivery by caesarean section.

- Prostaglandin is not contraindicated when there are no Doppler or fetal heart rate signs of compromise.

- Perform caesarean section if induction of labour is not successful.

- Fetal heart rate monitoring and close surveillance is mandatory during labour if growth restriction is suspected.

- Use the lower midline vertical uterine incision for delivery for fetuses more than 750 gm and over 24 weeks' gestation if lower uterine segment is poorly formed. Monitor fetal heart rate until just before skin incision.

- Consider general anaesthesia which is associated with less fetal acidaemia.

- In preterm fetuses with growth restriction, presence of pregnancy hypertension confers an advantage with reduced perinatal mortality. Perinatal mortality rises significantly after 40 weeks of pregnancy.

- A neonatologist must attend delivery as these babies have impaired metabolic adaptation, such as poor response to hypoglycaemic stress, and increased risk of necrotising enterocolitis and respiratory distress syndrome.

---

along the pelvic canal. It is, however, usual to notice disproportion at the pelvic brim (inlet disproportion), at the level of the ischial spine (mid-pelvic disproportion at the plane of least diameters) and at the pelvic outlet (outlet disproportion). Labour is prolonged whenever disproportion is present.

Management
- Perform vaginal examination to assess cervical status, station of the presenting part of the fetus, presence of caput and adequacy of the pelvis.

- Request erect lateral pelvimetry. Additional information concerning the shape of the sacrum and possible reasons for inlet disproportion may be obtained.

- Perform a caesarean section if absolute disproportion is diagnosed at the inlet, mid-pelvis or outlet. Absolute disproportion is present whenever any pelvic diameter is smaller than the biparietal diameter. For the average fetus a diameter of 9.5 cm is not adequate.

- Inlet disproportion is associated with a flat pelvis, spondylolisthesis, sacralisation of the fifth lumbar vertebra, pelvic deformity (rickets, osteomalacia) pelvic fracture or congenital defects (Naegele's or Robert's pelvis). If absolute disproportion is not evident (fetal head overlaps symphysis when an attempt is made to direct the head into the pelvis) and there is no contraindication to further labour, observe closely and review after two hours. Cord prolapse is a threat when the presenting part of the fetus is poorly applied. Delivery by caesarean section is usual.

- Mid-pelvic disproportion. Both the short, stocky, obese, hirsute woman and the tall athletic woman with boyish hips are susceptible. Malposition is common. If conditions are suitable for further labour, review after an interval of 2 hours. Deliver by caesarean section if there is no progress. If the cervix is fully dilated and there is no absolute disproportion, ventouse or forceps delivery by an experienced obstetrician may be attempted after correction of malposition.

- Outlet disproportion. This presents classically as delay in the second stage. The cervix is fully dilated with the presenting part below the mid-plane. A trial of forceps is acceptable if absolute disproportion is excluded. Outlet disproportion must be excluded in a breech delivery.

Deficient/delayed cervical dilatation (passage)

Poor cervical dilatation reflects or contributes to the slow progress of labour.

- The cervix dilates less well if the presenting part of the fetus is poorly applied.

- Occurs in 5% of primigravidae. It can be associated with poor cervical response to pregnancy changes. Assisted delivery or caesarean section is likely.

- Strong labour with poor descent can produce an oedematous cervix and gives the impression that dilatation is regressing.

- Poor dilatation can reflect weak or incoordinated uterine activity.

- Poor dilatation can be associated with disproportion.

- A scarred or fibrotic cervix (following cerclage or cone biopsy) may not dilate despite the descent of the presenting part to the introitus. If there is failure to dilate beyond 5 cm or more, make 2 cm incisions in the cervix at the 5 and 7 o'clock regions and deliver by forceps (Figure 14.2). Cervical incisions are seldom performed because further extension during delivery with resultant haemorrhage and damage to the lower uterine segment can occur. Do not incise if the cervix is not thinned out – deliver by caesarean section.

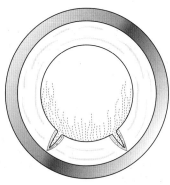

Figure 14.2 Cervical incisions.

CONSEQUENCES OF PROLONGED LABOUR

Fetus

The consequences for the fetus include trauma, acidosis, hypoxic damage, infection and increased perinatal mortality and morbidity.

Mother

The consequences for the mother are reduced morale, exhaustion, dehydration, acidosis, infection and risk of uterine rupture. The need for surgical intervention increases mortality and morbidity. Ketoacidosis by itself can result in poor uterine activity and prolonged labour.

General management

- Anticipate likelihood of this complication before the onset of labour or at the initial assessment in the labour suite.
- Determine the cause of prolonged labour. Treat correctable causes.
- Determine if there is justification for further continuation of labour. Fetal or maternal compromise precludes further labour.
- Continuing labour must be closely monitored. Support maternal morale and include the woman and her partner in discussion of the likely outcome.
- Anticipate the possibility of a caesarean section (required for 80% mothers not responding to oxytocics).

TRIAL OF LABOUR

All labour can be considered a trial. The term 'trial of labour' is reserved for situations where possible complications of labour are anticipated. The trial assesses the adequacy of the pelvis and the ability of the fetus or mother to withstand labour.

Contraindications

- Absolute disproportion.
- Malpresentations such as face and brow.
- Breech presentation. The trunk is the smaller or more compressible part of the fetus. The dangerous situation where the body is delivered with entrapment of the larger fetal head can occur.
- Fetal compromise.
- Maternal complications such as severe pre-eclampsia or severe cardiac disease.
- A uterus already weakened, for example by previous surgery or caesarean section.

Requirements

- Contraindications must be excluded.
- Presence of regular effective uterine contractions. The cautious augmentation of uterine activity by intravenous oxytocics may be required. The trial examines the outcome of contractions. It is not a trial to determine if contractions can be generated or maintained. If possible await spontaneous onset of labour.
- Rupture membranes once the fetal head engages and apply direct fetal heart rate monitoring.
- Close fetal and maternal surveillance is necessary.
- Assessment at 2–4 hour intervals should be made, preferably by the same person.
- There should be adequate analgesia.
- General anaesthesia and surgery may be required. Adjust oral intake and cross-match blood.
- Supportive nursing and full discussion of the situation with the woman must be maintained.

Failed trial of labour

The trial must be abandoned when:

- fetal distress develops
- maternal distress or complications arise
- there is no progress after 2–4 hours despite adequate uterine contractions.

If the anticipated problem is limited to the pelvic outlet and instrumental delivery is considered, the term trial of forceps or ventouse is used. Delivery is by caesarean section if the trial of labour or trial of instrumental delivery fails. Caesarean section is required for subsequent pregnancies if the fetal size is the same or larger.

TRIAL OF SCAR OR VAGINAL DELIVERY

This term is used when vaginal delivery is considered after a previous lower segment caesarean section, or on occasion, a hysterotomy where the midline incision is sited in the lower half of the uterus.

Contraindications

- Previous classic caesarean section.
- History of uterine damage or plastic reconstruction.
- Suspicion of disproportion.
- History of complications (e.g. infection) which might have affected healing after previous caesarean section or uterine surgery.
- Uterine tenderness when the uterine scar is palpated.

Requirements

Many obstetricians are loath to allow vaginal delivery after any caesarean section. Caesarean section is not without risk and when conditions are satisfactory vaginal delivery can be safer and provide the woman with an experience of normal childbirth. In less than ideal conditions attempts at vaginal delivery can result in uterine rupture. It is, therefore, important that:

- An experienced obstetrician assesses and decides on the mode of delivery.
- The pelvic diameters must be ideal.
- Labour is conducted in a properly equipped environment.
- Close surveillance of both fetal and maternal conditions are maintained.
- All attending staff are aware of the risks and signs of uterine rupture.
- Any expression of increased or continuous pain must be investigated, particularly when epidural analgesia is used. Scar tenderness necessitates suspension of the trial. Deliver by caesarean section.
- Impose a short second stage. Avoid excessive pushing by performing an episiotomy and the early use of instrumental delivery.
- An experienced obstetrician must supervise or conduct delivery.

The uterine scar may be weakened after each successive vaginal delivery. Repeated vaginal delivery after previous caesarean section must be conducted with extreme caution.

Bibliography

Adamson SL 1999 Arterial pressure, vascular input impedance, and resistance as determinants of pulsatile blood flow in the umbilical artery. European Journal of Obstetrics, Gynecology and Reproductive Biology 84:119–125

Alfirevic Z, Neilson JP 1995 Doppler ultrasonography in high risk pregnancies: systematic review with meta-analysis. American Journal of Obstetrics and Gynecology 172:1379–1387

CESDI, 5th Annual Report 1998 Maternal and child health research consortium. London

Chang TC, Robson FC, Spencer JA et al 1994 Prediction of perinatal morbidity at term in small fetuses: comparison of fetal growth and Doppler ultrasound. British Journal of Obstetrics and Gynaecology 101:422–427

Divon MY, Ajglund B, Niselo H et al 1998 Fetal and neonatal mortality in the post term pregnancy: the impact of gestational age and fetal growth restriction. American Journal of Obstetrics and Gynecology 178:726–731

Kiserud T, Eik-Nes SH, Vlaas HG et al 1994 Ductus venous blood flow velocity and the umbilical circulation in the seriously growth retarded fetus. Ultrasound Obstetrics and Gynaecology 4:109–114

Phelan JP, Clarke SL, Daiz MA et al 1987 Vaginal birth after Caesarean. American Journal of Obstetrics and Gynecology 157:1510–1515

Piper JM, Xenakis EM, McFarland M et al 1996 Do growth retarded premature infants have different rates of perinatal morbidity and mortality than appropriately grown premature infants? Obstetrics and Gynecology 87:169–174

Tyson JE, Kennedy K, Broyles S et al 1995 The small for gestational age infant: accelerated or delayed pulmonary maturation? Increased or decreased survival? Paediatrics 95:534–538

Chapter 15

Induction and augmentation of labour

David T Y Liu
Mentors: Sam Mukhopadhyay, Sabaratnam Arulkumaran

CHAPTER CONTENTS

Induction of labour as therapy 117
Indications for induction 117
    Maternal 117
    Fetal 117
    Fetus and mother 118
Induction of labour as prophylaxis 118
Induction: general considerations 118
Contraindications to induction 118
Requirements before induction of labour 118
Induction of labour: process 119
    Cervical ripening 119
    Induction of labour 119
    Bishop's score of 4 or less 119
    Bishop's score between 4 and 7 (favourable
        cervix) 119
    Induction of labour: artificial rupture of
        membranes 120
    Technique for low ARM (forewater rupture) 120
    Infusion of synthetic oxytocin (Syntocinon) 121
Risks of induction 121
Induction of labour: special situations 122
    Previous caesarean section 122
    Pre-labour rupture of membranes 123
        For term fetus (36 completed weeks) 123
        For 34 weeks' gestation to term 123
        Before 34 weeks' gestation 123
    Breech presentation 123
    Twin pregnancies 123
    Intrauterine fetal death 123
Key points in induction of labour 124
Augmentation of labour 124
    Augmentation before 3 cm cervical
        dilatation 124
    Augmentation after 3 cm cervical dilatation 124

Induction of labour is a process for initiation of uterine activity to achieve vaginal delivery. Induction rates between 10% and 25% reflects current policies, referral patterns and sometimes women's choice. Labour is initiated to benefit principally the mother, the fetus or both and as an elective prophylactic procedure. In the UK, women with uncomplicated pregnancies are offered induction of labour after 41 weeks.

INDUCTION OF LABOUR AS THERAPY

This is considered for the following reason:

- When it is safer for the woman not to continue pregnancy. Consider the woman's preferences and priorities.
- When the fetus is less at risk if delivered or when both mother and fetus benefit by delivery. Induction must be the most appropriate mode of delivery.

Close surveillance in labour is mandatory when induction is carried out to address fetal or maternal compromise. If fetal distress develops or labour is not progressing well early resort to caesarean section is advised.

INDICATIONS FOR INDUCTION

Maternal

Medical or obstetric conditions not responding to treatment and which threaten the woman's health, such as heart failure, severe pre-eclamptic toxaemia and deteriorating renal function or central nervous system disorders.

Fetal

Presence of progressive growth restriction, abnormality not compatible with life, or fetal death.

Fetus and mother

Where induction of labour benefits both the mother and fetus, such as in poorly controlled diabetes, following rupture of fetal membranes or when chorioamnionitis is evident. This indication is particularly pertinent in contemporary obstetric practice when women with medical conditions previously not considered suitable for pregnancy are now prepared to accept inherent risks to become mothers.

INDUCTION OF LABOUR AS PROPHYLAXIS

Induction of labour is also considered to anticipate potential complications. Examples are:

- Even in uncomplicated pregnancies, evidence suggests the fetus is best delivered by 2 weeks post term. Prophylactic induction reduces the incidence of caesarean section, instrumental delivery, fetal compromise during labour and perinatal mortality.
- To achieve better control after previous precipitated labour. (Labour less than 2 hours.)
- To avoid fetal demise in prior unexplained sudden death after fetal maturity.
- To avoid macrosomia and complications of shoulder dystocia especially in a diabetic woman.
- Occasionally induction is considered for logistic or psychosocial reasons such as difficult access to hospital because of distance.

INDUCTION: GENERAL CONSIDERATIONS

- Before formal induction, current practice suggests women should be offered membrane sweeping.
- Labour can subject both mother and fetus to stress. If there is significant compromise consider caesarean section as the preferred mode of delivery.
- When advice for induction of labour is declined close fetal and/or maternal surveillance is essential, e.g. scan for liquor volume, twice weekly cardiotocograph (CTG).

- When induction for fetal or maternal compromise fails deliver by caesarean section. When failure follows prophylactic indications, there is the option to reassess and repeat the process.

CONTRAINDICATIONS TO INDUCTION

Induction of labour should not be considered in the following situations:

- When vaginal delivery is not advised or possible, for example pelvic disproportion, placental praevia, cord presentation and in the presence of active infection such as genital herpes.
- Uterine contractions can cause uterine rupture after previous classic or inverted T uterine incision, after myomectomy or surgery which extends into the uterine cavity and where lower segment caesarean section is complicated by extension or infection. Review operation notes from previous caesarean sections. Palpate to exclude tenderness over previous lower segment caesarean section scar.
- Induction is contraindicated if labour threatens further compromise for mother and/or fetus.

Only proceed when the woman provides informed consent.

REQUIREMENTS BEFORE INDUCTION OF LABOUR

Review medical and obstetric history. Perform clinical examination to exclude contraindications for induction of labour. Ensure the woman and her partner are fully informed of the risk and benefits and consent to the intended programme. Provide written information.

Perform vaginal examination to assess adequacy of pelvis and determine cervical status. Cervical dilatation, cervical length, consistency, position and station of presenting part are combined into a score – Bishop's score (Table 15.1), often modified to describe cervical

Table 15.1 Modified Bishop's score

Cervical feature	Pelvic score			
	0	1	2	3
Dilatation (cm)	<1	1–2	2–4	>4
Length of cervix (cm)	>4	2–4	1–2	<1
Station (relative to ischial spines)	−3	−2	−1/0	+1/+2
Consistency	Firm	Average	Soft	–
Position	Posterior	Mid/Anterior	–	–

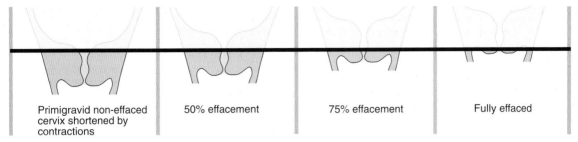

Figure 15.1   Cross-section of cervix to illustrate the degree of effacement.

status (Figure 15.1). A low score forewarns increased likelihood of induction failure and need for cervical preparation or ripening.

Cervical dilatation exerts twice the influence on successful induction compared with cervical consistency.

INDUCTION OF LABOUR: PROCESS

Cervical status governs choice for methods to induce labour. A low or unfavourable cervical score necessitates a ripening process for effacement and/or softening of the cervix to facilitate cervical dilatation. This is achieved by drugs, for example prostaglandins, which soften the cervix and produce uterine activity to draw up or create cervical effacement. Membrane sweeping releases prostaglandins and provides a biomechanical advantage to initiate or assist induction.

Cervical ripening

Pharmacological substances such as prostaglandins are prescribed to prepare or ripen the cervix. The current most clinically acceptable and effective is prostaglandin E_2 (PGE$_2$). PGE$_2$ given intravaginally as a pessary, as water soluble gel or more recently in the form of a slow-released hydrogel is associated with least systemic side effects. Vaginal pH, moisture, temperature, and infection can, however, all affect efficacy of the preparation. Do not use obstetric cream for vaginal examination if prostaglandins may be given. Where appropriate membrane sweep is returning as an acceptable procedure for uncomplicated pregnancies over 40 weeks. Both vaginal gel and vaginal tablets are equally effective and use is governed by cost.

Induction of labour

Auscultate fetal heart and perform CTG trace for 30 minutes prior to the induction process. Omit if induc-

tion is for fetal demise. If the trace is non-reassuring, discuss delivering by caesarean section.

Bishop's score of 4 or less

Administer 2 mg prostaglandin gel into posterior fornix. Give another 1 mg in 6 hours if needed. Review by experienced obstetrician 6 hours after second dose. Uterine activity usually starts 1 hour after administration of prostaglandin gel. Pharmacological effect lasts up to 4 hours. Continuous CTG monitoring is essential. When there is no urgency let the woman rest overnight and recommence the programme in the morning. The maximum total dose of PGE$_2$ used is 4 mg for primigravidae and 3 mg for multigravidae. Vaginal prostaglandin tablets are alternatives (3 mg PGE$_2$ vaginally and repeat once in 6 hours). With ruptured membranes consider vaginal prostaglandin or intravenous oxytocin.

Bishop's score between 4 and 7 (favourable cervix)

In primigravidae start with 1 mg prostaglandin gel. Repeat after 6 hours if indicated. Again if labour is not established review by experienced obstetrician 6 hours after second dose. A maximum of 4 mg PGE$_2$ is advised.

In multigravidae start with 1 mg prostaglandin gel and repeat in 6 hours if required. Review 6 hours after last dose if labour is not established. A maximum of 3 mg is advised.

Uterine hypertonus or hyperstimulation may occur. Close fetal surveillance is essential. Monitor fetal heart rate for at least 60 minutes after inserting prostaglandins. Watch out for signs of uterine rupture when there is a lower segment caesarean section scar. If labour is not established by evening, return the woman to the ward if appropriate and repeat the programme in the morning. If labour ensues recommence fetal heart rate monitoring. Repeat tracing when mother is warded. If artificial rupture of membranes (ARM) is not possible after a course of prostaglandins review the situation with a senior obstetrician.

Induction of labour: artificial rupture of membranes

With a Bishop's score of 8 or more the cervix is often sufficiently dilated to allow access to the fetal membranes. Options are:

- membrane sweep
- ARM or amniotomy
- rupture of fetal membranes and start oxytocin (Syntocinon).

Surgical induction of labour can be achieved by passage of an instrument through the cervical os to artificially rupture the fetal membrane. Drainage of amniotic fluid reduces the size of the uterine cavity and promotes more effective contractions by improving the myometrial length tension ratio. Prostaglandins are also released from the decidua. Onset of labour usually follows amniotomy in 6–12 hours. This interval before onset of labour is shortened by simultaneous use of intravenous infusion of an oxytocic such as Syntocinon.

Technique for low ARM (forewater rupture)

Make sure the woman and her partner give consent (verbal or written) and understand the reasons and steps for the procedure.

Place mother in the lithotomy position. Use sterile drapes and an aseptic technique. The fetal membranes in front of the presenting part can be ruptured using forceps such as Kocher's forceps or various designs of amniohooks (Figure 15.2).

If placenta praevia has not been excluded by ultrasound examination palpate the vaginal fornices carefully. Suspect placenta praevia if a thick spongy sensation is felt between the fornices and presenting part of the fetus (Figure 15.3). Insert a finger through the cervical os. Palpate the membranes through the internal os for a distance of 2 cm to exclude pulsating vessels associated with vasa praevia or cord presentation.

When amniotomy is not contraindicated insert a second finger (index and middle fingers are used). Guide the forceps between the fingers to the membranes (Figure 15.4). The membranes are picked up by the forceps and ruptured by wiping the index finger over the tip of the forceps. This technique allows good control of the amount of tear and the rate of escape of amniotic fluid. Record quantity and colour of liquor (blood stained, meconium or clear).

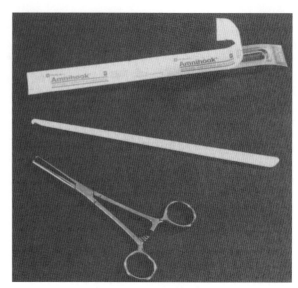

Figure 15.2   Instruments for low ARM.

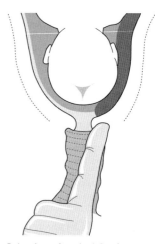

Figure 15.3   Palpation of vaginal fornices to exclude placenta praevia.

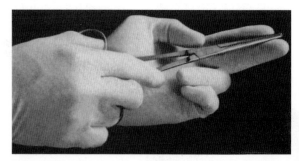

Figure 15.4   Technique for low ARM with Kocher's forceps.

Table 15.2 Oxytocin regimen for induction of labour (NICE 2001)

Time after starting (min)	Oxytocin dose (mU/min)	Volume infused (ml/h) Dilution 30 in 500 ml	Dilution 10 IU in 500 ml
0	1	1	3
30	2	2	6
60	4	4	12
90	8	8	24
120	12	12	36
150	16	16	48
180	20	20	60
210	24	24	72
240	28	28	84
270	32	32	96

Alternatively introduce an amniohook through the cervix. This is guided to a safe area of the presenting part of the fetus (for example, away from the fetal face). Approximate amniohook to the membrane by the index finger. The hook is withdrawn to tear the membranes. An advantage of this option is the need for less cervical dilatation, but the size of the tear is less predictable.

Infusion of synthetic oxytocin (Syntocinon)

Points to note with Syntocinon usage are:

- Myometrial sensitivity to oxytocin increases throughout pregnancy.

- Oxytocin increases both frequency, duration and amplitude of contractions. Use minimal dose which produces adequate uterine contractions. Maximum recommended dose is 20 mU/min.

- Prior treatment with prostaglandins potentiate action of oxytocin. Do not use oxytocin before 6 hours after last dose of PGE_2.

- Oxytocin at 30 IU in 500 ml of normal saline will give 1 mU/min if run at 1 ml/h.

- Intravenous oxytocin can be titrated to give better control of uterine contractions. Commence infusion using regulated drip set to deliver 2 mU/min and escalate dose at 2 mU/min every 30 minutes until contractions lasting 40 seconds recur every 4–5 times in 10 minutes. The dosage schedule recommended in the National Institute for Health and Clinical Excellence (NICE) guidelines is indicated in Table 15.2. Most women however, achieved adequate uterine contractions with 12 mU/min of Syntocinon. Once labour is established, maintain the same dose until delivery unless hyperstimulation warrants reduction in the dosage. Some women will continue labour when the dose is reduced to 8 mU/min. Infusion pumps should be used to control accurate delivery of the oxytocin infusion (Figure 15.5).

- After prolonged use of oxytocin maintain infusion for 1 hour after delivery to minimise the possibility of atonic postpartum haemorrhage.

- Side effects of Syntocinon usage include: uterine hyperstimulation, water retention due to an antidiuretic effect once the dosage exceeds 16 mU/min and maternal and fetal hyponatraemia. Water toxicity and hyponatraemia can cause maternal headache, nausea, psychosis and convulsions. Fetal adverse effects include lethargy, feeding difficulties, apnoea, cyanotic spells, respiratory distress and convulsions. Neonatal hyperbilirubinaemia has been described after oxytocin infusion.

- Start Syntocinon once membranes are ruptured particularly in the primigravida. Close monitoring of both mother and fetus is mandatory.

Doses in bold italics are quantities above those referred to in the summary of product characteristics of 20 mU/min (Table 15.2).

Figure 15.6 presents an algorithm for induction of labour depending on the presence or absence of complications in pregnancy.

RISKS OF INDUCTION

- Failed induction

This describes the situation when effective uterine activity is not established or maintained. Failure is less likely for gestations near term or when the Bishop's score is high. When membranes are ruptured there is the risk of infection. Deliver by caesarean section if there is fetal or maternal compromise.

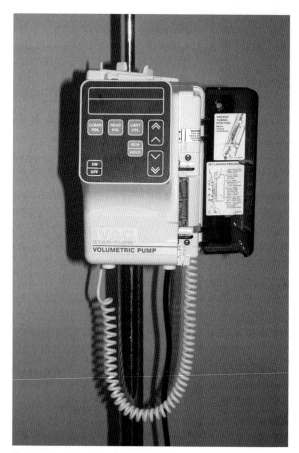

Figure 15.5   An infusion pump.

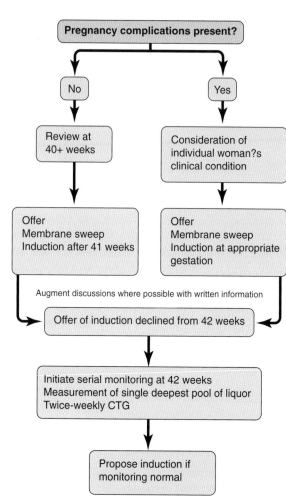

Figure 15.6   Algorithm for induction of labour (NICE 2001).

• Intrauterine infection

Once membranes rupture intrauterine and fetal infection is more likely. Some women such as those with diabetes are more susceptible. Where possible exclude active vaginal infection such as cervical herpes and presence of Group B streptococcus. Once membranes rupture monitor maternal pulse and fetal heart rate and maternal temperature. Aim to achieve delivery within 24 hours.

• Cord prolapse

Incidence of cord prolapse is 0.1–0.5% following membrane rupture. Exclude cord presentation before rupturing membranes. This complication is more likely when the fetal presenting part is not well applied to the cervix or when there is polyhydramnios.

• Uterine hyperstimulation

Pharmacological agents used to stimulate uterine activity can lead to excessive amplitude and frequency of contractions. Once the contraction frequency exceeds 5 per 10 minutes uterine activity becomes less efficient. Hyperstimulation follows use of high concentrations of oxytocics or where a woman is particularly sensitive to the drug. Hyperstimulation causes fetal hypoxia and threat of uterine rupture particularly in the grand multipara or in women with previous caesarean section scars. β-sympathomimetics such as ritodrine (50 µg to maximum of 350 µg per minute) or terbutaline, 250 µg subcutaneously or in 5 ml saline can be given intravenously to overcome hyperstimulation (20 µg/min should not be exceeded).

INDUCTION OF LABOUR: SPECIAL SITUATIONS

Previous caesarean section

• Induction of labour is contraindicated in a uterus with a classical, inverted 'T' or complex extended scar. This statement also applies to situations in which the uterine cavity was entered such as during myomectomy, when uterine infection caused poor uterine wound healing and after two previous caesarean sections.

- For high Bishop's scores with ruptured membranes titrate uterine activity with intravenous Syntocinon.

- For low Bishop's scores administer 1 mg prostaglandin E_2 (PGE$_2$) vaginally. The risk of scar dehiscence or rupture varies between 0.7% and 2.2%. Repeat doses of PGE$_2$ must be balanced against this risk.

- Watch out for signs of scar rupture and fetal distress.

Pre-labour rupture of membranes

- Membrane rupture carries risk of cord prolapse and intrauterine infection. Infective morbidity increases after 48 hours. More than 75% of women, however, labour spontaneously within 24 hours of membrane rupture.

- Take careful history, perform clinical examination to determine presence or absence of uterine activity or uterine tenderness. Confirm the presence of membrane rupture and exclude cord prolapse. Commence CTG monitoring.

For term fetus (36 completed weeks)
Induce labour immediately if there is threat or evidence of maternal or fetal infection. Deliver by caesarean section if CTG suggests evidence of fetal compromise.

If there is no risk of complication or fetal or maternal compromise discuss options with the woman. Conservative management for 24 hours to await spontaneous onset of labour is acceptable. Induce labour after 24 hours of ruptured membranes.

For 34 weeks' gestation to term
Allow pregnancy to continue. When obstetric risk is present such as infection or fetal compromise induce labour or deliver by caesarean section where appropriate.

If conservative management is acceptable take cervical swabs. Transfer to antenatal ward and commence 4 hourly recording of maternal pulse rate and temperature. Check abdomen for tenderness at the same time. Perform twice daily fetal CTG recordings and weekly ultrasound scan of the fetus. Deliver at 37 weeks or if fetal compromise becomes evident.

Before 34 weeks' of gestation
In the absence of contraindications such as infection give two doses of 12 mg dexamethasone at 12 hourly intervals. Dexamethasone can cause a transient rise in white cell count for 24–36 hours. The fetal heart rate change is difficult to interpret but fetal tachycardia is a useful guide for infection. Give appropriate antibiotics for pathogens. Deliver if chorioamnionitis is evident. Consider caesarean section if there is fetal risk.

Adopt the same criteria for induction as described above. Vaginal prostaglandin is not contraindicated.

Breech presentation

Contemporary practice advises attempts at external cephalic version when there is no contraindication and if this is unsuccessful deliver by caesarean section. The woman's informed opinion must be considered. Current evidence recommends that caesarean section for breech presentation is the safest approach.

Twin pregnancies

In the absence of obstetric complications induction of labour by amniotomy or use of prostaglandin is not contraindicated. Requirements for twin delivery must be satisfied. The first twin should be in cephalic presentation. Breech presentation of the first twin suggests the need for delivery by caesarean section.

Intrauterine fetal death

The main risks associated with intrauterine fetal death are infection, and if the dead fetus is retained more than four weeks coagulopathy may develop.

- Confirm fetal death by ultrasound scan.

- Convey the news with empathy and offer possible explanation for the death. Consult with all involved to arrange a mutually acceptable time for induction of labour. Immediate induction of labour after confirmation of intrauterine death may not be the most helpful psychological approach. Onset of coagulopathy can vary. Check platelet count and perform clotting screen.

- Administer prostaglandins as described above. Recently misoprostol, a cost-effective option has also been used.

- In very early pregnancies (before 24 weeks of gestation) extraamniotic prostaglandin delivered by placement of a size 12–14 Foley catheter through the cervix is an option. The balloon is inflated with 20–40 ml of saline to keep the catheter in place. An infusion pump is used to deliver PGE$_2$ 10 mg/ml at a rate of 0.5 ml/h. This can be increased by 0.5 ml hourly to a maximum dose of 3.0 ml/h. Augment with oxytocin (Syntocinon) if delivery is not achieved within 24 hours. Misoprostol 500 μg every 4 hours is the current alternative. Cervical laceration and uterine rupture are recognised complications. Examine the woman carefully and observe closely for 6 hours after delivery.

- When induction of labour is contraindicated (rarely) or carries substantial risk deliver by hysterotomy or caesarean section.

KEY POINTS IN INDUCTION OF LABOUR

- Make sure the woman and her partner are aware and accept the reasons, process and risk of induction.
- Decision and assessment for induction of labour must be made by an experienced obstetrician.
- Deliver by caesarean section instead of induction for severe maternal or fetal compromise.
- Deliver by caesarean section when induction for maternal and fetal compromise is unsuccessful.
- Oxytocin by intravenous infusion allows good control of uterine activity. Use the minimum dose which provides adequate uterine contractions.
- The pharmacological effect of oxytocin is potentiated after administration of prostaglandin.
- Once membranes are ruptured aim to deliver within 24 hours to reduce risk of intrauterine infection.
- Close maternal and fetal surveillance is mandatory.

AUGMENTATION OF LABOUR

This process describes enhancement of uterine contractions when progress of labour is slow. Before augmentation exclude malpresentation, gross disproportion and fetal or maternal compromise.

Decision to augment labour must follow assessment of situation by experienced obstetrician. This decision must be acceptable to the woman. Aim to achieve adequate contractions (frequency of four to five contractions per 10 minutes, each contraction lasting 40–60 seconds). Contractions should produce cervical dilatation and descent of the presenting part. A wide range of uterine activity can produce cervical dilatation averaging 1 cm/h.

Augmentation, like induction of labour, must be conducted with due care. This care includes nursing support, pain relief and close surveillance.

Augmentation before 3 cm cervical dilatation

In the latent phase of labour, augmentation is advised after 8 hours of painful contractions occurring at a frequency of 2 every 10 minutes if there is slow progress (World Health Organization (WHO) 1994). Exclude contraindications to labour.

Augmentation after 3 cm cervical dilatation

This is considered when cervical dilatation drifts 2–3 hours to the right of the alert line of the normal partogram (WHO 1994). Exclude contraindications to further labour. Rupture fetal membranes if these are still intact. The same Syntocinon regimen for induction of labour is used. Labour progress is measured both in terms of cervical dilatation and descent of the fetal head. Cervical dilatation without descent of the fetal head forewarns of possible disproportion.

Close surveillance is mandatory. If fetal distress develops or little change is detected after 4 hours of adequate contractions consider delivery by caesarean section. In the absence of contraindications 6–8 hours of oxytocin can result in optimal outcome.

Obstructed labour in primigravidae leads to incoordinate labour or cessation of uterine activity. In multigravidae the uterus attempts to overcome the obstruction by increasing frequency and intensity of contractions with resultant tetanic uterine activity and risk of uterine rupture.

References

National Institute of Clinical Excellence 2001 Induction of labour. Clinical Guideline D. NICE, London
World Health Organization 1994 Maternal Health and Safe Motherhood Programme. World Health Organization

Partograph in management of labour. Lancet 343:1399–1404

Bibliography

Arulkumaran S, Koh CH, Ingemarsson I et al 1987 Augmentation of labour. Mode of delivery related to cervimetric progress. Australian and New Zealand Journal of Obstetrics and Gynecology 27:304–308

Bakketeig LS, Bergsjo P 1989 Post-term pregnancy: magnitude of problem. In: Chalmers M, Enkin, M Keirse (eds) Effective Care in Pregnancy and Childbirth. Oxford University Press, Oxford

Bishop EH 1964 Pelvic scoring for elective induction. Obstetrics and Gynecology 24:266–268

Bouvain M, Iron O 2001 Sweeping the membranes for inducing labour or preventing post-term pregnancy (Cochrane Review). In: The Cochrane Library, Issue 1. Update Software, Oxford

Calder AA 1979 Management of unripe cervix. In: Keirse MNJC, Anderson ABM (eds) Human Parturition. Leiden University Press, Leiden, pp. 201–217

Confidential Enquiry into Stillbirths and Deaths in Infancy 1995 4th Annual Report Concentrating on Intrapartum related Deaths. Maternal and Child Health Research Consortium, London

Crowley P 1995 Elective induction of labour at 41 weeks' gestation (revised 5 May 1994). In: Enkin MW, Keirse MJBC, Renfrew MJ et al (eds). Pregnancy and children module. In: The Cochrane Database (database on disk and CD ROM). The Cochrane Library, Issue 2. Update Software, Oxford

Frait G, Daniel Y, Lessing JB et al 1998 Can labour with breech presentation be induced? Gynecological and Obstetric Investigations 46:181–186

Friedman EA 1954 The graphic analysis of labour. American Journal of Obstetrics and Gynecology 68:1569

Griffiths M 2003 A survey of current practice and opinion regarding methods for the induction of labour. Clinical report, Pharmacia, Milton Keynes, UK

Johnson TA, Greer IA, Kelly RW et al 1992 The effect of pH on release of PGE_2 from vaginal and endocervical preparations for induction of labour: an in vitro study. British Journal of Obstetrics and Gynaecology 99:877–880

Liu DTY, Kerr-Wilson R 1977 Cervical dilatation in spontaneous and induced labours. British Journal of Clinical Practice 31:177

MacKenzie IZ 1991 Prostaglandin induction and the scarred uterus. Second European Congress on Prostaglandins in Reproduction, The Hague 1991. Excerpta Medica, Amsterdam, pp 29–39

MacKenzie IZ, Magill P, Burns E 1997 Randomised trial of one versus two doses of prostaglandins for induction of labour. I Clinical outcome, II Analysis of cost. British Journal of Obstetrics and Gynaecology 104: 1062–1067

National Institute of Child Health and Human Development Research Planning Workshop 1997 Electronic fetal heart rate monitoring: research guidelines for interpretation. American Journal of Obstetrics and Gynecology 177:1385–1390

Nuutila M, Kajanoja P 1996 Local administration of prostaglandin E_2 for cervical ripening and labour induction: the appropriate route and dose. Acta Obstetrica et Gynecologica Scandinavica 75: 135–138

Royal College of Obstetricians and Gynaecologists 1998 Guidelines on induction of labour. London, RCOG Press

Royal College of Obstetricians and Gynaecologists 2001 Induction of labour. Evidence-based clinical guideline number 9. London: RCOG Press

Tarnow-Mordi, W, Shaw JCL, Liu DTY et al 1981 Iatrogenic hyponatraemia of the newborn due to maternal fluid overload: a prospective study. BMJ 283:639

Wing DA, Rahall A, Jones MM et al 1995 Misoprostol: An effective agent for cervical ripening and labour induction. American Journal of Obstetrics and Gynecology 172:1811–1816

Chapter 16

Assisted vaginal delivery and shoulder dystocia

David T Y Liu
Mentor: George S H Yeo

CHAPTER CONTENTS

Indications for instrumental assisted vaginal deliveries 127
  Maternal indications 127
  Fetal indications 128
  Labour indications 128
Requirements for assisted delivery 128
Forces operating in the second stage of labour 128
  Passage and passenger 128
  Powers 128
    Uterine contractions 128
    Maternal expulsive effort 128
    Fundal pressure 128
Assisted delivery 129
  Informed consent 129
  Instruments for assisted delivery 129
    Forceps 129
    Vacuum extractors 129
    Choosing between forceps and vacuum extraction for assisted deliveries 129
Traction procedures 132
  Before application of instruments 132
  During the use of instruments 132
  Delivery of the baby 133
  Procedures after delivery 133
Rotational procedures 135
  Requirements 136

Manual rotation 136
  Technique 136
Ventouse rotation 136
  Technique 136
Rotation by Kjelland's forceps 137
  Application by wandering anterior blade 137
  Application by the direct method 137
  Rotation and delivery 137
  Inherent dangers of Kjelland's forceps 138
Trial of forceps or vacuum 138
Maternal complications 139
Neonatal complications 139
Medicolegal issues 139
Symphysiotomy 140
  Precautions 140
Shoulder dystocia 140
  Management 140
    Antenatal 140
    Intrapartum 141
    Post partum 141
Haematomas 141
Bladder function and care during labour and after delivery 141
  In labour 142
  After delivery 142

INDICATIONS FOR INSTRUMENTAL ASSISTED VAGINAL DELIVERIES

The incidence of instrumental vaginal delivery should be between 8% and 10% of births.

Maternal indications

- Maternal exhaustion.
- To avoid excessive voluntary expulsive effort when increase in intra-abdominal, intrathoracic and

intracranial pressure is best avoided (e.g. maternal cardiac disease, poor respiratory reserves, or neurological disorders).

Fetal indications

- Fetal distress when there is good reserve and little calculated difficulty for assisted delivery.
- For the aftercoming head of the breech (by controlled delivery with forceps).

Labour indications

- Malposition (e.g. occipitoposterior and occipitotransverse).
- Prolonged second stage of labour (1 hour for multiparas, 2 hours for nullipara). Extra hour with regional anaesthesia.
- To expedite delivery.

REQUIREMENTS FOR ASSISTED DELIVERY

1. Thorough assessment of:
   a. the forces of the second stage of labour, in particular presence of dystocia
   b. the degree of difficulty of the assisted delivery.

2. The fetus – membranes are ruptured. The head is engaged (determined by abdominal palpation and vaginal examination). Position of the fetal head is defined and the station is at or below the ischial spines. The fetus's ears are always palpable to provide guidance for position of fetal head.

3. The mother – the cervix is fully dilated. There is adequate anaesthesia. Absolute disproportion is excluded.

4. Adequate communication between the woman, her partner and medical carers. Obtain informed consent.

5. The obstetrician is experienced or supervised by an experienced senior. There must be willingness to abandon the attempt if assisted delivery does not proceed easily. Ensure neonatal support and caesarean section facilities are available.

FORCES OPERATING IN THE SECOND STAGE OF LABOUR

Successful outcome for assisted delivery is governed by a dynamic balance between the passage, passenger and powers.

Passage and passenger

An accurate assessment of the passage and passenger begins with antenatal care and continues into the intrapartum period.

In the antenatal period, the fetus (or passenger) is continuously monitored for signs of intrauterine growth restriction or macrosomia. Fetal size, presentation, position, attitude and growth are assessed by a combination of abdominal and ultrasound examination.

The passage is assessed by clinical examination and magnetic resonance and radiological pelvimetry. Gross pelvic contracture can be detected, but usefulness of pelvimetry for predicting dystocia has been questioned.

Past obstetric history detailing modes of delivery for various birthweights allows estimation of fetal size against past performances to indicate likelihood of dystocia in the current pregnancy.

Gross cephalopelvic disproportion must be excluded before any attempt at assisted vaginal delivery. Minor degrees of disproportion are difficult to detect. Possible reduced pelvic diameters and/or a moderately big fetus forewarn likely borderline cephalopelvic disproportion and need for assistance.

Powers

Abdominal palpation and tocographic monitoring both detect frequency and duration of uterine contractions but not their intensity. Use of intrauterine pressure catheters for intensity of uterine contractions is not helpful in the management of dystocia.

The forces in the second stage for delivery are:

- uterine contractions
- maternal expulsive effort
- fundal pressure.

Uterine contractions
Uterine contractions will facilitate assisted delivery.

Maternal expulsive effort
Poor maternal effort is a common indication for assisted deliveries. Pushing is both exhausting and ineffective when it is not synchronised with uterine contractions Advise women to push to coincide with uterine contractions. They should rest between contractions to avoid getting tired.

Fundal pressure
Fundal pressure is used during caesarean births and assisted deliveries (see Figure 16.1). Pressure is applied at the uterine fundus (usually over the buttocks of the fetus) along its longitudinal axis to coincide with uterine contractions and maternal expulsive efforts. Fundal pressure should not be applied in between contractions particularly when maternal effort is absent.

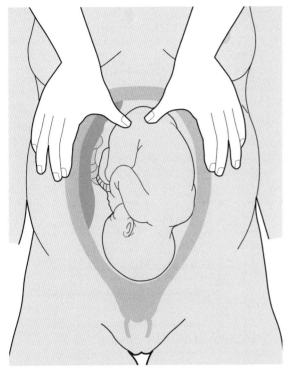

Figure 16.1   Application of fundal pressure: both hands are placed on the fundus of the uterus and a gentle push is applied during contraction.

ASSISTED DELIVERY

Assistance should be in synchrony with expulsive forces to overcome soft tissue resistance in the second stage of labour, usually for delivery of the fetal head. Resistance arises from individual difference in pelvic musculo-fascial soft tissue, perineal tissue compliance and to some degree moulding of the fetal head.

Informed consent

Assisted vaginal delivery is an operative procedure with attendant risks and complications, and therefore requires detailed discussion with the woman and her partner. Consent, usually verbal, is often obtained just before an emergency procedure from a distressed woman. Although necessarily brief, discussion and counselling are essential. A more detailed discussion should follow to debrief and answer questions.

Instruments for assisted delivery

Forceps
- Traction forceps
  - Long handles, e.g. Neville Barnes

- Short handles for outlet procedures or during caesarean section, e.g. Wrigley's
- Rotational forceps, e.g. Kjelland's.

Description of forceps   Each forceps has a left and right fenestrated blade. Each traction blade has a cephalic curve for the fetal head and a pelvic curve to accommodate the curvature of the maternal pelvis. When joined as a pair through a fixed lock, these blades form a protective cage which surrounds the fetal head without compression. When traction is applied, pressure transmitted to the fetus is safely contained by the firm fetal malar bones (Figures 16.2, 16.3).

Kjelland's rotational forceps differs from traction forceps. The shank is long and the blade is thin. The modest pelvic curve allows rotation through a much smaller circumference. The sliding lock allows application when asynclitism is present (see Chapter 19). Knobs on the handles point towards the occiput (also known as occipital knobs) (Figures 16.4–16.6).

Vacuum extractors
Rigid cups in use are:

- Malmstrom – anterior cup
- Bird – anterior and posterior cup
- O'Neill – anterior and posterior cup
- Mityvac – anterior cup
- Kiwi OmniCup – universal anterior and posterior cup

Soft cups in use are:

- Silc cup – anterior cup
- Silastic cup – anterior cup

Description of vacuum extractor   The principal components of the vacuum extractor are the pump, the pressure gauge, the traction piece and the cup used to raise the chignon for traction (Figure 16.7). Figure 16.8 shows a contemporary ventouse extraction and delivery system.

Choosing between forceps and vacuum extraction for assisted deliveries
Contemporary reviews found that vacuum extraction was associated with significantly less maternal trauma than forceps delivery. Fewer caesarean sections were carried out in vacuum extractor groups. However, the vacuum extractor was associated with an increase in neonatal cephalhaematoma and retinal haemorrhages. Forceps were associated with a lower failure rate. The chief disadvantage of forceps is a higher risk of significant maternal perineal injury, especially anal sphincter injuries.

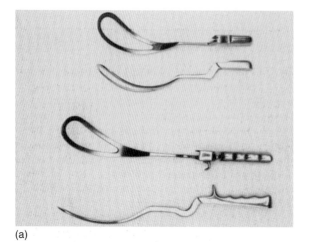

(a)

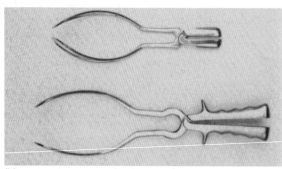

(b)

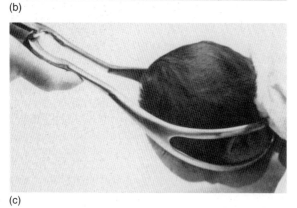

(c)

Figure 16.2 Large and small traction forceps (a) as separates, (b) as pairs and (c) applied.

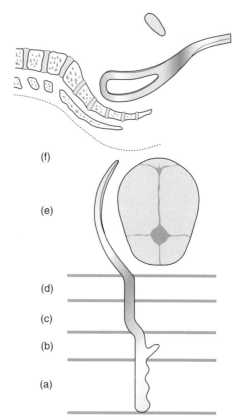

(f)

(e)

(d)

(c)

(b)

(a)

Figure 16.3 Traction forceps illustrating (a) handle (b) shoulder, (c) lock, (d) shank, (e) blade with cephalic curve and (f) pelvic curve.

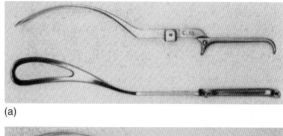

(a)

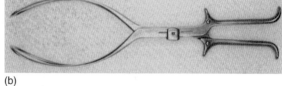

(b)

Figure 16.4 Kjelland's forceps (a) as separates and (b) as paired.

Neither instrument is superior for assisted vaginal deliveries. The forces and requirements for either form of assisted delivery are similar. The choice of instrument depends on the clinical scenario as well as the operator's experience, training and preferences. Both instruments are equally suited to most assisted deliveries. In circumstances where cephalopelvic disproportion is confidently excluded and speed is of

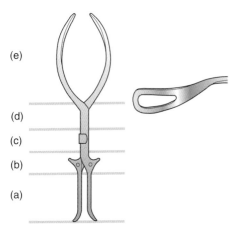

Figure 16.5 Components of Kjelland's forceps: (a) handle, (b) shoulder, (c) sliding lock, (d) shank and (e) blade.

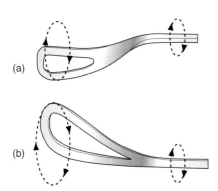

Figure 16.6 Rotation of Kjelland's forceps (b) is through a smaller circumference than with the traction forceps (a).

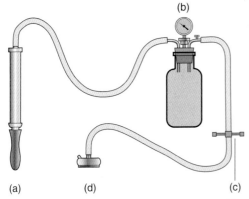

Figure 16.7 Components of the ventouse extractor: (a) pump, (b) container with pressure gauge, (c) traction piece and (d) cup.

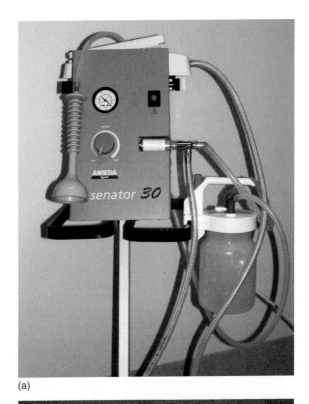

(a)

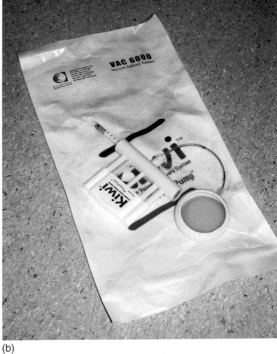

(b)

Figure 16.8 (a) Contemporary ventouse extractor. (b) Vacuum delivery system.

Table 16.1   Instrumental vaginal delivery

	Forceps	Vacuum
Popularity	Decreased	Increased
Preterm	Yes	Not before 36 weeks
Undilated cervix (around 9 cm)	Contraindicated	Yes
Anaesthesia	Yes	Need less
Failure to achieve delivery	Less likely	More likely
Tissue trauma	Possible	Less
Cephalhaematoma	Possible	More likely
Retinal haemorrhage	Possible	More likely
Postpartum perineal pain	Yes	Less

essence (e.g. ominous cardiotocographic tracing), forceps may be the instrument of choice for expediting delivery. The vacuum extractor may be preferred where asynclitism is present, when rotational delivery is needed and there is limited experience with forceps. There is no increased morbidity in completing a delivery by forceps when the vacuum fails provided that the requirements for assisted delivery are fulfilled. Table 16.1 shows a comparison between the two types of instrumental delivery. The long-term outcome is the same for mother and child.

TRACTION PROCEDURES

Box 16.1 describes the types of traction procedure used in assisted delivery.

Before application of instruments

- Indication and requirements – ensure that these have been met.
- Communication with colleagues – inform consultant (if appropriate), anaesthetist and operating theatre staff (if a trial of forceps in operating theatre is indicated), and neonatologist (especially if the indication is for fetal distress).
- Informed consent – obtain verbal consent after explaining to the woman and her partner the need for assisted delivery. Caution the woman that intense pressure and the sensation of pelvic separation may be felt at the moment of birth. This is the normal experience of childbirth. Unless forewarned, especially in a nulliparous woman, this frightening sensation could be wrongly attributed to the misuse of instruments or obstetric ineptitude.
- Position – the lithotomy position is favoured. The legs are suspended by stirrups or other means.

Box 16.1   Traction procedures used in assisted delivery

American College of Obstetricians and Gynecologists (ACOG) classification of forceps deliveries 2000

Outlet procedure refers to the application of the instrument when:

- scalp is visible at the introitus without separating labia
- fetal skull has reached pelvic floor
- sagittal suture is in anteroposterior diameter, or in the right or left occiput anterior or posterior position
- fetal head is at or on perineum
- rotation is less than 45°

Low procedure refers to the application of the instrument when:

- the leading point of fetal skull is at station +2 or more, and not on the pelvic floor. There are two subdivisions:
  rotation of 45° or less
  rotation of more than 45°

Mid-pelvic procedure refers to the application of the instrument when:

- the head is engaged but the station is between 0 and +2.
- with subdivisions as for low procedures.

Adopt a 15° left lateral tilt to overcome supine hypotension.

- Bladder – empty the bladder to avoid damage during traction and/or rotation.

During the use of instruments

1. Position of the obstetrician – the flexed forearm is at the level of the vulva or slightly lower (Figure 16.9).

2. Position of the mother – the perineum should slightly overhang the edge of the bed. There should be room below the buttock for assisted delivery, especially for rotational forceps.

3. Check the instrument. For forceps delivery check that both blades lock easily and are well lubricated. For vacuum assisted delivery: check that the traction chain and the tubings are airtight; check that the suction apparatus and the vacuum have

to detect inclusion of cervix and vagina into the vacuum.

- Apply traction during uterine contractions and bearing down efforts in line with the pelvic axis (Figure 16.14). Pajot's manoeuvre may be used with the forceps. Traction is applied perpendicular to the cup in the direction of the pelvic axis when the vacuum is used (Figure 16.15).
- No more than 15–20 kg of pull is required to achieve delivery.
- Apply traction for 20–30 seconds at a time. Delivery should be achieved with three or fewer pulls (Figure 16.16). More than 30 minutes of vacuum can result in scalp necrosis.
- An episiotomy is usually required as the vertex is crowning.
- Change direction of traction to 30° from the horizontal once the vertex (chin in face presentation) emerges beneath the symphysis. Failure to change direction is an important cause of trauma to the perineum (Figures 16.16, 16.17).
- After crowning ask mother to stop pushing and start panting. Panting will produce gentle intermittent intra-abdominal pressure which nudges the baby slowly out of the birth canal.

Delivery of the baby

1. Deliver the head slowly to avoid tears to the perineum or extension of the episiotomy.
2. Once the head is delivered, the blades of the forceps are disengaged (or the vacuum is released and the cup removed).

The rest of the delivery is the same as that for normal birth.

Procedures after delivery

1. Check arterial and venous cord pH and base excess.
2. Examine the pelvic structures to exclude damage. Locate the apex of the episiotomy to check for extension. Rotational deliveries are more likely to cause damage.
3. Jointly with the neonatologist conduct examination of the baby (including any soft tissue injuries). Communicate findings of the baby to the parents and reassure if appropriate.
4. Document fully findings, discussions with the mother and her partner, steps of the procedure and condition of the mother and baby after delivery (including Apgar score and cord pH).

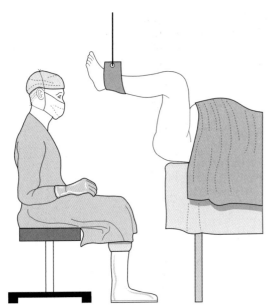

Figure 16.9 Position of an obstetrician for forceps delivery. The woman's legs are suspended by stirrups or other means.

been connected properly; and choose the appropriate cup size (the largest cup possible should be used).

4. Reassure the woman and her partner. Discourage pushing during insertion of the blades. The partner's prime role is support and not as a spectator.
5. Apply the instrument as described in Box 16.2.
6. Check application.

For forceps
- Ensure that the sagittal suture is in the midline, equidistant between the blades (Figure 16.13).
- The posterior fontanelle should be one finger's breadth above the shanks (for occipitoanterior position).
- The fenestrated blades should admit one finger between the heel of the blade and the fetal head.

For vacuum
- Ensure that the centre of the cup is over the sagittal suture and 3 cm anterior to the posterior fontanelle.
- Check that the woman's cervical and vaginal mucosa have been excluded from the cup before traction.
- Apply gentle traction. The vacuum cup is held against the fetal head with the thumb and index finger of the left hand to detect any tendency of the cup to separate. Check repeatedly with index finger

Box 16.2   Application of instruments

Forceps

1. Insert the left blade first
   a. Check that there is no uterine contraction and that woman is not pushing.
   b. Place the index and middle fingers of the right hand along the left side of the fetal head to exclude the vaginal walls (Figure 16.10).
   c. The left hand holds the blade vertical and by dropping the handles slips the forceps into position guided by the palmar aspects of the intravaginal fingers.
   d. The blade rests over the fetal ear and malar bones.

2. Repeat the procedure for the right blade.
   a. The right hand now holds the blades which are guided into position by the left index and middle fingers.
   b. The blades should fall together into position.

3. If resistance is felt, check to ensure that all the requirements for forceps delivery are met.

4. Lock the two blades – no undue force should be used. If the blades do not lock easily reassess situation. The blades are then reapplied.

Vacuum

1) Lubricate the cup.

2) Insert it sideways through the introitus (Figure 16.11). Aim to position the centre of the cup 3 cm anterior to the posterior fontanelle and over the sagittal suture. This will maintain the head in the optimal maximum flex attitude. Avoid placement over fontanelle.

3) Exclude cervix or folds of vaginal mucosa.

4) Create an initial vacuum up to 0.2 kPa over 1–2 minutes. Check again that cervix and vaginal mucosa have been excluded from the cup.

5) The vacuum pressure is raised to a working pressure of 0.8 kPa.

6) Once working pressure is achieved wait for 30 seconds for the chignon to form before applying traction (Figure 16.12).

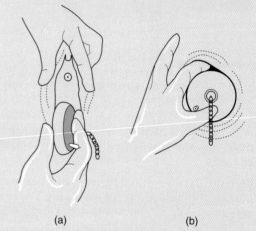

(a)   (b)

Figure 16.11   Insertion (a) and application (b) of cups.

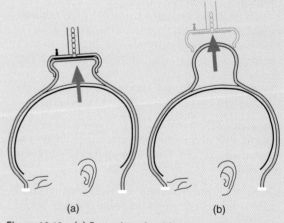

(a)   (b)

Figure 16.12   (a) Formation of a chignon to assist traction (b) with residue swelling persisting for 24–48 hours after cup is removed.

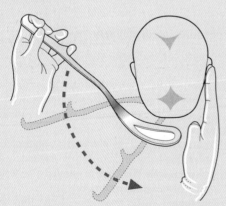

Figure 16.10   Application of traction forceps.

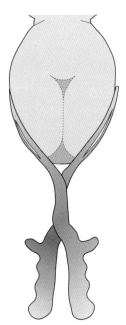

Figure 16.13   Position of sagittal suture with correct application of forceps.

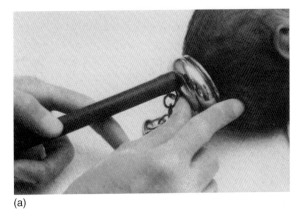

(a)

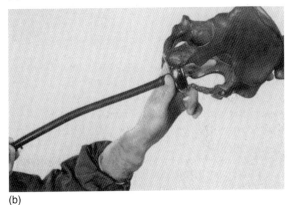

(b)

Figure 16.15   (a) Placement of intravaginal fingers and (b) direction of traction.

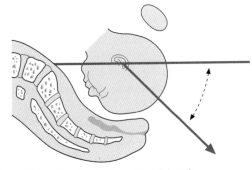

Figure 16.14   Traction in line with pelvic axis.

ROTATIONAL PROCEDURES

A wider diameter is presented when the vertex is in the occipitolateral or occipitoposterior position. Rotation into the anteroposterior diameter of the pelvic outlet may occur on the perineum or at any level between the ischial spines and the perineum. Delivery in the occipitoposterior position may increase perineal trauma unless carefully conducted.

The three most common techniques used for placing the vertex into the anteroposterior diameter of the pelvic outlet are:

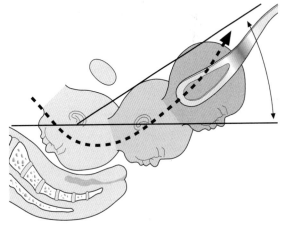

Figure 16.16   Delivery of head with forceps.

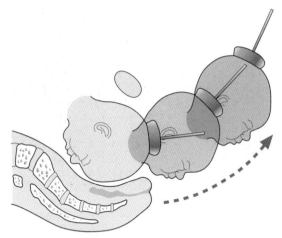

Figure 16.17   Delivery of the head with the Ventouse extractor.

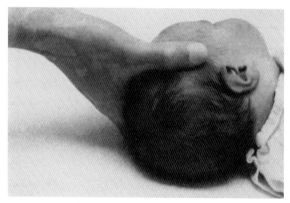

Figure 16.18   Position of hand for manual rotation.

- rotation by hand (manual)
- rotation with a vacuum extractor
- rotation with Kjelland's forceps.

Requirements

- Include requirements for assisted vaginal deliveries. Ensure adequate anaesthesia at level of rotation.
- A neonatologist should be in attendance.
- If any difficulty is anticipated, the procedure should be conducted in the operating theatre with provisions made for immediate caesarean section.

Manual rotation

This is a safe technique. Pressure on the fetal head is easy to judge and trauma to soft tissue is less likely. Check cervical dilatation and adequacy of pelvis.

Technique
1. Confirm the malposition.

2. Lubricate the traction forceps and place them within reach.

3. The left hand is used for right occipitolateral or posterior positions, the right hand is used for left occipitolateral or posterior positions.

4. Insert the hand into the vagina to grasp the fetal head across the parietal diameters with thumb uppermost. Use thumb, index and middle finger if access is limited (Figure 16.18).

5. Disimpact the fetal head and rotate the occiput anteriorly. Place the free hand over the woman's abdomen in the region of the anterior fetal shoulder. The shoulder is brought across the midline towards the opposite iliac crest to assist rotation at the same time as rotation of the vertex. An assistant can help prevent tendency of the shoulder to revert to its original position. Flexion with contraction is often evident with correct rotation.

6. While the vertex is held in the occipitoanterior position, the forceps blades are applied in the usual manner. Check correct alignment of the sagittal suture.

7. Difficulties in locking the blades suggest inadequate rotation and hence incorrect application of the forceps.

8. Apply traction only after application of the forceps is judged to be correct.

Ventouse rotation

Technique
1. Apply the cup well back on the fetal head so that traction corrects any deflexion which is usual in malposition.

2. Asynclitism (see Chapter 19) is almost always present in malposition and is corrected by a more posterior application of the cup.

3. Initial traction down towards the floor allows the vertex to descend and correct asynclitism. Rotation usually takes place at the pelvic floor level. The thumb and index finger in the vagina to ensure contact between cup and the scalp can also help rotation by directing cup in direction of turn.

4. After successful rotation, complete the delivery by maintaining traction perpendicular to the cup in line with the pelvic axis.

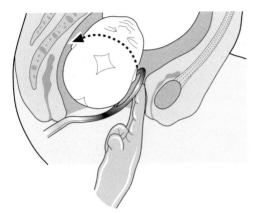

Figure 16.19 Application of anterior blade.

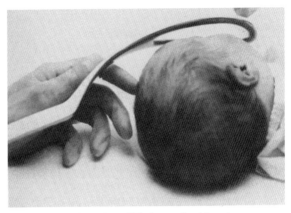

Figure 16.20 Direction of blade over fetal face by intravaginal fingers.

Rotation by Kjelland's forceps

Designed for rotation, the shank is long and the blade thin. There is no pelvic curve so rotation is through a smaller circumference. The sliding locks allow application when asynclitism is present (see Figures 16.5, 16.6).

Application by wandering anterior blade

1. Check placement of the blades by assembling them in front of the pelvis. Ensure that the directional knobs point towards the occiput.

2. Select the anterior blade (the blade which will be placed on the upper surface of the fetal head). The second and third fingers of the hand on the side of the fetal face are inserted into the vagina (Figure 16.19).

3. The anterior blade, held vertically by the free hand, is slipped into the vagina between the fetal face and the intravaginal fingers. The handle is depressed towards the floor at the same time. The face is chosen because the bitemporal diameter, being smaller than the biparietal diameter, provides for easier application.

4. When the blade is two-thirds of the way inside the vagina, the handle is nearly horizontal. The handle is rotated towards the floor from this position while the intravaginal fingers assist the passage of the blade across the fetal face. When the blade is positioned correctly over the ear and malar bone the handle is raised so that the blade will encompass the full length of the fetal head (Figure 16.20).

5. Sometime, the occiput rotates into the direct occipitoposterior position during the application of the

wandering blade. Kjelland's forceps can then be inserted directly with the knobs pointing towards the occiput.

6. If difficulty is encountered, withdrawing the blade by a short distance can help. Alternatively, apply the blade across the occiput.

Application by the direct method

1. The anterior blade is held vertically with the handle pointing towards the floor. The cephalic curve is placed in contact with the fetal head at the level of the ears and malar bones. Two intravaginal fingers guide placement of the blade as the handle is elevated.

2. The posterior blade is always applied directly to the head. Intravaginal fingers guide the blade into position. The tip of the blade is always kept close to the fetal head. When applied correctly there should be no difficulty in locking the blades. Presence of asynclitism would mean that the shoulders of the handles are not at the same level.

Rotation and delivery

1. When correctly applied, the handles are at 45° from the horizontal and in line with the pelvic axis. Vertical direction of the handles more than 45° indicates that the head is not fully engaged and it may be safer to abandon the procedure.

2. Correct asynclitism by adjusting the handles so that the shoulders of the blades are level. Sometimes this is easier during a contraction.

3. The blades are held by the shoulders. The fourth finger is interposed between the handles to remind the obstetrician not to compress them. This

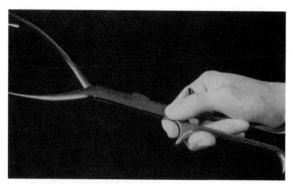

Figure 16.21   Grip technique for rotation.

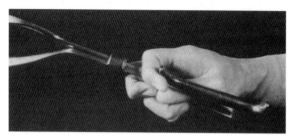

Figure 16.22   Grip technique for traction.

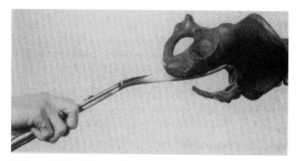

Figure 16.23   Axis traction.

particular grip for rotation prevents excessive force being used and is highly sensitive to the presence of unnecessary resistance (Figure 16.21).

4. The fetal head is rotated at the level of application of the forceps. The rotational force needed is usually not more than what is comfortably applied with two fingers. If difficulty is encountered, rotation may be achieved with descent during the next contraction. Occasionally moving the fetal head up a few centimetres allows rotation at the widest pelvic plain.

5. Once rotation is achieved, the grip is changed to facilitate traction (Figure 16.22). Traction must be

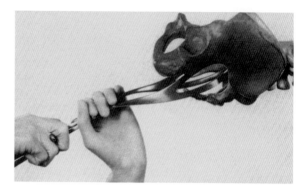

Figure 16.24   Axis traction with Pajot's manoeuvre to maintain traction in pelvic axis.

along the pelvic axis (Figure 16.23). Interpose the thumb between the handles. Pajot's manoeuvre can help (Figure 16.24).

6. An episiotomy is made in the usual manner. Do not make an episiotomy before rotation otherwise the spiral torque during rotation may cause extension of the episiotomy.

Inherent dangers of Kjelland's forceps
There are two inherent dangers in the design of the Kjelland's forceps. Firstly, the thin blades can cause considerable soft tissue trauma. Secondly, the wandering technique necessitates moving the blades over a large area of vagina. This increases the risk of trauma. Whether Kjelland's forceps should continue to be used is controversial.

Trial of forceps or vacuum

• All potentially difficult forceps or vacuum deliveries should be conducted as a trial by an experienced obstetrician.

• The trial should be conducted in the operating theatre with immediate access to caesarean section if the trial fails (remember prophylactic citrates, informed consent, intravenous line and grouped blood available at short notice). The neonatologist, anaesthetist and theatre staff must be in attendance. Do not perform episiotomy until vaginal delivery is assured.

• The trial fails when there is no advance or little descent with a moderate amount of traction. A trial of forceps after use of vacuum should only be performed if the operator is confident vaginal delivery is possible and the fetal head is deeply engaged. Only then is delivery accomplished without harm to the mother or baby. Note reason for failure with the first instrument. Check requirements for assisted delivery are met.

- Leave an indwelling catheter, disimpact the fetal head and place it above the level of ischial spines to facilitate delivery of the head by caesarean section when trial of vaginal delivery fails.

MATERNAL COMPLICATIONS

Assisted vaginal delivery is associated with the following maternal complications:

- Perineal and vaginal lacerations, extension of episiotomy, third degree tears and haematoma formation. A thorough examination must be performed after delivery is achieved. Injury to the urethralvesical angle and anal sphincter can lead to immediate problems such as difficulty with voiding or subsequent urinary and faecal incontinence.

- Vaginal haematoma formation and laceration can occur with spontaneous vaginal deliveries but are more likely after rotational instrument delivery. Severe laceration, particularly if the vaginal vault is involved, may require laparotomy and extended surgery hence an experienced obstetrician must be present. Haematomas following rupture of vaginal veins will need evacuation if large, painful or judged to be enlarging.

- Do not perform instrumental delivery unless the cervix is fully dilated. Exceptions include vacuum delivery for the second twin or when there is a need for urgent vaginal delivery at 9 cm cervical dilatation and requirements for easy delivery are met. Torn cervix leading to maternal death has been reported with use of the vacuum. Again experience is mandatory before attempting repair of cervical lacerations especially if there is extension into the fornix. Minor lacerations that are not bleeding can be managed expectantly.

- The lumbosacral nerves may be impinged upon by movement of the sacroiliac joints, compression by the fetal presenting part or use of forceps. Transient loss of sensory and motor function may result.

Following delivery:

- Consider thromboprophylaxis if there are risks for thrombosis.
- Debrief with woman. Ensure adequate analgesia and urinary output for 24 hours.
- There is a place for antibiotics.

NEONATAL COMPLICATIONS

Assisted vaginal delivery is associated with the following neonatal complications:

- Risk of perinatal trauma in instrumental vaginal delivery correlates with duration of attempt, level of the fetal head in the birth canal, need for rotation and condition of baby at start of procedure.

- Compared with forceps, the vacuum is associated with higher rates of neonatal trauma. These include cephalhaematoma with neonatal hyperbilirubinaemia needing phototherapy, scalp injuries and retinal haemorrhage.

- Chignon or swelling of the scalp, which develops when vacuum is applied, is seen when the cup is removed. This swelling, which diffuses within an hour to behave like a normal caput succedaneum, usually disappears over 1 or 2 days. Scalp markings or abrasions can last as long as 6 months after delivery.

- Subcutaneous haematomas resolve in a few days. Cephalhaematomas may take up to a few weeks to disappear. Reassure the parents.

- Neonatal jaundice is more common after vacuum extraction than after forceps or spontaneous delivery. There is no difference in the number of babies requiring phototherapy.

- Subgaleal haemorrhage associated with difficult instrumental delivery is more likely when fetal hypoxia or coagulopathy is present. This lifethreatening condition is a serious complication associated with vacuum extraction. Intracranial haemorrhage can also complicate difficult vacuum extractions.

- Retinal haemorrhage, more common after instrumental delivery than normal birth, is significantly more likely after vacuum extraction than after forceps delivery. This is a transient lesion.

MEDICOLEGAL ISSUES

Instrumental vaginal delivery followed by complications or poor fetal outcome is a ready situation for complaints and litigation. The following are important from the perspective of clinical governance and risk management:

- Appropriate assessment of the situation. Obstetric history, presence of maternal or fetal compromise, good appreciation of pelvic diameters and configurations, the woman's preference, available expertise and option for caesarean section are all important issues.

- The obstetrician must be adequately trained or supervised.

- The woman and her partner must be made aware of need, likely outcome and options. Obtain consent and maintain communication to inform and reassure.

- There is no place for instrumental delivery if the obstetrician cannot properly assess the pelvis and relate fetal head size to pelvic diameters and outlet.

- Be prepared to abandon the procedure when difficulty is encountered and when there is little descent with traction. Avoid repeated attempts and use of multiple instruments. Forceps can be considered after failure with the vacuum. The reverse sequence is not acceptable. Sequential use of instruments increase neonatal trauma.

- Detail documentation is essential. This includes indication, discussion with the woman and her partner regarding risks and options, any complication and remedial action, condition of mother and baby, cord arterial and venous values.

- Full explanation and prompt attention to complications. Offer apology where appropriate.

- Introduce audit for individual obstetrician and the labour ward as a whole to ensure continuous quality control.

SYMPHYSIOTOMY

This procedure is seldom used but can be effective for delivery if the aftercoming head of a normal live breech is stuck at the pelvic outlet. Requirements are:

- Lithotomy position.
- General, regional or local anaesthesia.
- Catheterised bladder. Leave catheter indwelling.
- Incise the skin above symphysis with a firm blade. Probe with the blade to identify non-bony joint.
- Displace the urethra from the midline by a finger in the vagina.
- Hold the blade at 30° from horizontal and advance vertically down towards the vagina. Use a sawing action until the tip of the blade is sensed by the intravaginal finger.
- Once the joint separates apply forceps and deliver the fetal head. An episiotomy is helpful.

Precautions

- Avoid wide separation of symphysis to protect sacroiliac joint and urethra.
- Insert drain if there is venous bleeding when arcuate ligaments are cut.
- Leave catheter in situ for 48 hours.
- Support pelvic girdle and nurse the mother on her side.

SHOULDER DYSTOCIA

The term shoulder dystocia describes difficulty with delivery of the shoulder after delivery of the fetal head. This unpredictable emergency occurs in 0.5–2% of vaginal deliveries. The complication is usually due to the anterior shoulder becoming stuck above the symphysis pubis (unilateral dystocia). Bilateral dystocia is when both shoulders are impacted above the pelvic inlet. Shoulder dystocia results from failure of the shoulder to rotate to the transverse diameter of the pelvic inlet followed by 90° rotation to the anteroposterior diameter of the outlet.

Risk factors include:

- Abnormalities of fetal chest or abdomen.
- Fetal macrosomia – the rate increases from 10% to 20% for birthweight between 4250 gm and 4750 gm.
- Diabetic women – the risk compared with non-diabetic women is increased by more than 70% for similar birthweight.
- Prolonged labour and long second stage. (70% are associated with normal labours.)
- Past history of shoulder dystocia. (Over 50% incidence of shoulder dystocia are in babies weighing less than 4000 gm.)
- Suspect when fetus descends with contractions than retracts between contractions (Turtle's sign) or if the fetal head extension is restricted during delivery.

Management

Antenatal
- Neither clinical nor ultrasound diagnosis of macrosomia is reliable.
- No evidence that induction at full term is helpful but benefit of earlier delivery at 37–38 weeks remains a subject for investigation.
- There is a place for elective caesarean section when estimated fetal weight is more than 4500 gm, when likely macrosomia accompanies diabetes and for a definite history of previous difficulty with shoulder dystocia.

- Forewarn at risk women to ensure their delivery is in hospital. Document clearly to alert labour ward staff.

Intrapartum

All labour ward medical staff must be regularly 'drilled' to become practised in managing this emergency. Assess all women admitted for delivery. If risk is suspected make sure an experienced obstetrician attends delivery. When this emergency arises activate the following steps.

1. Recruit help from an experienced midwife, a senior obstetrician, an anaesthetist and a paediatrician.

2. Adopt McRoberts' manoeuvre. Flex the woman's thighs against abdomen and chest. Offer assistance if she cannot do this herself. The manoeuvre straightens the lumbosacral angle and rotates the symphysis superiorly thus opening the pelvic outlet. This manoeuvre alone is effective in resolving 80% of this emergency. The posterior shoulder is often pushed over the sacral promontory into hollow of the sacrum.

3. The left lateral position is seldom used. Squatting or knee chest 'on all fours' position achieves the same advantages but delivery in this position requires experience.

4. Perform an episiotomy to remove soft tissue resistance and allow better access for subsequent steps.

5. Apply suprapubic pressure with flat of hand to free the shoulder, to adduct and reduce the biacromial diameter and direct the shoulder beneath the symphysis into the anteroposterior widest diameter of the pelvic outlet. This step improves delivery rate by an additional 3%.

6. If delivery is not achieved adopt Woods cork screw manoeuvre. Insert appropriate hand into posterior vagina and rotate posterior shoulder clockwise or anticlockwise 180°. This will bring the impacted anterior shoulder to below the level of the symphysis to allow delivery.

7. If the above steps fail employ Mazzanati's procedure to deliver the posterior arm. Flex arm at the elbow. The hand or forearm is grasped and swept across the baby's chest and face. The anterior shoulder is disimpacted and slides out beneath the symphysis. The baby's clavicle or humerus may be fractured (18% risk). The biacromial diameter can be reduced by breaking the clavicle (clavicular osteotomy).

8. Impaction of both anterior shoulder against the symphysis and the posterior shoulder in the sacral promontory necessitate resort to Zavanelli's option. Rotate baby's head into the anteroposterior position. Flex the head and push it into the pelvis. Deliver by caesarean section. Maternal morbidity must be considered.

Points to remember
- If one manoeuvre fails move quickly to the next to avoid delay.
- Brachial plexus injury follows excessive or prolonged traction to the baby's neck, e.g. Erb's palsy.
- Keep detailed records of all procedures and outcomes.

Post partum
- Enlist the neonatologist's assistance. Check for presence of injury to baby and mother.
- When appropriate discuss events with the woman and her partner to answer questions and agree plans for future pregnancies.

HAEMATOMAS

A shearing action between the vagina and deeper tissues during normal, assisted or rotational delivery can rupture the vaginal plexus of veins to form a haematoma. If extensive, this will involve the paravaginal space, the labia, urethra and even extension into the broad ligament. Inadequate haemostasis following episiotomy repair or closure of the caesarean section wound also result in haematoma formation.

- Presents as pain, bruising, urinary retention and, if extensive, hypovolaemic consequences.

- Vaginal examination and if indicated ultrasound scan will help diagnosis.

- Small haematomas can be managed conservatively. Catheterisation is required if the urethra is involved.

- For large haematomas an experienced obstetrician must attend to assess the situation. Surgery, on occasion laparotomy, may be required to evacuate the clots and secure haemostasis. Transfusion may be necessary. Leave drains after surgery if oozing is anticipated.

BLADDER FUNCTION AND CARE DURING LABOUR AND AFTER DELIVERY

Labour and particularly delivery can potentially affect pelvic floor musculature and nerves causing urinary and bowel dysfunction. Contributory factors include nulliparity, prolonged labour, epidural anaesthesia with bladder overdistension, instrumental delivery and vaginal or perinatal trauma.

In labour

- Encourage voiding every 3 or 4 hours.
- If unable to void obtain consent and intermittently catheterise. Record output.
- Normal bladder capacity is 300–500 ml. A residual volume of more than 700 ml will warrant urological follow-up.
- Following delivery ensure women are advised about the importance of bladder function and care.

After delivery

- Make sure women can void before leaving the labour ward. Communicate bladder function and care to postnatal carers.
- Prevention of urinary retention is part of good labour care.
- Indwelling catheter until the woman is ambulatory may be necessary after assisted delivery. Seek the woman's consent and offer clear explanation.
- If voiding difficulties persist, intermittent self-catheterisation is the current usual advice.

References

American College of Obstetricians and Gynecologists 2000 Operative vaginal delivery: use of forceps and vacuum extractors for operative vaginal delivery. ACOG Practice Bulletin Number 17, Washington DC

Bibliography

Acker DB, Sachs BB, Friedman EA 1985 Risk factors for shoulder dystocia. Obstetrics and Gynecology 66:762–766

Bahl R, Strachan B, Murphy DJ 2004 Outcome of subsequent pregnancy three years after previous operative delivery in the second stage of labour – cohort study. BMJ 328:311–314

Cardozo L, Gleeson C 1997 Pregnancy, childbirth and continence. British Journal of Midwifery 5:277–281

Chan CCT, Malathi I, Yeo GS 1999 Is the vacuum extractor really the instrument of first choice? Australian and New Zealand Journal of Obstetrics and Gynaecology 39:305–309

Cheung YW, Hopkins IM, Caughey AB 2004 How long is too long: does a prolonged second stage of labour in nulliparous women affect maternal and neonatal morbidity? American Journal of Obstetrics and Gynecology 191:933–938

Drife JO 1996 Choice and instrumental delivery. British Journal of Obstetrics and Gynaecology 103:608–611

Dupuis O, Madelenat P, Rudigoz RC 2004 Faecal and urinary incontinence after delivery: risk factors and prevention. Gynaecology Obstetrics Fertility 32:540–548

Eustice S 2004 Management of voiding difficulties associated with pregnancy. Nursing Times 100:50–53

Fortune PM, Thomas RM 1999 Sub-aponeurotic haemorrhage: a rare but life-threatening neonatal complication associated with ventouse delivery. British Journal of Obstetrics and Gynaecology 106:868–70

Gherman RB, Goodwin TM, Soutar I et al 1997 The McRoberts' manoeuvre for elevation of shoulder dystocia: how successful is it? American Journal of Obstetrics and Gynecology 176:656–661

Gonen R, Spiegel D, Abend M 1996 Is macrosomia predictable, and are shoulder dystocia and birth trauma preventable? Obstetrics and Gynecology 88:526–529

Gonen O, Rosen DJ, Dolfin Z et al 1997 Induction of labour versus expectant management in macrosomia: a randomised study. Obstetrics and Gynecology 89:913–917

Johanson RB, Heycock E, Carter J et al 1999 Maternal and child health after assisted vaginal delivery: five year follow up of a randomised controlled study comparing forceps and ventouse. British Journal of Obstetrics and Gynaecology 106:544–9

Johnstone FD, Myerscough PR 1998 Shoulder dystocia. British Journal of Obstetrics and Gynaecology 105:811–815

Jolley S 1997 Intermittent catheterisation for post operative urinary retention. Nursing Times 93:46–47

Leaphart WL, Meyer MC, Capeless EL 1997 Labour induction with a perinatal diagnosis of fetal macrosomia. Journal of Maternal-Fetal Medicine 6:99–102

Leather AT 1993 The management of shoulder dystocia. Contemporary Reviews in Obstetrics and Gynecology 5:61–64

Louise DF, Raymond RC, Perkins MB et al 1995 Recurrence rate of shoulder dystocia. American Journal of Obstetrics and Gynecology 172:1369–1371

Luria S, Benarie A, Hugay Z 1994 The ABC of shoulder dystocia management. Asia Oceania Journal of Obstetrics and Gynecology 20:195–197

Morales R, Adair CD, Sanchez-Ramos L et al 1995 Vacuum extraction of preterm infants with birthweights of 1,500–2,499 grams. Journal of Reproductive Medicine 40:127–130

Nesbitt TS, Gilbert WM, Herrchen B 1998 Shoulder dystocia and associated risk factors with macrosomic infants born in California. American Journal of Obstetrics and Gynecology 179:476–480

Petroikovksy B 1998 Emergency symphysiotomy: too little too late. American Journal of Obstetrics and Gynecology 178:631–632

Rane A, Frazer M 1999 Intrapartum and post partum bladder care. Journal of Obstetrics and Gynaecology; 1:311–313

Schwartz BC, Dixon DM 1958 Shoulder dystocia. Obstetrics and Gynecology 11:468–471

Sultan AA, Johanson RB, Carter JE 1998 Occult anal sphincter trauma following randomised forceps and vacuum delivery. International Journal of Obstetrics and Gynaecology 61:113–119

Towner D, Castro MA, Eby-Wilkens E et al 1999 Effect of mode of delivery in nulliparous women on neonatal intracranial injury. New England Journal of Medicine 341:1709–14

Vacca A 1999 The trouble with vacuum extraction. Current Obstetrics and Gynaecology 9:41–45

Vasket TF, Allen AC 1995 Perinatal implication of shoulder dystocia. Obstetrics and Gynecology 86:142–147

Yips K, Sahota D, Pang MN et al 2004 Post partum urinary retention. Acta Obstetrica et Gynaecologica Scandinavica 85:881–891

Chapter 17

Caesarean section

David T Y Liu
Mentor: Alexander Omu

CHAPTER CONTENTS

Indications for caesarean section   145
Preoperative care   146
Postoperative care   146
Types of incision   146
   Abdominal incisions   146
      Subumbilical midline incision   146
      Transverse (Pfannenstiel's) incision   147
   Uterine incisions   147
      Lower segment caesarean section   147
      Classical caesarean section   147
      Krönig–Gellhorn–Beck incision   147
      Other situations   148
Operative steps for caesarean section   148
Caesarean section: specific issues   148
   Communication   148
   Vaginal birth after caesarean section   148
   Signs of uterine scar rupture   149
      Management for uterine rupture   150
   Caesarean section after intrauterine fetal
      death   150
   Difficulty with delivery of the fetal head   151
   Caesarean hysterectomy   151
   Classical caesarean section   152
   Holding stitch   152
   Bleeding lower segment uterine angles   152
   Sterilisation   152

Caesarean section describes the surgical procedure for delivery of the fetus by incisions through the abdomen and uterus. The attendant risk of a surgical procedure must be considered. In the UK direct deaths following all caesarean sections is 82.3 per 1 000 000. For elective procedures this is 38.5 per 1 000 000. Death rate following vaginal delivery is 16.9 per 1 000 000 maternities (Department of Health (DoH) 2001). Pulmonary embolism, hypertension haemorrhage and sepsis continue to be salient causes of mortality. Inappropriate delegation, inadequate facilities and poor communication contribute to substandard care and necessitate improvement.

Sequelae of vaginal birth such as rectal and urinary incontinence, the question of choice, increased safety for caesarean section, more older women having babies and ready redress to litigation for complications with operative vaginal deliveries are factors leading to an increase in the rates of caesarean sections.

INDICATIONS FOR CAESAREAN SECTION

Caesarean sections can be subdivided into elective, scheduled or planned of varying emergency, unplanned emergency and peri-mortem and post-mortem categories to facilitate audit. Clearly complications and mortality attributed to the surgical procedure must be distinguished from contributions by obstetric complications and maternal medical problems.

Caesarean sections are performed to:

- overcome cephalo-pelvic disproportion and abnormal uterine activity
- expedite delivery for maternal or fetal reasons
- reduce fetal trauma (for example the small pre-term breech) and fetal infection (for example risk of transmitting herpetic infection or the human immunodeficiency virus (HIV))

- reduce maternal risk (for example certain cardiac disorders, intracranial lesions or cervical malignancy)
- allow women to exercise their informed choice.

PREOPERATIVE CARE

- Ensure reasons for surgery are valid. There should be input by senior colleagues and clear discussion with the woman and her partner. Document clearly for medicolegal reasons.
- Past obstetric and medical history must be reviewed. Check gestation (usually not before 39 weeks if elective surgery).
- Discuss mode of anaesthesia with the anaesthetist and the woman. Ideally, mode of anaesthesia or analgesia should be discussed in advance at a joint clinic with the anaesthetist. Regional anaesthesia is safer for the woman and the baby.
- Inform the paediatrician in good time.
- Check that cross-matched blood is available. Most labour wards now reserve 2 units of 0 Rhesus negative blood for emergencies. Cross-match 4 or more units if increased bleeding is likely, e.g. placenta praevia. Use cell saver for heavy loss or women refusing blood transfusion.
- Give an antacid (see Chapter 9).
- Obtain written consent. This includes discussion of need and procedure, risks, inadvertent damage to bladder and fetus.
- Introduce indwelling catheter.
- Administer prophylactic antibiotics. This is particularly relevant in emergency caesarean sections. Assess need for prophylaxis against thromboembolism following recommendations from the Royal College of Obstetricians and Gynaecologists' Working Party Report (Department of Health 1995). Women with three or more moderate risk factors such as age more than 35, obesity of more than 80 kg, para 4, gross varicose veins, concurrent infection, pre-eclampsia, 4 days immobility prior to surgery, labour over 12 hours, major medical disease, extended pelvic surgery, personal or family history of venous thrombosis or pulmonary embolism (thrombophilia) and presence of antiphospholipid antibody will need heparin prophylaxis and leg stockings.

POSTOPERATIVE CARE

Presence of obstetric or medical complications mean some women will need close observation following caesarean section. The labour ward can serve as an area for recovery and care. Intensive or high dependency care facilities must be readily available in the same hospital. General care for all women includes:

- Assess vital signs at regular intervals (15 minutes). Make sure condition is stable.
- Watch fundal height, any bleeding from wound and amount of lochia. This is particularly important if the labour is prolonged, when the uterus has been distended by polyhydramnios or multiple pregnancies and where there is a threat of coagulation defects, for example, after antepartum haemorrhage and pre-eclamptic toxaemia. Infuse oxytocin for 4–6 hours.
- Maintain fluid balance.
- Ensure adequate analgesia. Continued use of epidural analgesia is particularly useful.
- Address specific requirements which prompt indication for caesarean section, e.g. medical conditions such as diabetes.
- Early physiotherapy and ambulation if there is no contraindication.
- Remember thrombo-prophylaxis. Early ambulation and attention to hydration suffice for low risk women with uncomplicated pregnancies and no risk factors. Avoid use of dextran 70. Subcutaneous heparin or mechanical methods are required where risk is considered moderate. Where risk of thromboembolism is high, heparin and leg stockings should be used for 5 days following surgery or until full mobilisation. For past histories of venous thromboembolism in pregnancy or the puerperium thrombo-prophylaxis should be continued for 6 weeks post partum.
- Before discharge an opportunity should be made available to examine events and address questions.
- Schedule an opportunity for postnatal review to ensure complete recovery, to discuss subsequent pregnancies and ensure follow-up care for medical conditions.

TYPES OF INCISION

Abdominal incisions

Essentially these are the subumbilical midline and transverse lower abdominal incisions (Figure 17.1).

Subumbilical midline incision

This incision is easy and quick. Access is good with minimal bleeding. It is useful when access to the lower segment is difficult, for example severe kypho-

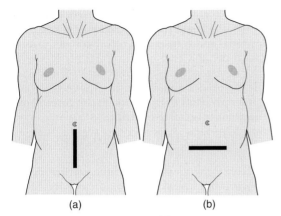

Figure 17.1 Abdominal incisions: (a) subumbilical midline and (b) transverse 'Pfannenstiel's'.

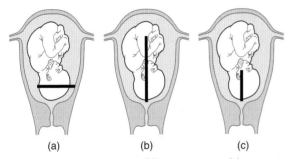

Figure 17.2 Uterine incisions: (a) lower segment (b) classical and (c) Krönig–Gellhorn–Beck.

scoliosis or anterior lower segment fibroid. The scar however, is unsightly, there is more postoperative discomfort and dehiscence is more likely compared with transverse incisions.

Where extension upwards into the abdomen is likely a left or right paramedian incision can be performed.

Transverse (Pfannenstiel's) incision

This is the current incision of choice. It is cosmetically pleasing, is less likely to dehisce and being less uncomfortable, allows better postoperative mobility. The incision can be technically more difficult especially in repeat surgery. It can be associated with greater blood loss and poorer access.

Variations include the Joel Cohen incision (placed higher up the abdomen) and Misgav Ladach (emphasises preservation of anatomical structures).

Uterine incisions

Entry into the uterus can be through a midline or a transverse lower segment incision (Figure 17.2).

Lower segment caesarean section (Figure 17.2a)

This is the most common approach. The transverse incision is placed in the lower segment of the gravid uterus behind the uterovesicle peritoneum. Advantages include:

- The site is less vascular hence less blood loss.
- It contains spread of infection into abdominal cavity.
- It is in the less contractile part of the uterus hence scar rupture in subsequent pregnancies is less likely.
- Healing is better with fewer postoperative complications such as adhesions.
- Implantation of the placenta over the uterine scar is less likely in subsequent pregnancies.

Disadvantages include:

- Access may be limited.
- Proximity to the bladder increases risk of damage particularly in repeat procedures.
- Extension into the lateral angles or behind the bladder can increase blood loss.

Classical caesarean section (Figure 17.2b)

This incision is placed vertically in the midline of the uterine body. Indications for use include:

- Early gestation, when the lower segment is poorly developed.
- When access to the lower segment is prevented by adhesions or uterine fibroids.
- When the fetus is impacted in the transverse position.
- Where the lower segment is vascular because of an anterior placenta praevia.
- When there is cervical carcinoma.
- When speed is essential, for example following death of the mother.

Disadvantages include:

- Haemostasis is more difficult with a thick vascular incision.
- Adhesions to surrounding organs are more likely.
- The anterior placenta may be encountered during entry.
- Healing is impaired because of myometrial involution.
- There is more risk of uterine rupture in subsequent pregnancies.

Krönig–Gellhorn–Beck incision (Figure 17.2c)

This is a midline incision in the lower segment. It is used in preterm deliveries where the lower segment is poorly formed or in situations where extension into the upper uterine segment is anticipated to provide more access. It has fewer of the complications associated with a classical Caesarean section. This incision need not preclude vaginal delivery.

Other situations

An inverted T incision or a J incision may on occasion be required when access is found to be inadequate despite a lower segment incision.

These incisions are best avoided. Like classical caesarean sections subsequent pregnancies will need to be delivered by elective caesarean section.

OPERATIVE STEPS FOR CAESAREAN SECTION

1. Open the abdomen through a midline or transverse Pfannenstiel's incision. In the Pfannenstiel approach a transverse skin incision is placed above the symphysis pubis. This is followed by division of the rectus sheath and separation of the rectus muscles prior to opening the abdominal peritoneum.

2. After opening the abdomen a Doyen retractor is inserted to hold the incision open for access into the lower uterine segment. Check the rotation of the uterus.

3. Identify and pick up loose peritoneum (Figure 17.3a) over the lower uterine segment and open transversely (Figure 17.3b). Replace the Doyen retractor to displace the peritoneum and bladder away from the intended uterine incision. Avoid excessive dissection behind the bladder otherwise troublesome venous bleeding may occur.

4. Incise the lower uterine segment transversely over an area of 2–3 cm until the amniotic cavity or membranes are identified. Extend the incision laterally with fingers until there is adequate room for delivery (Figure 17.3c). Bleeding is common when the lower segment is incised and care is needed to avoid fetal damage.

5. Remove the retractor. Insert a hand into the uterine wound below the breech or the fetal head. The presenting part is gently brought out (Figure 17.3d) through the uterine and abdominal incision. A characteristic hiss may be heard when the vacuum effect is lost. Facilitate delivery by fundal pressure (use the free hand or that of an assistant). An impacted presenting part can be dislodged by an assistant gently pushing through the vagina.

6. Once the fetal head is delivered, clear the airways (mouth first). Carefully deliver the shoulders to avoid further extension of the incision at the lateral angles. Syntocinon (5 units) or ergotamine (0.25 mg) is given. Clamp and cut the cord. Take arterial and venous cord blood samples to assess fetal pH and base excess. (Particularly relevant for emergency caesarean sections.) The placenta is removed manually. Ensure the uterine cavity is empty. Pass a digit through the cervical os to facilitate discharge of lochia.

7. Identify the lateral angles and secure bleeding vessels with clamps.

8. Identify the lower edge of the uterine incision, secure the lateral angles and close the uterine wound in two layers with continuous sutures (Figure 17.3e).

9. Exteriorise the uterus if needed to facilitate uterine wound closure (warn the anaesthetist if a spinal or epidural is used for anaesthesia). When haemostasis is achieved close the peritoneum with continuous suture.

10. Remove blood and clots from the peritoneal cavity. Check normality of salpinges and ovaries. Remove abdominal packs if used. Use a drain if oozing is a cause for concern.

11. Close the abdominal wound in layers. Current practice does not require closure of the parietal peritoneum. Likewise when there is no bleeding, the subcutaneous layer need not be sutured. Catgut is not used in contemporary surgery.

12. All steps of the procedure should be clearly documented. All complications must be highlighted to support counselling for subsequent pregnancies.

See Box 17.1 for a summary of the dos and do nots of caesarean section.

CAESAREAN SECTION: SPECIFIC ISSUES

Communication

Apart from issues of consent and good practice of forewarning team members such as anaesthetists and neonatologists it is important to define the degree of urgency for need to deliver the baby. In an emergency the current accepted decision to delivery interval is 30 minutes or less. This is however, not an evidence-based standard. Regular drills will ensure smooth assembly for urgent surgical delivery.

Vaginal birth after caesarean section (VBAC)

Vaginal delivery is contraindicated after a classic caesarean section and if there is need to extend the transverse uterine incision (T, J incisions). Where there is no recurrent indication for caesarean section, vaginal

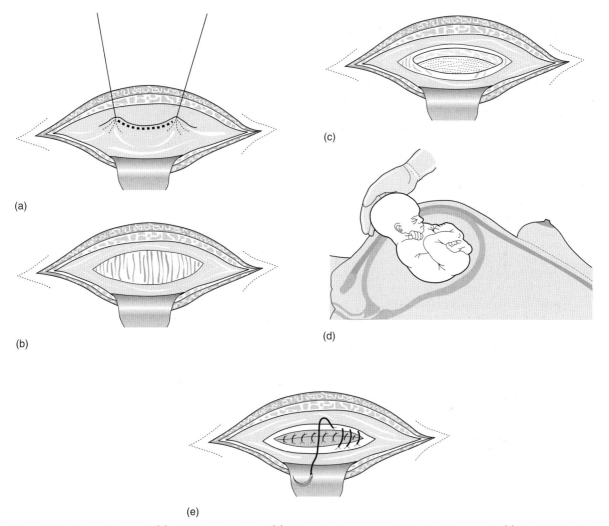

(a)

(b)

(c)

(d)

(e)

Figure 17.3 The peritoneum is (a) picked up and opened (b) before the lower segment is incised transversely (c). The fetal head (d) is delivered and the uterine wound is closed in two layers (e).

delivery reduces maternal mortality and morbidity. There is however, a 0.3% rate of uterine rupture associated with trial of scar. There is 25% perinatal mortality and a 25% need for hysterectomy following uterine rupture. Although a quarter to a third of women with prior caesarean section can successfully deliver vaginally, the following must be satisfied.

- The woman gives informed consent.
- The woman is well and there is no obstetric complication. The fetus is of normal size.
- The pelvis is adequate. A trial of labour is not acceptable.
- There is no complication following the previous caesarean section, e.g. extension of uterine scar or infection following surgery.

- Delivery must be conducted in a safe environment where appropriate care and continuous surveillance such as fetal heart rate monitoring is available.
- A successful vaginal delivery following caesarean section need not indicate reduction in risk for a second vaginal delivery.
- The second stage should not be prolonged.
- No new complication develops (after mutually agreed VBAC).

Signs of uterine scar rupture

Mothers with a classic uterine scar may experience uterine rupture prior to onset of labour. The low vertical uterine incision does not contribute an

---

Box 17.1 Dos and do nots of caesarean section

Do

- Place the woman in a 15° left lateral tilt (using a wedge) to overcome caval compression.
- Check the fetal heart before surgery. Operation may be contraindicated if the fetus is dead.
- If possible place the fetus into a longitudinal lie by external version.
- Once the fetus is delivered quickly the safety of the mother and her subsequent obstetric career must govern the tempo of surgery.
- The average blood loss is 400–600 ml. Consider replacement of blood if there is excessive bleeding.
- Ensure lochia can drain especially after elective caesarean section. Pass a finger or artery forceps from above through the cervix before closing the uterine incision.
- Insert drains if haemostasis is considered unsatisfactory or oozing is anticipated.
- If uterine infection is suspected take uterine swabs for culture.
- Ensure there is adequate width of the abdominal wound in a repeat transverse incision. Scar tissue is less compliant compared with normal tissue and may not stretch to allow easy delivery of the fetus.

- A thorough toilet of the abdominal cavity reduces the risk of postoperative ileus.
- Make sure the uterus is contracted.
- Clean the vagina. This procedure removes a nidus for infection and allows early recognition of postoperative bleeding.
- Document clearly difficulties encountered or complication with the surgery. A plan for management of subsequent deliveries should be included.
- Wear double gloves if the woman has a viral infection, e.g. HIV.
- Encourage early contact of mother and baby.

Do not

- Conduct trial of labour after a caesarian section.
- Vaginal delivery is usually contraindicated after two caesarean sections.
- Do not hesitate to use a subumbilical midline incision if a previous transverse lower abdominal incision is considered unsatisfactory.
- Do not place the uterine lower segment incision too close to the bladder.

---

increased risk to uterine rupture compared with the low transverse uterine incision. Signs of uterine rupture are:

- Fetal heart rate – signs of compromise.
- Suprapubic pain present between contractions and often felt despite presence of epidural analgesia.
- There is exquisite tenderness on palpation of the lower uterine segment.
- The presence of a rising maternal pulse rate.
- There is intrapartum vaginal bleeding.
- Sudden cessation of uterine contractions.
- Abdominal palpation detects malpresentation and fetal parts are easily palpable.
- Vaginal examination may reveal the presenting part has moved up into the pelvis.
- There may be maternal shock and collapse.

Management for uterine rupture

Maternal mortality for uterine rupture was 2.3 per 1 000 000 maternities (Confidential Enquiries into Maternal Deaths in the United Kingdom, 1994–1996). Correct planning of delivery and induction (judicious prostaglandin usage after one dose), delivery in an appropriate setting, and involvement of experienced obstetric staff in intrapartum care can contribute to improved outcome.

When scar rupture is suspect:

- Perform immediate laparotomy.

- Following assisted delivery or where manual removal of the placenta is required the lower segment following a previous caesarean section can be examined by an experienced surgeon. The lower segment is identified by locating the thick upper uterine segment and then withdrawing the examining finger towards the cervix. Integrity of the loose thinner lower segment is best examined by running the finger gently from side to side (Figure 17.4). For small dehiscence with no bleeding no further action is necessary apart from close observation. Future deliveries must be by elective caesarean section. For large rupture, especially when bleeding continues, laparotomy and repair are necessary.

Caesarean section after intrauterine fetal death

This is necessary when vaginal delivery is not feasible (for example impacted shoulders, fetal abnormality)

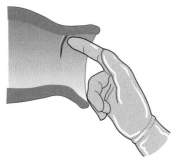

Figure 17.4   Examination for uterine scar integrity.

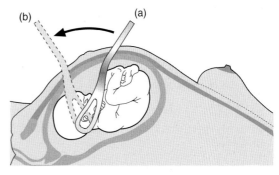

Changing the position and lifting head through uterine wall

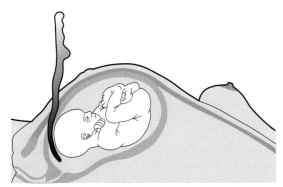

Figure 17.5   Use of single forceps blade to assist delivery of the fetal head.

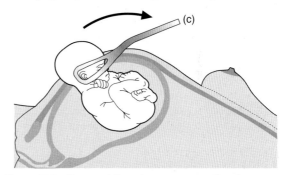

Figure 17.6   Forceps delivery in caesarean section: forceps such as Wrigley's are applied to the fetal head in the direct occipitoposterior position (a), changing to position (b) to lift head through the uterine wound and complete delivery by directing forceps towards the mother's head (c).

or for the mother's welfare (for example abruptio placentae, with severe bleeding and fetal death). Exclude coagulation defects. Additional psychological support will be required.

Difficulty with delivery of the fetal head

Caesarean section following a trial of labour or trial of forceps may find the fetal head impacted or deep in the pelvis. Delivery of the presenting part is facilitated by:

- Displacement of the presenting part up into the pelvis by an assistant pushing through the vagina.
- Turning the fetal head into the occipitoposterior position.
- Wrigley's forceps. A single blade can be employed as a lever (Figure 17.5) or both blades can be applied to effect delivery (Figure 17.6). Forceps are useful to bring a high head through the uterine incision.
- Extended uterine incision, e.g. inverted 'T' (Figure 17.7).

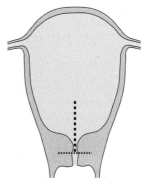

Figure 17.7   Inverted T incision.

Caesarean hysterectomy

Indications include gross uterine rupture or uncontrollable haemorrhage. The woman's condition is usually compromised hence speed and experience are required. Consider the following:

- Time is saved if the uterus is removed before tying the pedicles.

- There may be difficulty in differentiating between the oedematous lower segment, the cervix and surrounding tissues. A subtotal hysterectomy is advised when damage and bleeding are confined to the uterine body.
- Bilateral ligation of the internal iliac artery may be required.
- Repair the ruptured uterus if the mother is stable, surgical expertise is available and fertility has to be preserved.

Classical caesarean section

Remember to check the rotation of the uterus. If possible start at the lower half of the upper uterine segment and extend if required. The uterine wall should be closed in three layers. The herringbone suture technique for closure of the superficial layer minimises oozing.

Holding stitch

- Rate of fetal scalpel laceration is about 2%.

- A holding stitch can help lift the lower segment away from tight application to the fetus. Traction on the stitch will allow incising without damage to the fetus (Figure 17.8). The stitch can also help identify the distal lower segment flap if difficulty is anticipated.

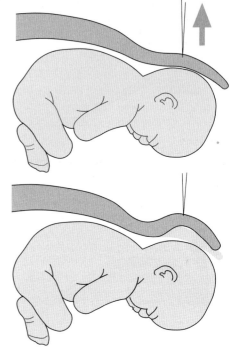

Figure 17.8 A holding stitch.

Bleeding lower segment uterine angles

- A drier field and better control of bleeding is achieved if the uterus is delivered through the abdomen wound. Warn the anaesthetist if this procedure is intended.

Sterilisation

- Consent for this procedure from both partners should be obtained well in advance. Use of an epidural or spinal anaesthesia will allow opportunities for discussion at time of surgery.
- The couple should be fully counselled in terms of irreversibility of the procedure, increased failure rates and technique used.
- The isthmic portion of salpinges are usually excised and the cut ends ligated. The excised segments should be dispensed for histological verification. Clips are less reliable because the salpinges are enlarged by pregnancy.

References

Department of Health 2001 Report on Confidential Enquiries into Maternal Deaths in the United Kingdom 1997–1999. HMSO, London

Department of Health 1998 Report on Confidential Enquiries into Maternal Deaths in the United Kingdom, 1994–1996. HMSO, London

Royal College of Obstetricians and Gynaecologists 1995 Report of the Working Party on Prophylaxis Against Thromboembolism in Gynaecology and Obstetrics. London: RCOG Press

Bibliography

Appleton B, Targett C, Rasmussen M et al 2000 Vaginal birth after Caesarean section. An Australian Multicentre Study. VBAC Study Group. Australian and New Zealand Journal of Obstetrics and Gynaecology 40:87–91

Bergsjo P 1993 Quality assurance: a concept rediscovered. Acta Obstetrica et Gynecologica Scandinavica 72:143

Caughev AB, Shipp TD, Repke JT et al 1999 Rate of uterine rupture during a trial of labour in women with one or two prior Caesarean deliveries American Journal of Obstetrics and Gynecology 181:872–876

Chazotte C, Cohen WR 1990 Catastrophic complications of previous Caesarean section. American Journal of Obstetrics and Gynecology 163:738–742

Donald I 1979 Practical Obstetric Problems. Lloyd-Luke (Medical Books) Ltd, London

Duff P 1987 Prophylactic antibiotics for Caesarean delivery. A simple cost-effective strategy for the prevention of post-operative morbidity. American Journal of Obstetrics and Gynecology 157:794–798

Gregory KD, Korst LM, Cane P et al 1999 Vaginal birth after Caesarean and uterine rupture rates in California. Obstetrics and Gynecology 94:985–989

Guise JM, McDonagh MS, Osterweil P et al 2004 Systemic review of the incidence and consequences of uterine rupture in women with previous Caesarean section. BMJ 329:1–7

Malkasian GD 1990 The conscience of the specialty. Obstetrics and Gynecology 75:1–4

Martens MG, Faro S, Philips LE et al 1987 Postpartum endometritis in high risk C section patients. Surgical Infections 6:96–99

Miller DA, Fidelia GD, Paul RH 1996 Vaginal birth after Caesarean section. New England Journal of Medicine 335:689–695

Molmgren G, Sjoholm L, Stark M 1999 The Misgav Ladach method for Caesarean section: method description. Acta Obstetrica et Gynecologica Scandinavica 78:615–621

Royal College of Obstetricians and Gynaecologists 1998 Guideline 15: Peritoneal closure. RCOG, London

Royal College of Obstetrician and Gynaecologists 2004 Guideline 4: Male and female sterilization. RCOG, London

Shipp TD, Zelop CM, Repke JT et al 1999 Intrapartum rupture and dehiscence in patients with prior lower uterine segment. Vertical and transverse incisions. Obstetrics and Gynecology 94; 735–740

Smith GC, Pell JP, Pasupathy D et al 2004 Factors predisposing to perinatal death related to uterine rupture during attempted vaginal birth after Caesarean section: retrospective cohort study. BMJ 329;275–379

Sood AK et al 2000 Pregnant women with cervical cancer should be delivered by caesarean section. Obstetrics and Gynecology 95:832–838

Sood AK, Sorosky JI, Mayr N et al 2000 Cervical cancer diagnosed shortly after pregnancy: Prognostic variables and delivery routes. Obstetrics and Gynecology 95:832–838

Chapter 18

Emergencies in the immediate puerperium

David T Y Liu
Mentor: Charles Rodeck

CHAPTER CONTENTS

Postpartum haemorrhage   155
    Complications   156
    Diagnosis   156
    Predisposing factors   156
    Management   157
    Bimanual compression   158
    Alternative procedures   158
Retained placenta   158
    Diagnosis   158
    Management   158
    Pathologically adherent placenta   160
Acute uterine inversion   160
    Precipitating factors   160
    Outcome   160
    Management   161

The exertions of labour and delivery subject women to potential risks (summarised in Table 18.1) because:

- Strong contractions threaten uterine rupture in any scarred uterus. Pelvic vein thrombi may be dislodged to cause pulmonary embolus and increased intrauterine pressure can squeeze amniotic fluid into the venous sinuses to produce amniotic fluid emboli. Following delivery uterine retraction injects up to 500 ml of sequestrated blood into the circulatory system. Women with restricted cardiac output may develop pulmonary oedema.

- Increased intra-abdominal, intrathoracic and intracranial pressures are associated with pushing efforts during delivery. Aneurysms (e.g. splenic or intracranial) or lung bullae (following chronic lung disease) can rupture.

- Placental and membrane separation expose a large area with open venous sinuses. Some bleeding is inevitable but postpartum haemorrhage can result if the myometrium fails to contract or is prevented from doing so. Occasionally a vacuum is created after expulsion of the placenta and air can be sucked in to produce air emboli.

- Women may react adversely to the administration of drugs such as opioids or oxytocics.

- Stress and exertion can aggravate existing medical conditions, such as epilepsy or adrenal insufficiency. A difficult labour can have psychological sequelae.

POSTPARTUM HAEMORRHAGE

Bleeding in excess of 300 ml after delivery is considered excessive. By convention, a loss of 500 ml or more is described as a haemorrhage. True postpartum

Table 18.1 Complications resulting from strong uterine contractions

Condition	Predisposition	Signs and symptoms	Management	Prophylaxis
Uterine rupture	Uterine scarring	Range from asymptomatic to collapse and haemorrhage	Resuscitate, explore extent of damage and repair if indicated or perform hysterectomy	Anticipate, care with oxytocics, reduce pushing in second stage, consider elective caesarean section
Pulmonary thromboembolism	History of prolonged bed rest Pelvic infection or trauma	Range from asymptomatic to pleuritic pain, blood stained sputum, dyspnoea, cyanosis and collapse	Resuscitate, ventilate confirm diagnosis and treat with anticoagulation ECG, blood gases and ventilation perfusion scans are helpful	Heighten index of suspicion in at-risk mothers Aim for spontaneous delivery and short second stage Give heparin for at risk mothers
Amniotic fluid embolism	Polyhydramnios, excessive pushing, early placental separation, misuse of oxytocics	Collapse, dyspnoea, cyanosis, coagulation defect	Resuscitate, ventilate, hydrocortisone to treat coagulation disorder Antibiotics	Avoid long labour and excessive pushing in mothers with predisposition Care needed with induction of labour
Air embolism	Uterus fails to contract following rapid delivery of placenta	Sudden collapse, dyspnoea, cyanosis, cardiac arrest and 'machinery murmur'	Resuscitate, ventilate, occasionally air in right cardiac auricle or ventricle may be aspirated	Control delivery of placenta Ensure uterine contraction
Pulmonary oedema	Restriction in cardiac output	Acute heart failure	Oxygen, digitalis, diuretics, occasionally venesection	Avoid ergometrine in at-risk mothers Care needed if there is output obstruction

haemorrhage is bleeding after delivery of the placenta, an academic point of little practical value. Bleeding is further classified as primary (within 24 hours of birth) and secondary (after 24 hours after birth).

Complications

- Hypovolaemic shock and death (still a major cause of maternal mortality).
- Pituitary infarct and necrosis (Sheehan's syndrome).
- Anaemia.
- Anxiety. Haemorrhage is a frightening experience and all women and their partners appreciate a full explanation and reassurance.
- Pulmonary thromboembolism (see Box 18.1 for more details).

Diagnosis

- The presence of continuous fresh blood loss, torrential bleeding or collapse.

- Blood may collect in an atonic uterus with little evidence of excess external loss but fundal height increases.

Predisposing factors

- Poor maternal health.
- History of antepartum or postpartum haemorrhage.
- Prolonged labour especially after the use of oxytocics.
- Poor uterine contraction/retraction, for example in a grand multipara (more than four babies), or where the uterus is previously overdistended, for example a multiple pregnancy or polyhydramnios).
- Blood dyscrasias or inherited bleeding tendencies, for example von Willebrand's disease.
- Birth trauma, surgery and uterine inversion.
- Retained placenta or partial separation of a placenta accreta.

This complication remains a major cause of maternal mortality hence prevention and correct management is important.

- Identify at-risk women.

- Prevention is by subcutaneous heparin 5000–10 000 IU preoperation and then twice daily (maintain anti-factor Xa levels below 0.3 IU/ml) or equivalent such as Fragmin 2500 IU subcutaneously 1-hours before surgery and then daily until fully mobile to cover labour or caesarean section. Bleeding is more likely if prothrombin time is more than 2.5 times control or the heparin level exceeds 0.5 IU/ml. Pre-eclampsia, renal impairment and aspirin ingestion reduce heparin requirements.

- Women with anti-thrombin III deficiency are at particular risk. During labour and the early puerperium give anti-thrombin III infusions or equivalent. Heparin is not useful because its action depends on anti-thrombin III.

- Women with mitral valve disease or prosthetic heart valves are usually given intravenous heparin before delivery at levels of 0.8 IU/ml. Reduce levels to one-third during labour and raise again in the puerperium.

- Pulmonary embolism is often symptomless. If possible confirm diagnosis. Treatment is by heparin 40 000 units daily by intravenous infusion (anti-factor Xa levels of 0.5–1.5 IU/ml; partial thromboplastin time of 1.5 to 2.5 times control) for 1 week before changing the regimen.

- Contraindication or caution with heparin usage includes uncontrolled hypertension, haemorrhagic disorders, peptic ulcers and advanced renal or hepatic diseases.

- An episiotomy can contribute up to 150 ml of blood loss. Episiotomies must be repaired quickly to reduce blood loss.
- Placenta praevia.
- Uterus with multiple fibroids.

Management

- Anticipate. Set-up intravenous infusion and reserve cross-matched blood for at-risk women. Ergometrine, 0.25 mg intravenously, encourages uterine

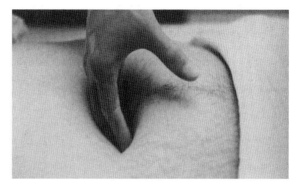

Figure 18.1   Uterine massage to encourage contraction.

contraction. Following antepartum haemorrhage coagulation defects must be excluded before delivery or surgery.

- An experienced person should conduct the delivery of at-risk women. Active management of third stage is suggested.

- Treat shock. Untreated severe shock for more than 30 minutes will result in Sheehan's syndrome in 40% of mothers. Select crystalloid, colloid, cross-matched bloods or O negative blood (emergency) in sequence.

- Calculate blood loss and ensure adequate replacement. Note consistency and ability of blood to clot. If necessary correct coagulation defects. Maintain haemoglobin above 100 g/l, blood pressure above 100 systolic/50 diastolic mmHg and pulse below 100 beats per minute.

The dictum 'an empty and contracted uterus does not bleed' is worth remembering. Check size and consistency of the uterus. Removal of a blood clot in the uterine cavity may be all that is necessary. Uterine atony is the most common cause of postpartum haemorrhage.

- If the uterus is poorly contracted massage gently to encourage contraction. Place four fingers of one hand behind the fundus of the uterus with the thumb in front and massage with a circular motion (Figure 18.1). Give 0.25 mg ergometrine or one ampoule of Syntometrine intravenously if there are no contraindications such as hypertension. Maintain contraction by intravenous oxytocics (Syntocinon) for 6–8 hours. A useful regimen is 40 IU of Syntocinon in 500 ml of physiological saline administered at 20 drops or more per minute.

- An alternative drug that produces powerful and prolonged uterine contraction is misoprostol.

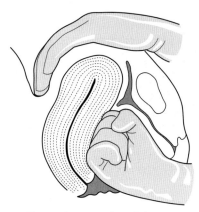

Figure 18.2 Bimanual compression of the uterus.

Rectal administration 1000 µg is usually highly effective.

- Intramyometrial injection of prostaglandin (PG) F$_2\alpha$ (250 µg, repeated in 15 minutes) can also be tried. Maximum total dose is 2 mg (eight doses). Do not use if the woman is asthmatic.

- If the uterus is well contracted, conduct an exploration under adequate epidural or, preferably, general anaesthesia. Exclude vaginal, cervical or uterine lacerations. Ensure that the uterus is empty (no clots or placenta). Women must be observed closely for 4–6 hours after an exploratory procedure.

- Classical manoeuvres, described below, can be tried.

Bimanual compression

- Ensure adequate anaesthesia.
- Place a fist vaginally in the anterior fornix while the abdominal hand compresses the uterus against the fist (Figure 18.2). This is still worth considering as a temporising measure in torrential bleeding. It is physically exhausting and cannot be maintained for any length of time.

Alternative procedures

- External aortic compression can be tried. Lift uterus out of pelvis, grasp and compress lower segment with one hand while the fundus is pushed against the aorta with the other hand.

- Hydrostatic balloon.

- A urological catheter can be inserted into the uterine cavity and injected with 500 ml warm saline to exert hydrostatic pressure. Infuse Syntocinon to maintain uterine contraction.

Box 18.2   Management of women who refuse blood transfusion

- Give oxygen, infuse colloid, e.g. Haemaccel.
- Exclude retained products of conception or trauma.
- Give Syntometrine. If hypertensive, give 10 U IV of Syntocinon.
- Misoprostol (PGE$_1$ analogue) 600 µg orally; 800 µg intrauterine or 1000 µg rectally.
- Uterine packing.
- Brace suture.
- Hysterectomy.

Postpartum
- IV iron sucrose (Venofer) if anaemic.
- Erythropoietin 300 U/kg three times weekly subcutaneously helps erythropoiesis.

- On occasion the uterus can be packed.

- Perform laparotomy if severe bleeding continues. Deliberation can lead to maternal decompression.
  - Inspect to exclude trauma or rupture. Repair where required.
  - Stepwise ligation of vessels, uterine, ovarian and internal iliac if appropriate.
  - Brace sutures to compress the uterus.
  - Hysterectomy. In a sick mother, subtotal hysterectomy is justified.

Box 18.2 describes the approach to the situation in which women may refuse a blood transfusion.

RETAINED PLACENTA

The placenta is retained if it is not delivered within 30 minutes after the birth of the fetus. The placenta may be:

- separated but trapped by the cervix
- partially separated
- pathologically adherent (placenta accreta, increta, percreta).

Diagnosis

- A high fundus.
- Postpartum haemorrhage.
- Absent signs of placenta separation.

Management

The placenta should be removed manually (Box 18.3) if it is retained. Immediate removal is mandatory if there is haemorrhage. A hysterectomy may be required

Box 18.3 Manual removal of placenta

- Cross-match blood. Set up drip.

- Use epidural or general anaesthesia.

- Use the lithotomy position and aseptic technique. Catheterise bladder.

- Perform a vaginal examination with liberal use of obstetric cream.

- A placenta protruding through the cervix is readily removed.

- Manual dilatation is necessary if the cervix is clamped down.
  - Appose the tips of all five fingers of examining hand to form a cone (Figure 18.3).
  - Insert the tips of the fingers through cervix (Figure 18.4)
  - Spread the fingers repeatedly rotating hand at same time and ease the hand through the cervix (Figures 18.5, 18.6). Stabilise the fundus with the external hand.

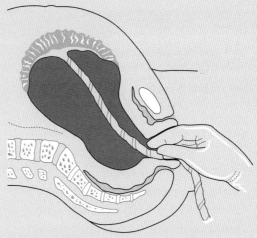

Figure 18.4 Manual dilatation of the cervix.

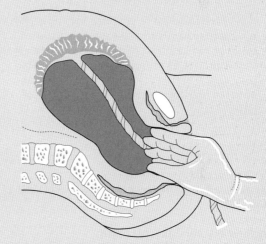

Figure 18.5 Easing hand through the cervix.

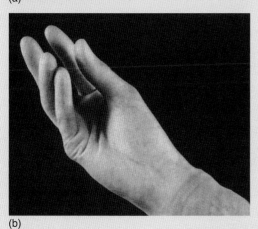

(a)

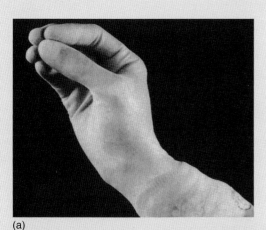

(b)

Figure 18.3 Apposed fingers (a) spread repeatedly (b) to dilate cervix.

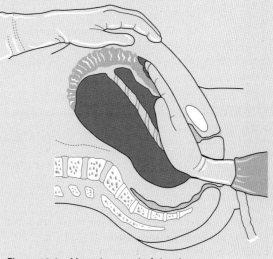

Figure 18.6 Manual removal of the placenta.

Box 18.3 *Continued*

- Once inside the uterine cavity, locate the placenta by following the umbilical cord to its insertion.

- The placenta is separated by sliding the open hand between the placenta and the uterine wall. The abdominal hand stabilises the uterus and acts as a guide to prevent damage to the thin myometrium (Figure 18.7).

- Remove the placenta only when it is totally separated.

- Examine the placenta for missing cotyledons. Re-explore the uterine cavity.

- Close observation for 4–6 hours after manual removal is necessary. Make sure that the uterus is well contracted. Leave indwelling catheter.

- If the placenta cannot be separated from the uterine wall, hysterectomy is often the safest option when bleeding continues. If there is no bleeding maintain close watch and await spontaneous expulsion after some days. A pathologically adherent placenta can be left to reabsorb spontaneously. Consider use of methotrexate.

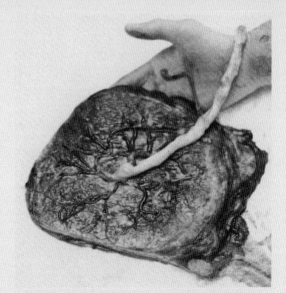

Figure 18.7 Technique for separation of the placenta.

for a pathologically adherent placenta when bleeding continues.

Pathologically adherent placenta

- Incidence is around 1 in 7000 pregnancies.
- Magnetic resonance imaging (MRI) or transabdominal colour Doppler sonography can detect some placenta accreta and assist preoperative planning.
- When there is no bleeding, conservative management with methotrexate and close observation is an option.

ACUTE UTERINE INVERSION

The whole spectrum ranging from a dimple in the uterine fundus to complete protrusion through the introitus can present (Figure 18.8).

Precipitating factors

- Incorrect use of fundal pressure.
- Cord traction when the uterus is not well contracted and the placenta not separated.
- Fundal insertion of the placenta.
- Uterine laxity.

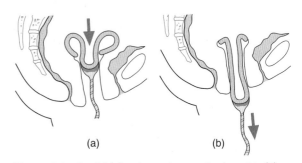

Figure 18.8 Partial (a) and complete uterine inversion (b).

- Pathological attachment of the placenta.
- Severe bearing-down efforts.
- A short cord.

Outcome

- Shock.
- Severe dragging pain.
- Haemorrhage.
- The normal shape and position of the fundus is lost. The fundus may not be palpable but vaginal examination will confirm suspicion.

Management

- Anticipate the possibility in at-risk women (grand multipara, polyhydramnios).

- Prevent by proper management of the third stage of labour.

- Inversion occurring during delivery of the placenta – if the placenta is still attached replace placenta/uterus immediately. Firm pressure is applied to push the whole mass first into the vagina then through the cervix and finally into its normal position. Do not remove the placenta unless it is congested and obstructs replacement. Attempts to remove the placenta at this stage waste time, may cause severe bleeding or may not be possible because of pathological adherence.

- Treat shock and replace blood.

- If immediate replacement is not possible general anaesthesia is necessary once the mother's condition is stabilised. Reduce the inversion gradually by applying pressure to the dependent part of the uterus, and simultaneously pressing with the other hand on all the parts of the uterus which inverted last (Figure 18.9).

- O'Sullivan's technique. The dependent part of the uterus is replaced into the vagina. Five or more litres of physiological saline is deposited into the posterior fornix of the vagina. An assistant holds the vulva against the operator's wrist or forearm to

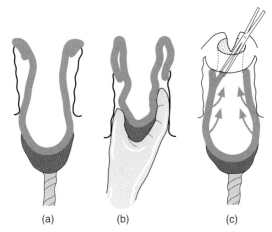

(a)   (b)   (c)

Figure 18.9 Replacement of inverted uterus manually (a, b) and at laparotomy (c).

effect a watertight seal. Hydrostatic pressure replaces the uterus.

- Once the uterus is reduced, attempt to remove the placenta. Administer oxytocics to encourage contraction.

- If all attempts fail laparotomy is necessary. Incise the posterior ring of the inverted uterus to overcome resistance to replacement. Restoration to the normal position can be achieved by traction on the parts of the uterus just inside the inverted ring (Figure 18.9c). Vaginal effort by an assistant pushing from below will help.

Bibliography

AbdRabbo SA 1994 Stepwise uterine devascularization: a novel technique for management of uncontrolled postpartum hemorrhage with preservation of the uterus. American Journal of Obstetrics and Gynecology 171:694–700

B-Lynch C, Coker A, Lawal AH, Abu J, Cowen MJ 1997 The B-Lynch surgical technique for the control of massive postpartum haemorrhage: an alternative to hysterectomy? Five cases reported. British Journal of Obstetrics and Gynaecology 104:372–375

Chou MM, Ho ESC 1997 Prenatal diagnosis of placenta praevia accrete with power amplitude ultrasonic angiography. American Journal of Obstetrics and Gynecology 177:1523–1525

Chou MM, Ho ES, Lee YH 2000 Prenatal diagnosis of placenta praevia accreta by transabdominal colour Doppler ultrasound. Ultrasound in Obstetrics and Gynecology 15:28–35

Griffiths D, Howell C 2003 Massive obstetric haemorrhage. In: Johanson R, Cox C, Grady K, et al (eds). Managing Obstetric Emergencies and Trauma; the MOET Course Manual. RCOG Press, London

Hansch E, Chitkara U, McAlpine J et al 1999 Pelvic arterial embolisation for control of obstetric haemorrhage: a five year experience. American Journal of Obstetrics and Gynecology 180:1454–1460

Johanson R, Kumar M, Obhrai M et al 2001 Management of massive postpartum haemorrhage: use of a hydrostatic balloon catheter to avoid laparoscopy. British Journal of Obstetrics and Gynaecology 108:420–422

Lemercier E, Genebois A, Descargue G et al 1999 MRI evaluation of placenta accreta treated by embolisation. Apropos of a case. Review of the literature. Journal of Radioliogy 80:383–387

Maier RC 1993 Control of postpartum haemorrhage with uterine packing. American Journal of Obstetrics and Gynaecology 169:317–323

Miller DA, Chollet JA, Goodwin TM 1997 Clinical risk factors for placenta praevia-placenta accreta. American Journal of Obstetrics and Gynecology 177:210–214

O'Brien P, El-Refaey H, Gordon A et al 1998 Rectally administered misoprostol for the treatment of post partum haemorrhage unresponsive to oxytocin and ergometrine: a descriptive study. Obstetrics and Gynecology 91:212–214

Royal Australian and New Zealand College of Obstetricians and Gynaecologists. Statement: Placenta accreta. 2003 Statement no C-Obs 20

Vedantham S, Goodwin SC, McLucas B et al 1997 Uterine artery embolisation: an underused method of controlling pelvic hemorrhage. American Journal of Obstetrics and Gynecology 176:938–948

Chapter **19**

Malpresentation and malpositions

David T Y Liu

CHAPTER CONTENTS

Definitions   163
  Malposition   163
  Malpresentation   163
    Associations   164
    Labour   164
Deflexed head   164
  Delivery   164
Occipitoposterior positions   164
  Diameters for consideration   164
  Types   164
  Diagnosis   164
    Palpation   164
    Vaginal examination   165
    Course of labour   165
    Uterine activity   165
    Gynaecoid and other adequate pelvis   165
    Anthropoid (ellipsoid) pelvis   165
    Android pelvis   165
    Occipitoposterior position and deflexion of
      the head   165
  Management   166
Face presentation   166
  Types   167
  Diagnosis   167

    Primary face   167
    Secondary face   167

  Management   167
    Mentoanterior position   167
    Mentolateral position   167
    Mentoposterior position   167
Brow presentation   168
  Types   168
  Diameters for consideration   168
  Diagnosis   168
    Primary brow   168
    Secondary brow   168
  Management   168
Compound presentation   168
  Management   168
Parietal presentation   168
  Anterior asynclitism   168
  Posterior asynclitism   168
Shoulder presentation (transverse or oblique lie)   169
  Diagnosis   169
    Abdomen   169
    Vaginal   169
  Prognosis   169
  Management   169

DEFINITIONS

Malposition

This describes a vertex presentation which is not in the fully flexed anterior position, for example a deflexed head, and occipitolateral and occipitoposterior positions. The occiput is the denominator. A higher incidence is seen in mothers of African and Chinese origin.

Malpresentation

This describes all presentations which are not vertex, for example: face, brow, shoulder and breech presentation.

Associations
- Fetus: abnormal, large, preterm, multiple.
- Uterus: abnormal, polyhydramnios, poor uterine tone, pendulous abdomen.
- Pelvis: abnormal, disproportion (contracted or capacious pelvis).

Labour

During pregnancy attention is drawn to these complications when the fundal height does not correspond to gestational dates, the lie is not longitudinal or the fetal head is not engaged. The fetal head may appear large because it is abnormal, or is in malposition. Before, or following labour, some of these complications may resolve spontaneously.

Labour in these women may:

- in certain circumstances produce these complications as a secondary feature (rotation from occipital anterior)
- be complicated by early membrane rupture and risk of cord prolapse
- be prolonged or become arrested
- require medical intervention assisted delivery or caesarean section.

An experienced obstetrician should be called to confirm the diagnosis and then to decide about labour and supervise the mode of delivery.

Diagnosis of malpositions signals need to anticipate operative delivery.

DEFLEXED HEAD

This describes a vertex presentation where the fetal head is not fully flexed to present the most advantageous biparietal diameter of 9.5 cm. This situation arises when:

- the fetus is small in relation to the pelvis, e.g. preterm birth
- congenital abnormalities are present
- the dimensions of the pelvis are marginal. This is particularly likely in occipitoposterior positions
- fibroids or tumours interfere with normal labour.

Labour is prolonged or may be arrested. Deflexion can progress to a brow or face presentation.

Delivery

Labour may be delayed in the second stage. Delivery may require an episiotomy, manual flexion of the fetal head or the application of forceps.

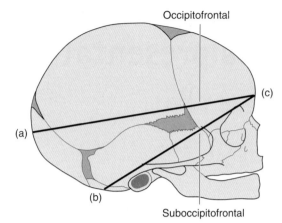

Figure 19.1 Diameters for consideration in occipitoposterior positions: occipitofrontal (a–c) and suboccipitofrontal (b–c).

OCCIPITOPOSTERIOR POSITIONS

These describe the situation where the occiput is in the posterior part of the pelvis. This position is found in 10–13% of all vertex presentations. Contributory factors include:

- a large baby
- an android or anthropoid (ellipsoid) pelvis
- pelvic brim contracture or flat sacrum
- anterior low-lying placenta
- a deflexed head
- malrotation.

Diameters for consideration

- Flexed occipitoposterior: presents the suboccipitofrontal which is 10 cm (Figure 19.1: b–c).
- Deflexed occipitoposterior: presents the occipitofrontal which is 11.5 cm (Figure 19.1: a–c).

Types

- a) Right occipitoposterior (ROP) is the most common – the occiput lies opposite the right sacroiliac joint.
- b) Left occipitoposterior (LOP).
- c) Direct occipitoposterior – the occiput lies in the hollow of the sacrum (Figure 19.2).

Diagnosis

Palpation

The fetal limbs are anterior and give a hollowed appearance to the woman's lower abdomen. The head is not engaged and the sinciput is felt superficial to the

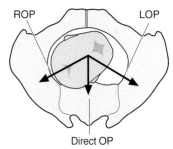

Figure 19.2 Types of occipitoposterior position: ROP, LOP and direct OP.

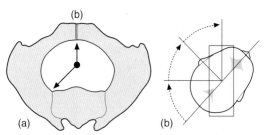

Figure 19.4 Rotation of occiput through the long arc (a) to deliver in the occipitoanterior position through the anteroposterior diameter of the outlet (b).

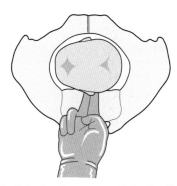

Figure 19.3 Palpating the ear as guide to direction of occiput.

occiput on palpation when the woman is lying horizontally. The fetal shoulder and loudest heart sounds are located well lateral to the midline.

Vaginal examination
The presenting part is poorly applied to the cervix. Deflexion is common. The anterior fontanelle is easily felt beneath the symphysis. If diagnosis presents difficulty, pass a finger alongside the fetal face and locate the ear. Running the fingers across the root of the ear will show that the pinna points in the direction of the occiput (Figure 19.3).

Course of labour
This depends on the quality of uterine activity, whether disproportion is present and the type of pelvis.

Uterine activity
Strong regular contractions encourage flexion, engagement and rotation to an occipitoanterior position. Labour tends to be longer because the application of the presenting part of the fetus to the cervix is poor. In about two-thirds of such women, rotation through an arc of 135° from an occipitoposterior to an

occipitoanterior position will be achieved (Figure 19.4). Extra time in labour is required to achieve this.

Gynaecoid and other adequate pelvis
Descent and flexion of the head occurs. Long rotation to the occipitoanterior position takes place at the level of the pelvic floor. Subsequently delivery is normal.

Anthropoid (ellipsoid) pelvis
Rotation to the occipitoanterior position is not favoured because the transverse diameter of the pelvis is narrow. The vertex rotates posteriorly a short distance, through 45° to deliver in the persistent occipitoposterior position. Deflexion is common, hence the presenting diameter is the wider occipitofrontal (11.5 cm) position. The head delivers by flexion followed by extension to allow the brow and the face to appear beneath the symphysis. The wider presenting diameter of the fetal head causes more trauma to the vagina, hence an episiotomy is necessary to prevent tearing. Assistance with forceps or ventouse extraction to complete the delivery is commonly required.

Android pelvis
Rotation to an anterior position becomes progressively more difficult with descent because the pelvis is narrow anteriorly, and the walls of the lower part of the android pelvis converge towards the outlet. Spontaneous rotation to an anterior position is possible if the pelvis diameters are adequate. In a marginal-sized pelvis, failure to rotate can occur at any level of the pelvis. The vertex can remain in the occipitoposterior position or rotation may be arrested with the head in the transverse position. When failure to rotate or descend occurs high in the pelvis, this situation is termed deep transverse arrest (DTA) (Figure 19.5). Delivery will require assistance.

Occipitoposterior position and deflexion of the head
In a marginal-sized pelvis partial deflexion will present wider fetal diameters and hence obstruction

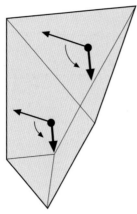

Figure 19.5 Schematic illustration of increasing difficulty for rotation to occipitoanterior in an android pelvis.

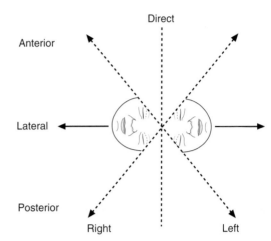

Figure 19.6 Mentum (chin) in the right and left posterior, lateral and mentoanterior positions together with direct mentoposterior and mentoanterior.

to progressive labour. With a capacious pelvis deflexion can produce a brow or face presentation.

Management

- Ensure good uterine contractions.

- Provide adequate analgesia. Epidural analgesia is useful for long labours and operative delivery. Relaxation of the pelvic floor muscles may hinder anterior rotation.

- Assess the pelvic diameters carefully. If necessary use X-ray or magnetic resonance imaging to anticipate and evaluate any likely problems.

- Avoid maternal ketosis.

- Institute close fetal surveillance.

- Examine every 2–4 hours to assess progress. Failure to progress before full cervical dilatation necessitates caesarean section. Examine immediately after membranes rupture to exclude cord prolapse.

- If the presenting part of the fetus is on the perineum in an occipitoposterior position, it is acceptable and possibly safer to deliver as an occipitoposterior with the help of an episiotomy and forceps or ventouse extractor.

- When occipitoposterior or transverse position causes delay in the second stage the following procedures should be adopted:
  - if the presenting part of the fetus is low down assist delivery by rotation to occipitoanterior or posterior position depending on the pelvic type and ease of manoeuvre

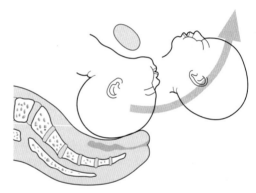

Figure 19.7 Delivery of head in mentoanterior by flexion.

  - if the presenting part of the fetus is at the midcavity, conduct a trial of forceps rotation and delivery with preparation for caesarean section in case of failure.

FACE PRESENTATION

The incidence of face presentation is 1 in 500 deliveries. The diameter for consideration is the submentobregmatic, which is 9.5 cm. The denominator is the chin or mentum which may be found in any one of eight positions (Figure 19.6). During labour the chin is the lowest point or leading part. Seventy-five per cent of face presentations are in the mentolateral or mentoanterior positions. Rotation in the lower half of the pelvis to the direct mentoanterior position usually occurs if the pelvis is adequate. The head is delivered by flexion. Assisted delivery is necessary for mentoposterior positions. Forceps rotation may be tried, but

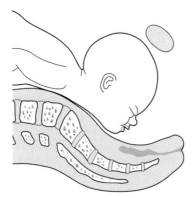

Figure 19.8   Face presentation provides a situation for a low presenting part with the impression of a non-engaged head.

caesarean section is usually required for delivery (Figure 19.7).

Types

* Primary: face presentation before the onset of labour.
* Secondary: face presentation during the course of labour.

Diagnosis

Primary face
This is diagnosed when there is a non-engaged head, the head feels large or when the extended head is felt on the same side of the uterus as the fetal back. Radiology or ultrasound scanning is carried out to confirm suspicion. Assess adequacy of pelvis and exclude any abnormalities (fetal and maternal).

Secondary face
Suspect this diagnosis if the presenting part of the fetus appears low yet a large part of the head is palpable suprapubically. The eyes, nose, supraorbital and alveolar ridges, and the mouth can be felt on vaginal examination. Unlike the anus, the mouth does not grip the examining finger and firm fetal gums are felt. Ultrasound scan can confirm the diagnosis (Figure 19.8).

Management

* Exclude any abnormalities. An ultrasound scan is useful.
* Assess carefully the size of the fetus and the pelvis. The face does not mould and safe vaginal delivery is not likely unless pelvic diameters are ideal.

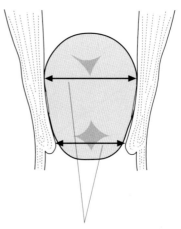

Figure 19.9   Schematic illustration of presentation of diameter 9.5 cm twice to the cervix: once with submentobregmatic then with the biparietal.

* Ensure adequate analgesia; epidural analgesia is particularly useful.
* Maintain close surveillance. Fetal distress is likely because of the long labour and unfavourable neck positions.

Mentoanterior position
Labour is prolonged. The presenting part is poorly applied. The engaging diameter 9.5 cm (submento-bregmatic) is at a lower level than the biparietal (9.5 cm) diameter. The diameter of 9.5 cm is thus presented twice at 90° to the cervix (Figure 19. 9). In ideal conditions spontaneous delivery can occur. Usually an episiotomy and assistance with forceps is required for vaginal delivery. The ventouse extractor is contra-indicated. Failure to progress in the first stage of labour necessitates a caesarean section.

Mentolateral position
In an adequate pelvis, expect rotation to the mentoan-terior position and an assisted vaginal delivery. Rotation occurs at or below the level of the ischial spines. Manual or forceps rotation may be required. If the pelvic outlet is suspect or spontaneous rotation is arrested in mid-pelvis, deliver by caesarean section.

Mentoposterior position
Unless the fetus is very small or the pelvis capacious, the shoulder and vertex cannot be accommodated at the same time. Obstruction is inevitable. Attempting rotation to the mentoanterior position is seldom advised. Deliver by caesarean section. If the fetus is dead consider delivery by craniotomy and forceps (only if the operator is experienced). Facial oedema and bruising is usual.

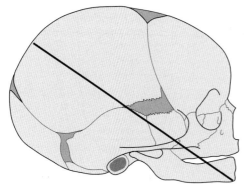

Figure 19.10 The mentovertical diameter in brow presentation.

BROW PRESENTATION

Brow presentation has an incidence of approximately 1 in 2000 or more deliveries.

Types

- Primary: presentation before labour. The position is usually transient and reverts to the occipitoposterior or face positions when labour starts. Exclude fetal abnormalities and inlet disproportion.
- Secondary: develops during labour. This usually follows deflexion of an occipitoposterior position.

Diameters for consideration

The fetus presents by the mentovertical diameter (13.5 cm) which is greater than the largest pelvic diameter of 12.5 cm (Figure 19.10).

Diagnosis

Primary brow

Abdominal palpation reveals a large non-engaged head. Exclude fetal abnormality and disproportion. Await onset of labour.

Secondary brow

Application to the cervix is poor. The presenting part may be felt high behind the bag of forewaters. The anterior fontanelle, supraorbital ridge and the nose can be felt. Confirm by ultrasound scan or radiology.

Management

- If the fetus is alive and of normal size, presentation by the brow can only be safely delivered by caesarean section. Unless practised expertise is

available, manipulative correction of the presentation is seldom justified.

- If the fetus is small or preterm, spontaneous delivery can occur. If assistance is necessary convert the brow to a face (mentoanterior) or occipitoposterior position before delivery by forceps.

COMPOUND PRESENTATION

This describes a situation when the hand or forearm accompanies the presenting part of the fetus. It is usually associated with poor application of the presenting part and a small or preterm infant in a large pelvis.

Management

- If compound presentation is found during labour, the hand can be pushed up behind the presenting part.
- If this is not possible, await full cervical dilatation, ensure adequate analgesia, disimpact the limb and deliver by forceps or ventouse extraction.
- If prolapse of the whole forearm obstructs labour, caesarean section is required.

PARIETAL PRESENTATION

In a flat pelvis the vertex engaging in the occipitolateral position will have to tilt (attitude of asynclitism) sideways to swivel past the sacral promontory and the symphysis.

Anterior asynclitism

This is when the parietal eminence in front tilts behind the symphysis. This is a favourable presentation and once the biparietal eminences swivel past the sacral promontory and symphysis, rotation to occipitoanterior or posterior is the usual course (Figure 19.11).

Posterior asynclitism

This is when the parietal eminence at the back enters the pelvis first by slipping past the sacral promontory. This is less likely to succeed because unlike anterior asynclitism in which the fetal body can lean anteriorly to assist engagement of the anterior parietal eminence, in posterior asynclitism the mother's spinal column prevents this action of the fetal body. Failure of either anterior or posterior asynclitism to engage the fetal head means that caesarean section is necessary for delivery (Figure 19.12).

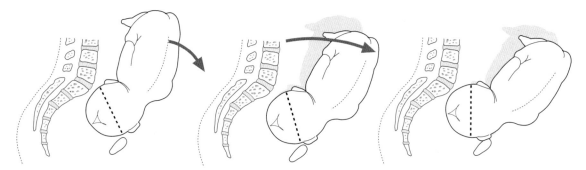

Figure 19.11   Anterior asynclitism illustrating position of fetal body to assist entry of the biparietal diameter into the pelvis.

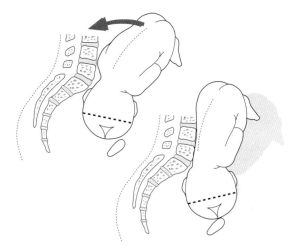

Figure 19.12   Posterior asynclitism illustrating restriction of fetal body movement to assist entry of biparietal diameter into pelvis.

Table 19.1   Causes of shoulder presentation

Maternal	Fetal
Relaxed multigravid uterus (most common cause)	Abnormality Twins
Pelvic contracture	Prematurity
Uterine abnormality	Fetal death
Obstruction by intra or extrauterine masses	Polyhydramnios Placenta praevia

Vaginal

No vaginal examination should be performed until placenta praevia is excluded. Avoid membrane rupture and risk of cord or arm prolapse. If the membranes have ruptured, examine immediately to exclude cord prolapse. The pelvis feels empty with the ilium and/or shoulder presenting. The fetal ribs give a characteristic 'washboard' feel.

SHOULDER PRESENTATION (TRANSVERSE OR OBLIQUE LIE)

In both transverse and oblique lie, the shoulder is the most common presenting part. In an oblique breech the ilium may present. The causes of shoulder presentation are listed in Table 19.1.

Diagnosis

Abdomen

The fundal height appears small for dates (unless there is multiple gestation or polyhydramnios). The uterus appears broad with fullness in the flanks. No presenting part is palpable in the pelvis. The head or breech is felt opposite the iliac crest or at right angles to the mid-line.

Prognosis

This is a dangerous situation for both the fetus and the mother. Spontaneous delivery is not possible unless the fetus is very small. The risk of cord prolapse, shoulder impaction, uterine rupture and the need for classical caesarean section all increase maternal and fetal mortality and morbidity.

Management

- The onset of labour with increased uterine tone may rectify the situation and convert an oblique to a longitudinal lie. This is most likely in a multigravid mother with a lax uterus.

- Identify the cause of malpresentation. Radiology or sonar examination is useful.

- Elective caesarean section is performed if vaginal delivery is contraindicated. This applies to the majority of primigravid mothers.

- If the mother is not in labour and vaginal delivery is suitable:
  - manoeuvre fetus (external version) to longitudinal lie. This is performed in a theatre prepared for caesarean section
  - set up intravenous oxytocin to generate and maintain uterine contractions
  - perform amniotomy, drain liquor slowly and guide the presenting part into the pelvis.

- If the mother is in early labour with ruptured membranes perform vaginal examination to exclude prolapse of the limbs or cord.

- Attempt to encourage a longitudinal lie if vaginal delivery is considered possible. If this is not successful deliver by caesarean section. A midline abdominal incision followed by a low vertical incision in the uterus is advised when fetal lie is fixed. Convert the vertical uterine incision to a classic incision if necessary.

- Impacted shoulders – whether the fetus is alive or dead, deliver by caesarean section. Destructive procedures in inexperienced hands may result in uterine rupture.

- Spontaneous expulsion of the fetus can only occur if the fetus is macerated or is very small.

Bibliography

Gardber GM, Tuppurainen M 1994 Persistent occiput posterior presentation – a clinical problems. Acta Obstetrica et Gynecologica Scandinavica 73: 45–47

Gardber GM, Laakkonen E, Salevarra M 1998 Sonography and persistent occiput posterior position:a study of 408 deliveries. Obstetrics and Gynecology 91: 746–749

Holmberg NG, Lilieqvist B, Magnusson S 1977 The influence of the bony pelvis in persistent occiput posterior position. Obstetrica et Gynecologica Scandinavica Supplement 66:49–54

To WW, Li IC 2000 Occipital posterior and occipital transverse positions: reappraisal of obstetric risks. Australian and New Zealand Journal of Obstetrics and Gynaecology 40:275–279

Chapter 20

Breech

David T Y Liu
Mentor: Pamela Loughna

CHAPTER CONTENTS

Diagnosis   171
  Vaginal examination   171
Classification   172
  Extended (frank)   172
  Flexed (complete or full)   172
  Footling or knee (incomplete)   172
Antenatal assessment   172
Spontaneous breech delivery   173
  Dangers in breech delivery   173
  Labour   174
  Dos and do nots with breech delivery   176
Breech in the second twin or triplet   176
Delivery by caesarean section   177
Special situations   178

The presenting part of the fetus is the breech with the sacrum as the denominator. It is more common before 28 weeks (20%) than at term (3%). Associated causes such as disproportion, obstructing pelvic masses (e.g. fibroids, ovarian cysts), uterine abnormalities (e.g. septate uterus), hydramnios, fetal prematurity or abnormalities and multiple gestation will influence the management of labour. Breech presentation is a marker for potential fetal handicap as it is more common in preterm and structurally abnormal fetuses.

DIAGNOSIS

- The fetal head is palpated above the umbilicus.
- Fetal heart sounds are heard most easily above the umbilicus, or if heard suprapubically, the heart sound becomes louder as one progresses towards the uterine fundus.
- Fetal movements are felt maximally away from the fundus.
- Diagnosis is confirmed by ultrasonography or vaginal examination (provided placenta praevia is excluded).

Vaginal examination

- Palpate the soft buttocks and three firm areas: the fetal sacrum and two ischial tuberosities.
- In labour, once the membranes are ruptured, the baby's feet may be felt. Differentiate from the hand by feeling five even-length digits at the end of the limb and by recognising the heel.
- Unlike the mouth, the fetal anus, when gently depressed, will grip the examining finger. Meconium may be present when the finger is withdrawn.

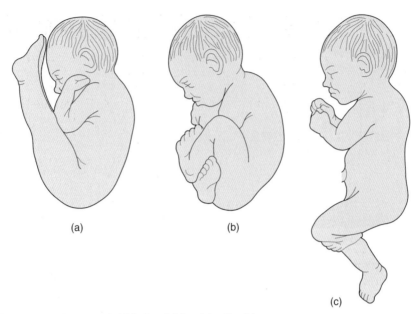

Figure 20.1   Breech presentation: extended (a), flexed (b) and footling (c).

CLASSIFICATION

The presentation is governed by the position of the lower limbs. Sometimes the lie may be more oblique than longitudinal.

Extended (frank) (Figure 20.1a)

This is the most common, occurring in 75% of primigravid and 50% of multigravid breeches. Good application to the cervix is possible but the extended legs may act as splints affecting the lateral flexion of the body. Delivery of the legs requires assistance.

Flexed (complete or full) (Figure 20.1b)

This occurs mainly in multigravid women with good pelvic diameters or in multiple gestation. There is a risk of cord prolapse. Spontaneous or easy delivery of lower limbs is likely.

Footling or knee (incomplete) (Figure 20.1c)

This is uncommon. There is poor application to the cervix, hence a higher risk of cord prolapse. It may indicate difficulty in engagement, thus delivery by caesarean section is recommended.

ANTENATAL ASSESSMENT

- Confirm presentation by ultrasound. This will permit description of the type of breech presentation. Vaginal delivery is acceptable only for frank or complete breech.

- Perform ultrasound biometry to gain an estimated fetal weight. Check for fetal abnormality, liquor volume and placental site. Exclude hyperextension of the fetal head.

- If gestation is uncomplicated, 37 weeks or more and not in labour, offer external cephalic version (ECV) (see Box 20.1). This involves turning the baby to a cephalic presentation by gentle manual rotation, with or without tocolysis. If the procedure is performed on a Rhesus negative woman, anti-D should be administered. ECV is most likely to be successful in a flexed breech that is not engaged in the pelvis, when liquor is adequate and in multiparous women. Facilities for immediate caesarean section must be available. Epidural anaesthesia can increase success rates of ECV.

- If ECV is declined or unsuccessful, the mode of delivery needs to be discussed. Factors which should be considered include the estimated fetal weight, clinical pelvimetry, relative risks of caesarean section versus vaginal breech delivery (see below), and the woman's informed options.

- ECV for preterm breech is not justified.

- In preterm breech delivery seek informed opinion of the woman and her partner to determine mode of delivery. There is insufficient evidence to support use of caesarean section for all preterm deliveries.

- Where appropriate vaginal delivery of the non-vertex second twin is acceptable.

Box 20.1   External cephalic version (ECV)

- Vaginal term breech delivery is associated with perinatal mortality and morbidity rates between 1% and 2%. The calculated excess risk of neonatal death is about 4 per 1000. Some 70% of term breeches are delivered by caesarean section.

- Between 60% and 70% (range 50–80%) ECV at term are successful. Up to 75% of these can deliver vaginally in cephalic presentation. ECV can reduce the overall caesarean section rate by 1%.

Contraindications
- Intrauterine growth restriction
- Multiple pregnancies
- Maternal obstetric complications
- Fetal compromise
- Oligohydramnios (amniotic fluid below 5 cm)
- Polyhydramnios (amniotic fluid over 25 cm)
- High body mass index
- Previous caesarean section
- Established labour or ruptured membranes
- Nuchal cord
- Conditions necessitating caesarean section

Procedure for ECV
1. Ensure gestation is 37 or more weeks.
2. Provide detail counselling. Obtain consent.
3. Perform ultrasound scan and exclude contraindications
4. Obtain cardiotocographic trace.
5. Dispense tocolytic (ritodrine 0.3 mg intravenously 2–3 minutes) if necessary.
6. Check maternal heart rate is less than 120 beats per minute if ritodrine is used.
7. Place the woman in a 30° lateral tilt.
8. Use gentle pressure to direct fetal head into pelvis. Apply pressure for 5 minutes at each attempt. Auscultate to check heart rate. Abandon procedure if the woman complains of discomfort.

Post procedure
1. Administer anti-D (500 IU) for Rhesus negative mothers (up to 5% small feto-maternal bleeds) if indicated by Kleihauer test.
2. Repeat ultrasound scan and trace fetal heart rate for 30 minutes (some 8% may show transient fetal heart rate changes). If trace suspicious ensure further monitoring.
3. Mother can go home if there is no complication.
4. Perform check scan in a week to determine fetal presentation and lie.
5. If ECV failed re-discuss mode of delivery. There is a place for elective caesarean section as vaginal delivery is more hazardous.

SPONTANEOUS BREECH DELIVERY

The widest part of the pelvic brim is usually the transverse diameter whereas the anteroposterior diameter is the widest part of the pelvic outlet. In spontaneous delivery the three fetal diameters, the bitrochanteric, bisacromial and anteroposterior of the fetal head, enter in sequence through the pelvic brim in the transverse or oblique diameter and are then guided by the levator ani muscles to fit the anteroposterior diameter of the outlet (see Figure 20.3).

The breech enters the pelvis with the trochanters aligned in the transverse or oblique diameter of the brim. Rotation takes place so the bitrochanteric diameter delivers through the anteroposterior diameter of the outlet. Once delivered, the breech rotates to the sacroanterior position so that the shoulders enter in the transverse diameter of the brim. Internal rotation allows the delivery of the shoulders in the anteroposterior position of the outlet and the passage of the head through the brim in the occipitolateral position. Following delivery of the shoulders (anterior shoulder delivers first) aided by lateral flexion of the trunk, the sacrum again rotates anteriorly so the posteroanterior diameter of the head (with the occiput beneath the symphysis pubis) delivers by flexion in the anteroposterior diameter of the pelvis. Figure 20.2 shows the possible positions of breech presentation.

Figure 20.3a shows the delivery of the breech and rotation of the sacrum anteriorly to assist the entry of the shoulders through the brim whereas Figure 20.3b shows the restitution of the sacrum to the lateral position to allow the shoulders to deliver in the anteroposterior diameter of the pelvic outlet. Meanwhile the fetal head enters the transverse diameter of the brim. Figure 20.3c shows that after delivery of the shoulders the back rotates to the anterior position again to allow anteroposterior diameters of the fetal head to deliver through the anteroposterior diameter of the outlet.

Dangers in breech delivery

- Perinatal morbidity and mortality is up to nine times higher than that for spontaneous vertex delivery. The incidence of trauma and hypoxic damage is particularly high in the small preterm babies (under 1.5 kg) and in big babies (over 3.5 kg). It must be remembered that more preterm and abnormal babies present by the breech.

- The likelihood of cord prolapse (5%) and cord compression is increased.

- The head is the widest and least compressible part of the fetus. The head may be trapped if the cervix is not fully dilated (especially in preterm infants) or if there is outlet contracture of the pelvis leading to hypoxia. There is little or no time for moulding hence the pelvic diameters must be more than just adequate to ensure safe delivery.

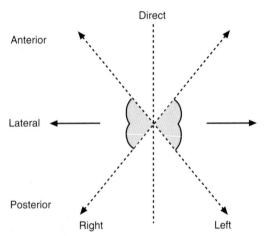

Figure 20.2   Breech presentation in the eight positions of right and left sacroanterior, lateral and posterior together with direct sacroanterior and posterior.

- There is an increased likelihood of placental separation in the second stage because of traction on the cord.

- There is increased maternal risk. If an epidural anaesthetic is not in place there is increased requirement for general anaesthesia. Assistance with delivery is more likely (see Box 20.2 for assisted breech delivery).

There is an increasing trend for breeches to be delivered by elective caesarean section, with the result that the number of operators skilled in vaginal delivery are reduced. However, the steps employed in the delivery of a breech at caesarean section are similar to those employed in vaginal delivery hence caesarean section deliveries provide some teaching opportunities.

Labour

- Careful monitoring of fetal wellbeing and progress of labour are important. Direct fetal heart rate monitoring is feasible by the application of a fetal scalp electrode to the fetal buttock, taking care to avoid the external genitalia.

- Cord compression or cord entanglement is more common. Cord compression patterns are therefore likely. Fetal blood sampling can be performed if indicated, with the region around the ischial tuberosity being the best site for blood sampling. It is often necessary to press the blade firmer to ensure a flow of capillary blood.

- Epidural anaesthesia may facilitate maternal co-operation during the second stage.

- Induction and augmentation of labour is acceptable in selected situations.

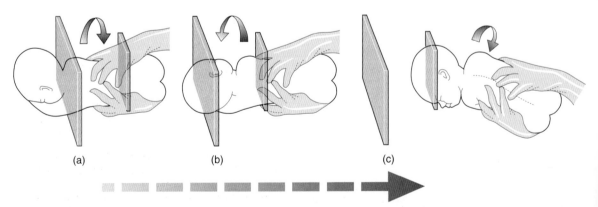

Figure 20.3   Geometric representation of breech delivery through the wide transverse/oblique diameter at the brim and the anteroposterior of the outlet. Delivery of the bitrochanteric (a), the bisacromial (b) and sagittal suture (c) as shown in sequence.

Box 20.2   Assisted breech delivery

- It is useful for the operator to have an assistant who is scrubbed.
- Most breech deliveries require minimal gentle assistance by the operator.
- The woman should be placed in the lithotomy position, with her bottom just overlapping the edge of the bed. She should be encouraged to push as for vertex presentation.
- An episiotomy is usually necessary, but should not be performed until the fetal anus is visible on the perineum.
- If there is any delay in spite of good maternal effort apply gentle groin traction. The operator's fingers must be directed into the groin to avoid fracturing the thigh or dislocating the hips (Figure 20.4a).
- Allow the trunk to deliver in the sacrolateral position until the tip of the anterior scapula appears beneath the symphysis. The operator should support the breech rather than apply traction.
- The legs will deliver spontaneously or readily with a little help. For extended legs deliver the anterior leg first (Figure 20.4b). Abduct the thigh, flex the knee, secure the foot and guide it out of the pelvis by bringing it across the fetal trunk. Repeat this manoeuvre for the posterior leg. Free a loop of cord to avoid tension on it.
- Place a towel or dry cloth over the baby's pelvis to prevent the hand slipping. Grasp the pelvis with both hands. Place the hands low down to avoid damage to the fetal liver or spleen. The thumbs are placed over the sacrum.
- Apply Lovset's manoeuvre to deliver the arms. Firm downward traction is applied while rotating the fetal

trunk through 180° to bring the posterior shoulder to lie anteriorly. When the elbow appears beneath the symphysis, that arm and hand is delivered by sweeping it across the fetal body. While maintaining gentle downward traction rotate 180° in the reverse direction to deliver the second shoulder. These manoeuvres may need to be repeated.

- Figure 20.5a shows Lovset's manoeuvre to deliver the posterior shoulder, and Figure 20.5b,c show

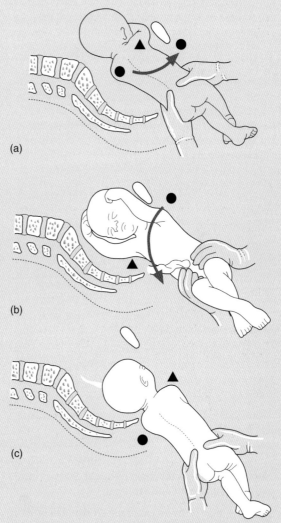

(a)

(b)

(c)

Figure 20.5 Lovset's manoeuvre to deliver the arms. The technique depends on the presence of a short symphysis in spite of a long curved sacrum. Rotation through 180° and traction delivers the posterior shoulder (a), second rotation (b) in reverse direction delivers the anterior shoulder (c). Repeat manoeuvre if necessary.

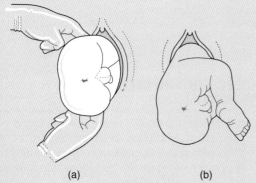

(a)   (b)

Figure 20.4 Groin traction (a) and delivery of anterior leg (b).

Box 20.2 *Continued*

delivery of the anterior shoulder. Lovset's manoeuvre depends on a short symphysis and a long curved sacrum. Traction and 180° rotation delivers the point (●). Further traction and reverse rotation through 180° delivers point (▲).

- Once the shoulders are delivered maintain progress by gentle traction on the ankles with both hands, until the hairline appears. Raise legs through an arc until the body is vertical to the maternal spine. This technique (Burns–Marshall) flexes the fetal head and places it in the anteroposterior diameter of the pelvic outlet (Figure 20.6). The baby's head may deliver spontaneously with this manoeuvre so care should be taken to anticipate delivery.

- If the head is not delivered, clear airways. Suck out the pharynx first. Forceps can be applied directly to assist the delivery of the head (after-coming head) (Figure 20.7). Mauriceau–Smellie–Veit manoeuvre may be used as alternative method for delivery of the fetal head (Figure 20.8).

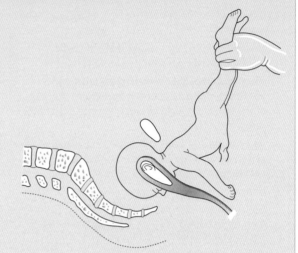

Figure 20.7 Delivery of the after-coming head with forceps.

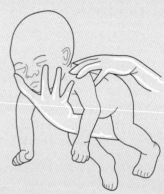

Figure 20.8 Placement of hands in the Mauriceau–Smellie–Veit technique. The baby's body is straddled on the forearm with index and middle fingers placed on malar processes to encourage flexion. Place free hand over shoulders, allowing middle finger to press on the occiput to assist flexion. Apply downward pressure and lift body upwards when occiput appears beneath symphysis to deliver the face, brow and vertex.

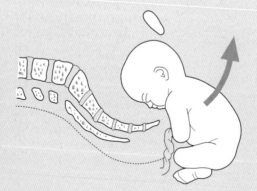

Figure 20.6 Burns–Marshall technique. Grasp legs, apply gentle traction, lift through an arc.

- Suboptimal care is the most frequent cause of intrapartum fetal death and stillbirth.

- Delivery must be by an experienced member of staff. Maintain competence by breech delivery drills.

Dos and do nots with breech delivery

Box 20.3 summarises the dos and do nots of breech delivery

BREECH IN THE SECOND TWIN OR TRIPLET

- It is acceptable to deliver the breech second twin vaginally if conditions are satisfactory.
- After delivery of the first twin the assistant places the breech or non-vertex positions into longitudinal lie (external version).
- Ensure continuing uterine contractions with an oxytocin (Syntocinon) infusion if necessary. If the

Box 20.3   The dos and don'ts of breech delivery

Do

- Learn how to deliver a breech. To perform a caesarean section just because the second twin is a breech is bad obstetric practice.

- Follow the dictum – breech plus obstetric complication justifies caesarean section.

- Use lithotomy position. The woman's bottom should just overlap the edge of the bed. Have serum grouped and saved. Both the anaesthetist and the paediatrician should be present before delivery commences.

- If the woman wishes a vaginal delivery and clinical measurements are suspect request pelvimetry (magnetic resonance imaging (MRI)) or a computed tomography (CT) scan.

- Consider delivery of the preterm breech (<1500 g) or a fetus with an estimated fetal weight of more than 3500 g by caesarean section. The perinatal mortality doubles with vaginal breech deliveries over 3600 g and increases with increasing weight. Below 1500 g the mortality is halved if caesarean section is used.

- Vaginal breech deliveries must be managed to minimise risk of hypoxia. Once the breech is delivered to the umbilicus the rest of the fetus should be delivered in 10 minutes or less. Monitor the fetal heart rate closely during all breech deliveries.

- Perform a vaginal examination once the membranes have ruptured to exclude cord prolapse.

- Realise that, although descent of the presenting part may be slow, in an adequate pelvis total labour time should be similar to that in cephalic presentation.

- Observe progress of the labour carefully if oxytocics are used. Augmentation of labour without due care is associated with increased perinatal mortality and morbidity.

- Consider a caesarean section for dysfunctional uterine activity associated with breech presentation.

Do not

- Do not conduct trial of labour in a breech if pelvis diameters are suspect. Caesarean section is the safest mode of delivery in such cases.

- Do not attempt delivery without some experience or without supervision by an experienced obstetrician.

- Do not let the breech hang from the vulva after delivery of the shoulders. This procedure is of little value and increases the risk of hypoxic insult to the fetus.

- Delay in descent of the breech after full cervical dilatation (i.e. delay in the second stage) is an indication for caesarean section. Do not use oxytocics. Breech extraction is rarely justified, except in the delivery of a second twin which is equal or smaller in size compared with the first twin.

- Do not attempt breech extraction unless experienced.

- Do not apply traction on the jaws in the Mauriceau–Smellie–Veit technique as dislocation or fracture of the mandible may result.

---

breech is at the level of the ischial spine or lower, rupture the membranes between contractions and allow the liquor to drain.
- Spontaneous breech delivery is anticipated in the next few contractions.
- If the breech is high in the pelvis or still in an oblique position, rupture the membranes, locate and bring the anterior leg down (internal podalic version, see Figure 20.9)
- Delivery is accomplished by breech extraction in which the obstetrician actively passes the breech through the steps required for delivery.

DELIVERY BY CAESAREAN SECTION

- Check that the breech is in longitudinal lie.

- For a footling breech first deliver the anterior then the posterior leg.

- In a flexed or extended breech, the baby's bottom is lifted out through the uterine incision with the breech in the sacrolateral position. Groin traction is then applied to deliver the trunk until the tip of the anterior scapula is visible. Extended legs are delivered as previously described.

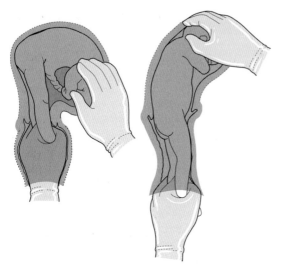

Figure 20.9   Internal podalic version.

- Lovset's technique is used to deliver the arms.

- After delivery of the arms the obstetrician faces the woman's head and places the baby in longitudinal lie with the back uppermost. The ankles are grasped and while tension is maintained the trunk is directed through a 90° arc similar to the Burns–Marshall technique. Do not hyperflex the neck. Clear the airways.

- While one hand holds the baby in the upright position, the baby's head can be lifted out with the free hand. If difficulty is encountered the assistant holds the breech while Wrigley's forceps are applied directly to the after-coming head to effect delivery.

- In preterm infants of 30 weeks' or less gestation the fetal head may be considerably larger than the trunk. The lower uterine segment is poorly formed and a transverse incision in the lower segment of the uterus may not be adequate for atraumatic delivery of the preterm breech. The low vertical uterine incision (Krönig's incision) is advised. Classical caesarean section may be considered.

SPECIAL SITUATIONS

- The cervix is not fully dilated – this usually occurs in preterm deliveries. Deliver by firm downward traction with the baby's back uppermost. Digital pressure on the malar processes assists flexion. Consider using forceps. In extreme circumstances, it may be necessary to cut the cervix at 10 and 2 o'clock positions (avoiding the lateral blood vessels)

> **Box 20.4   Preterm breech**
>
> - 25% incidence between 24 weeks' and 32 weeks' gestation.
>
> - Higher incidence of congenital abnormality, poor growth, lower fetoplacental ratio and perinatal complications.
>
> - Perform ultrasound scan to confirm diagnosis, exclude congenital abnormality, assess fetal weight and check placental site.
>
> - Determine if delivery is imminent, essential or can be delayed by tocolytics for corticosteroid administration or transfer to specialist centres.
>
> - Discuss fully options, risks and merits of delivery modes with women and their partners.
>
> - Occipital disasters with resultant cerebellar damage; intra or periventricular damage following haemorrhage or ischaemia, trauma to body, limbs and internal organs can occur with vaginal delivery or caesarean section.
>
> - Deliveries should be attended by an experienced obstetrician, anaesthetist and paediatrician.
>
> - Vaginal delivery needs particular attention to umbilical cord prolapse (especially if footling breech presentation) and incomplete cervical dilatation trapping fetal head (delivery by flexion of the head or rarely cervical incisions at 10 and 2 o'clock or 4 and 8 o'clock. Use of forceps for the after-coming head is controversial.
>
> - Caesarean section may need a lower segment midline incision (Krönig's or DeLee's incision) or classic section because the lower uterine segment is poorly formed. Women must be made aware of increase morbidity following midline or classic section and need for repeat caesarean section to avoid threat of uterine rupture.
>
> - Competency of neonatal support must be considered when mode of delivery is discussed.

using scissors. The cervix is sutured after delivery is completed.

- When there is disproportion of the fetal head, e.g. in the hydrocephalic baby, vaginal delivery can be achieved after decompression of the head. If the baby is normal and alive, symphysiotomy or caesarean section are the only avenues for a live birth.

- Face to pubes position – gently rotate the baby through 180° to bring the occiput to the anterior position and deliver as previously described. If the head is well down rotation may exert too much pressure on the fetal neck. Apply forceps to the head after the Burns–Marshall manoeuvre.

Box 20.4 describes the management of preterm breech.

Bibliography

Bewley S, Robson SC, Smith M, et al 1993 The introduction of external cephalic version at term into routine clinical practice. European Journal of Obstetrics, Gynecology and Reproductive Biology 82: 306–312

Bingham P, Lilford RJ 1987 Management of the selected term breech presentation: assessment of the risk of selective vaginal delivery versus Caesarean section for all cases. Obstetrics and Gynaecology 69:965–978

Cheng M, Hannah M 1993 Breech delivery at term: a critical review of the literature. Obstetric and Gynaecology 82:605–618

Danielian PJ, Wang J, Hall MH 1996 Long term outcome by method of delivery of breech presentation at term: population-based follow up. BMJ 312:1451

Grant A, Glazener CMA 2005 Elective caesarean section versus expectant management for delivery of the small baby. Cochrane Database of Systematic Reviews, Issue 1

Hannah ME, Hannah WJ, Hewson SA et al 2000 Planned Caesarean section versus planned vaginal birth for breech presentation at term: a randomised multicentre trial. Lancet 356:1375–1383

Hofmeyr GJ 1991 ECV at term; how high the stakes? British Journal of Obstetrics and Gynaecology 93:1–3

Hofmeyr GJ, Hannah MG 2005 Planned caesarean section for term breech delivery. Cochrane Database of Systematic Reviews, Issue 1

Hofmeyr GJ, Kulier R 2005 External cephalic version for breech presentation at term Cochrane Database Systematic Review, Issue 1

Hytten FE 1982 Breech presentation is it a bad omen? British Journal of Obstetrics and Gynaecology 89:879–880

Laros RK, Dattel BJ 1988 Management of twin pregnancy: the vaginal route is still safe. American Journal of Obstetrics and Gynaecology 158:1330–1338

Lau TK, Lo KWK, Wan D et al 1997 The implementation of external cephalic version at term for singleton breech presentation – how can we further increase its impact? Australian and New Zealand Journal of Obstetrics and Gynaecology 27:393–396

Mancuso KM, Yancey MK, Murphy JA et al 2000 Epidural analgesia for cephalic version: a randomised trial. Obstetrics and Gynaecology 95:648–651

1995 Recommendations of the International Federation of Gynaecology and Obstetrics (FIGO) Committee on perinatal health on guidelines for the management of breech delivery. European Journal of Obstetrics, Gynaecology and Reproductive Biology 58:89–92

Rosen MG, Debanne S, Thompson K et al 1985 Long term neurological morbidity in breech and vertex births. 151:718–720

Royal College of Obstetricians and Gynaecologists 1998 Pelvimetry – Clinical Indications. Guideline Number 14. London RCOG Press

Saunders NJ St G 1996 Breech delivery in the United Kingdom at the end of this century. Contemporary Review in Obstetrics and Gynaecology 8:82–85

Society of Obstetricians and Gynaecologists of Canada 1994 Policy statement: the Canadian consensus on breech management at term. Journal of the Society of Obstetricians and Gynaecologists of Canada 16:1839–1858

Viegas OAC, Ingemarsson I, Low PS et al 1985 Collaborative study on preterm breeches: vaginal delivery versus Caesarean section. Asia Oceania Journal of Obstetrics and Gynaecology 11:349–355

Wallace RL, Schifrin, BS, Paul RH 1984 The delivery route for very low birthweight infants. Journal of Reproductive Medicine 29:736–740

Wigglesworth JS, Husemeyer RP (1977) Intra cranial birth trauma in vaginal breech delivery: the continued importance of injury to the occipital bone. British Journal of Obstetrics and Gynaecology 84:684–691

Chapter 21

Twins and multiple deliveries

David T Y Liu

CHAPTER CONTENTS

Types   181
   Monozygotic or monochorionic twins   181
   Dizygotic twins   181
   Other multiples   182
Diagnosis   182
Presentation at delivery   182
   Frequency of combinations of presentation   182
Complications of twin pregnancy and delivery   182
   First twin   182
   Second twin   182
Vaginal delivery or caesarean section   183
Surveillance in labour   184
Special problems   184
   Conjoined twins   184
   Undiagnosed second twin   184
   Locked twins   184
   Triplets and higher multiples   185
   Antepartum fetal death of one twin   185

Multiple pregnancy is the term used when there is more than one fetus in the uterine cavity. Twins describes two fetuses, triplets for three fetuses and so on. The incidence of twinning is 40 per 1000 births for West Africans, 12 per 1000 for Caucasians and 6 per 1000 for Asians. The twinning rate is higher in fertile and older multiparous women. The advent of assisted fertility therapy has increased the incidence of multiple pregnancies.

TYPES

Monozygotic or monochorionic twins (uniovular/monovular/identical)

These are produced when one ovum divides to form two fetuses (Figure 21.1a). They can be dichorionic diamniotic, monochorionic diamniotic or monochorionic monoamniotic. The monozygotic twinning rate of 3–5 per 1000 is similar for all ethnic groups (the fetal sex is always the same). Complications such as hydramnios, fetal abnormality, discrepancy in fetal weight and fetal transfusion syndrome, are more likely, as are intrapartum complications and poor perinatal outcome. When one twin dies in utero there is a 25% risk of neurological and renal lesions and even intrauterine death in the survivor.

Dizygotic twins (binovular, non-identical)

With dizygotic twins, two ova are shed, usually in the same menstrual cycle and fertilised by two different sperms (Figure 21.1b). The fetal sex can differ. Twinning rate differs in different ethnic groups and is influenced by the use of fertility drugs to induce ovulation.

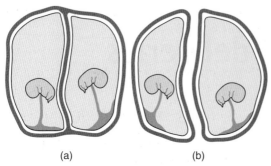

Figure 21.1   Monozygotic twins (a) and dizygotic twins (b).

(a)   (b)

Other multiples

These are seldom monovular, they usually follow multiple ovulation or combinations of monovular and multiple ovulation.

DIAGNOSIS

Diagnosis before delivery is important. Undiagnosed twins present additional risks to the mother and to the second fetus.

Perform ultrasound scans for all mothers with a family history of twins or where fertility drugs have been prescribed. The following factors should alert the obstetrician to the possibility of twin pregnancy:

- The uterus is large for dates or there is a history of acute hydramnios (complicates 12% of twin pregnancies).

- The mother describes fetal movement felt all over the uterus.

- Palpation of more than two fetal poles (head and breech), a small head in a large uterus or multiple fetal parts.

- Simultaneous detection of two fetal heart beats with rates differing by 10 beats or more per minute.

- Preterm labour where the uterus is larger than dates. Twins are five times more likely to be born preterm than singletons especially before 32 weeks.

- When multiple pregnancy is suspected confirm by sonar scanning. Undiagnosed twins are unlikely when there are programmes of routine antenatal ultrasound scanning. Chronicity should be determined. This is 100% accurate in first trimester and 80–90% in mid-trimester.

PRESENTATION AT DELIVERY

Malpresentation and malposition especially in the second twin are common hence the high incidence of assisted or operative deliveries. In 75% the first twin presents by the vertex, but abnormal presentation occurs in over 50% of twin deliveries.

Frequency of combinations of presentation

- Vertex/vertex – 45%
- Vertex/breech – 25%
- Breech/vertex – 10%
- Breech/breech – 9%
- Vertex/transverse – 11%
- Breech/transverse – 11%
- Transverse/transverse – 11%

COMPLICATIONS OF TWIN PREGNANCY AND DELIVERY

Pre-eclampsia (20%) uterine atony, anaemia and a large placenta increase the likelihood of postpartum haemorrhage. Cross-match and reserve blood when the woman is admitted into the labour ward. An increased rate of congenital abnormalities (twice as common and include cardiac anomalies, bowel atresia, neural tube defects) intrauterine growth retardation (30%) and preterm labour and delivery (10% before 34 weeks, 40% before 37 weeks) contribute to the higher perinatal mortality of 3–5%. Up to three-quarters of perinatal losses are due to delivery before 34 weeks. Compared with singleton pregnancies cerebral palsy is eight times greater in twin and 47 times greater in triplet pregnancies.

First twin

First twin has a higher perinatal mortality than with singleton births because of prematurity, cord prolapse, fetal abnormality and birth injury (double the singleton rates).

Second twin

With the second twin malpositions, malpresentations, prolonged delivery interval, likelihood of placental separation and greater need for operative delivery result in lower Apgar scores. The neonatal mortality, mainly due to birth trauma, is twice that of the first twin. The danger of hypoxia increases the risk of cerebral palsy in the second twin.

In general the perinatal mortality rate of twins is four to five times that of singletons. Mortality due to asphyxia is five times that of singletons. Risk of still-birth between 37 and 42 weeks is 6–9 per 1000 births. Induction at 38 weeks is advised.

VAGINAL DELIVERY OR CAESAREAN SECTION

The high incidence of prematurity together with the risk of hypoxia and damage in the second twin mean that vaginal delivery is only safe when conditions are ideal. Accurate knowledge of gestational dates and the fetal weight is important. Ultrasound examination forewarns of fetal abnormalities. A lateral erect pelvimetry or better still magnetic resonance imaging of the pelvis is advised if clinical pelvic assessment suggests reduced pelvic diameters. In general vaginal delivery is preferred for vertex–vertex presentation.

Vaginal delivery may be contemplated if:

* there is no obstetric complication.
* reliable monitoring of both fetal heart rates is achieved.

* gestation is 32 weeks or the fetal weight is 1500 g or more.

Caesarean section is advisable if:

* there are obstetric complications or evidence of poor intrauterine growth, particularly in the second twin.
* the first twin is in a breech presentation and/or gestation is less than 32 weeks.
* there is abnormal presentation of the first twin.
* maternal pelvic diameters are reduced.
* after a previous caesarean section.

For the breech second twin, if acceptable to the informed woman, vaginal breech delivery is only advised if conditions are suitable and an experienced obstetrician is present. Likewise for the non-vertex second twin internal podalic version followed by breech extraction when conditions are suitable is the advised primary procedure. Elective caesarean section is a recognised option.

Box 21.1 describes the procedure for delivery.

Box 21.1   Delivery of twins

* Place the woman in the lithotomy position with a left lateral tilt.

* Forceps and ventouse extractor should be available, especially if the second twin presents by the vertex.

* Consider an intravenous drip with oxytocin (Syntocinon) (e.g. 5 units in 500 ml of normal saline).

* An episiotomy is usually advisable.

* Maintain continuous monitoring of the second twin in the second stage.

* Deliver the first twin in the normal fashion for vertex position. If presentation is occipitoposterior, rotation to occipitoanterior may be difficult hence may necessitate delivery as a direct occipitoposterior presentation. The fetus is frequently smaller and delivery as a direct occipitoposterior presentation gives little difficulty.

* After delivery of the first twin clamp the cord, palpate the abdomen, and ensure that the second twin is in the longitudinal lie. Perform external version if appropriate (60% success especially with epidural anaesthesia when presenting part is in pelvis).

* Run Syntocinon at 20–40 drops/min to maintain uterine contractions.

* Perform internal podalic version if vaginal delivery is considered expeditious and appropriate. Palpate to identify lie. Locate fetal foot/feet with intrauterine hand. Grasp foot/feet and pull down steadily. Use external hand to direct lie into longitudinal. When buttocks are in the pelvis deliver as for breech. If not already ruptured, rupture membranes after foot is firmly grasped.

* If presenting parts (cephalic or breech) are well down the pelvis, rupture membranes of second sac.

* The vertex or breech presentation usually delivers readily with the next few contractions. A delivery interval of longer than 30 minutes between the first and second twin increases the latter's perinatal mortality and morbidity.

* When cord prolapse or heavy intrapartum bleeding occurs after delivery of the first twin, expeditious breech extraction or if vertex application of a ventouse extractor can bring the head into the pelvis.

* Deliver the placenta by controlled cord traction. Assess carefully the total amount of blood loss and ensure the uterus is well contracted. Delivery of the first placenta before the second twin, if not associated with bleeding, need not cause anxiety.

* Repair the episiotomy, replace blood if necessary and continue with Syntocinon if the uterus shows any tendency to relax.

* Examine the placenta for chorionicity.

Box 21.2   Points to consider in delivery of twins

Do

- Nurse the woman on her side as supine hypotension is more common with the larger uterus.

- Do consider epidural anaesthesia. This will facilitate manipulative delivery for the second twin.

- Ensure anaesthetist, paediatrician and experienced obstetrician are present for the delivery.

- Assess carefully if progress of labour is slow. The total length of labour should not be prolonged. Twin pregnancies enter labour with more cervical dilatation and hence a shorter latent phase; however the active phase may be lengthened.

- Consider intravenous Syntocinon to ensure adequate uterine activity and it should be available for use after delivery of the first twin.

- Assess carefully the suitability for vaginal delivery by considering the weaker fetus and the biggest twin.

- Use different clamps on the cords to identify first from second twin.

Do not

- Do not miss the diagnosis of twins. Undiagnosed twins impose unnecessary risk for the mother and fetuses.

- Avoid having to perform caesarean section for the second twin after vaginal delivery of the first twin. Proper assessment of suitability for vaginal delivery should obviate this complication. Some 5% of second twins are delivered by caesarean section after vaginal delivery of the first twin. Reasons for this include fetal distress in the second twin, cord prolapse, transverse lie of the second twin or the second twin remaining as a high breech.

- If the second twin is presenting by breech and is much larger than the first twin deliver by caesarean section. The partially dilated cervix which allowed delivery of the smaller first twin may present difficulty and delay delivery of the larger second breech. A compromise is cephalic version and delivery with a ventouse extractor.

- If the first twin is presenting by the breech consider delivery by caesarean section.

- For the extremely premature second twin consider delay if appropriate to dispense steroids.

SURVEILLANCE IN LABOUR

Monitoring the fetal heart rate by scalp electrode for the first twin and by ultrasound for the second twin is the current most satisfactory way of intrapartum surveillance. Fetal blood sampling should be performed to assess signs of distress in the first twin. Clear signs of fetal distress in the second twin necessitate delivery by caesarean section. Deliver by caesarean section if continuous monitoring of the second twin proves difficult.

Box 21.2 lists further points to consider in delivery of twins.

SPECIAL PROBLEMS

Conjoined twins

Suspect this condition when both fetuses are always at the same level and presentation. During labour conjoined twins may present as failure to progress. Radiology or ultrasound scan will help make the diagnosis. Delivery is by a midline abdominal incision and classic caesarean section.

Undiagnosed second twin

Oxytocics may have been given before a diagnosis of twin pregnancy is made. The fetus is endangered because of the contracting uterus and the reduced placental blood supply.

- Correct the lie and rupture the membranes.
- Forceps/ventouse for a vertex presentation or a breech extraction is the most expeditious mode of delivery.
- If the fetus is alive and trapped by an undilated cervix deliver by caesarean section.
- If the fetus is dead convert to a longitudinal lie and await vaginal delivery.

Locked twins

This occurs when the head of the first twin delivering as a breech is obstructed by the head of the second twin descending into the pelvis (incidence 1 in 600). If fetal head cannot be dislodged deliver by classic or lower segment caesarean section. Decapitation of the first dead twin can be considered. This condition can be avoided if all first twin breeches are delivered by elective caesarean section but if criteria are correct vaginal delivery need not be contraindicated.

Triplets and higher multiples

The increased risk to the fetus of prematurity, hypoxia and trauma with manipulative delivery supports the use of caesarean section for all deliveries. The placenta covers a large proportion of the uterus, hence placental damage during incision of the uterus is likely with resultant fetal blood loss. Reserve a unit of O negative blood to anticipate need for fetal transfusion. Compared with singleton pregnancies perinatal morbidity

and mortality, rates of low birthweight and cerebral palsy are much increased.

Antepartum fetal death of one twin

This may occur as in the twin–twin transfusion syndrome. The surviving twin may suffer cerebral and renal lesions and is at risk of intrauterine death. After 20 weeks, death of one twin may result in 20% risk of death in surviving twin with 4% morbidity if dichorionic and 30% morbidity if monochorionic. Expect and encourage parents to grieve loss of one of the twins. Parents should know fetal complications may exist before delivery.

Bibliography

Adam C, Alexander CA, Vaskett TF 1991 Twin delivery: influence of the presentation and method of delivery on the second twin. American Journal of Obstetrics and Gynecology 165:23–27

Caulkwell S, Murphy DJ 2002 The effect of mode of delivery and gestational age on neonatal outcome of the non-cephalic presenting second twin. American Journal of Obstetrics and Gynecology 187:1356–1361

Doherty J 1988 Perinatal mortality in twins, Australia 1973–1980. Acta Geneticae Medicae et Gemellologiae 37:313–319

Feldman GB 1992 Prospective risk of stillbirth. Obstetrics and Gynaecology 79:547–553

Fusi C, Gordon H 1990 Twin pregnancy complicated by single intrauterine death: Problems and outcome with conservative management. British Journal of Obstetrics and Gynaecology 97:511–516

Gocke SE, Nageotte MP, Garite T et al 1989 Management of the non-vertex second twin: primary Caesarean section, external version, or primary breech extraction. American Journal of Obstetrics and Gynecology 161:111–114

Grant A, Glazener CMA 2003 Elective Caesarean section versus expectant management for delivery of the small baby. The Cochrane Library, Issue 4. Wiley, Chichester

Jeffery RL, Watson A, Bowes JR et al 1974 Role of bed rest in twin gestation. Obstetrics and Gynaecology 43:822–826

Johanson R, Cox C, Grady K et al 2002 Managing obstetric emergencies and trauma. The MOET course manual. RCOG Press, London, Chapter 25 Twin Pregnancy

Kelsick F, Minkoff H 1982 Management of the breech second twin. American Journal of Obstetrics and Gynecology 144:783–786

Kleinman JC, Fowler MC, Kessel SS 1991 Comparison of infant mortality among twins and singletons; United States 1960–1983. American Journal of Epidemiology 133:133–143

Little J, Bryan E (1986) Congenital anomalies in twins. Seminars in Perinatology 10:50–64

Newman RB, Hamer C, Millar MC 1989 Outpatient triplet management: A contemporary review. American Journal of Obstetrics and Gynaecology 161:547–555

Petrikovsky BM, Vintzilees AM 1989 Management and outcome of multiple pregnancy of high fetal order: literature review. Obstetrical and Gynecological Survey 44:578–584

Petterson B, Nelson KB, Watson L et al 1993 Twins, triplets and cerebral palsy in births in Western Australia in the 1980s. BMJ 307:1239–1243

Rabinovici J, Barhai G, Reichman B et al 1988 Internal podalic version with unruptured membranes for the second twin in transverse lie. Obstetrics and Gynecology 71:428–430

Ramsey PS, Repke JT 2003 Intrapartum management of multifetal pregnancies. Seminars in Perinatology 27:54–72

Roopnarinesingh AJ, Sirjusingh A, Bassaw B et al 2002 Vaginal breech delivery and perinatal mortality in twins. Journal of Obstetrics and Gynaecology 22:291–293

Winn HN, Cimino J, Powers J et al 2001 Intrapartum management of non-vertex second-born twins: A critical analysis. American Journal of Obstetrics and Gynecology 185:1204–1208

Wolff K 2000 Excessive use of caesarean section for the second twin? Gynecologic and Obstetric Investigation 50:28–32

Chapter **22**

Medical complications

CHAPTER CONTENTS

(i) Haematological, coagulation, respiratory and neurological disorders 188
Haematological problems 188
  Sickle cell disease 188
    Labour and delivery 188
  Thalassaemia 188
  Inherited disorders of coagulation 189
    Labour 189
  Platelet disorders 189
    Pregnancy 189
    Labour 189
Respiratory problems 190
  Asthma 190
  Respiratory problems 190
Neurological conditions 190
  Epilepsy 190
  Raised intracranial pressure 191
  Neuromuscular disease 191
    Multiple sclerosis 191
    Myasthenia gravis 191
    Myotonic dystrophy 191
(ii) Endocrine disorders 192
Adrenal insufficiency 192
  Labour and delivery 192
  Fetus 192
Thyroid 192
  Hypothyroid 192
  Thyrotoxicosis 192
  Labour and delivery 192
  Thyroid storm 192
    Management 193
  Fetus 193
Diabetes 193
  Labour and delivery 193
    Induction of labour 193

Other common insulin regimens 193
Spontaneous labour 194
Caesarean section 194
Management of women not requiring insulin 194
Post delivery 194
Fetus 194
Medical emergencies 194
(iii) Cardiac disease 195
Labour 195
  Delivery 195
Fetus 195
Acute pulmonary oedema 195
  Management 196
Myocardial infarction 196
Hypertension 196
Pre-eclampsia 196
  Management of pre-eclampsia: investigation and assessment 197
    Antihypertensive therapy 197
    Anticonvulsant therapy 197
    Fluid balance 198
    General management 198
Eclampsia 198
Renal failure 198
  Procedure 198
(iv) Infections 199
  Bacterial 199
  Maternal signs 199
  Fetal signs 199
  Bacteraemia and septic shock 199
    Organisms 199
    Symptoms 199
    Septic shock 199
    Management 199

Labour and delivery 199
Haemolytic streptococcus group B 200
  Management 200
Listerosis (*Listeria monocytogenes*) 200
  Maternal symptoms 200
  Diagnosis 200
  Management 200
Chlamydia trachomatis 200
  Diagnosis 201
  Management 201
Syphilis 201
  Diagnosis 201
  Management 201
Viral 201
  Genital herpes 201
    Diagnosis 201

Management 201
Chronic bloodborne viruses 202
  General measures 202
  Hepatitis B 202
  Hepatitis C 202
  Human immunodeficiency virus 202
  Varicella zoster (chicken pox) 203
(v) Psychiatric illness 204
  Drug misuser 204
  Opioid user 204
  Cocaine user 205
  User of benzodiapines (temazepam or
    diazepam) 205
  Amfetamine user 205
  Cannabis user 205

(i) HAEMATOLOGICAL, COAGULATION, RESPIRATORY AND NEUROLOGICAL DISORDERS

Lucy Kean

HAEMATOLOGICAL PROBLEMS

Sickle cell disease (HBSS; HBSC; HB THAL)

- Sickle cell haemoglobin (HBS) a β-chain haemoglobin which affects women from Africa, Middle East and the Indian subcontinent can present as persistent anaemia.

- Hypoxia, cold, acidosis, dehydration and infection can precipitate a sickling crisis (Box 22.1) with resultant tissue infarction and pain. Sickling crisis complicates some 35% of pregnancies. Urinary tract infection, pneumonia and puerperal sepsis are more likely. Pulmonary infection or lung infarction can cause an acute chest syndrome characterised by fever, tachypnoea, pleuritic chest pain and leucocytosis. Other causes of chest pain include pulmonary thrombosis, thromboembolism and bone marrow embolism.

Box 22.1   Management of sickling crisis

- Enlist haematologist to provide team care.
- Ensure the woman is well oxygenated, hydrated and kept warm.
- Provide adequate analgesia.
- Monitor haemoglobin levels. Transfuse if indicated.
- Treat infection.

- Obstetric complications include increased incidence of preterm labour, early-onset preeclampsia, intrauterine growth retardation and antenatal and intrapartum fetal distress. Maternal and perinatal mortality is increased four to six times and morbidity is also increased.

Labour and delivery

- Keep the woman warm, oxygenated (keep oxygen saturation at 97% and monitor by pulse oximetry) and hydrated (intravenous fluids). Maintain this support for 24 hours post partum.
- Epidural anaesthesia is appropriate.
- Perform caesarean section for obstetric indications.
- Take cord blood for electrophoresis.
- Consider prophylactic antibiotics, for example metronidazole and cephradine for 7–14 days post partum.
- Administer stockings and heparin (Fragmin 5000 units subcutaneously daily) as a prophylaxis for thromboembolism even if delivery is vaginal.

Thalassaemia

Condition affects women from areas where historically malaria was prevalent, for example South East Asia (thalassaemia A and B) Middle East, India and the Mediterranean (mainly thalassaemia B). Most women are thalassaemia B trait with anaemia as the main risk factor. (Low mean corpuscular volume and mean cell haemoglobin with normal mean corpuscular haemoglobin concentration). Diagnosis is by globin chain analysis. Active management of the third stage to limit blood loss is important.

Inherited disorders of coagulation: haemophilia, von Willebrand's disease and factor IX deficiency

von Willebrand's disease (VWD) a result of inherited deficiency in von Willebrand's factor (VWF) affects 0.8–1.3% of women. Type I (70% of VWD) women produce less VWF with resultant defect of factor VIII. Type II is associated with defective VWF and thrombocytopenia. The rare but severe type III has low levels of both VWF and factor VIII.

- Haemophilia A (deficiency in factor VIII) with a prevalence of 1 in 10000 in the population is five times more common than haemophilia B (deficiency in factor IX).
- Inheritance of haemophilia is through sex linkage with carrier women having factor VIII or IX levels about 50% of normal.
- Bleeding can occur when levels are below 50% of normal and severity of bleeding is proportional to the degree of deficiency.
- Factor VIII levels tend to rise in pregnancy, as does von Willebrand's factor.

Labour
- Correct low (<50 IU/dl at 36 weeks) levels of factor VIII or IX before labour.
- Notify haematologist when the woman is admitted in labour. Site intravenous cannula. Take blood for full blood count, clotting studies and cross-match 4 units of blood.
- Administer relevant blood products in conjunction with haematological advice in any potentially affected fetus.
- Fetal risks include bleeding, cephalhaematoma, subgaleal and intracranial haemorrhage. Do not use scalp electrodes or perform fetal blood scalp sampling. Ventouse or mid-cavity rotational forceps are contraindicated but a simple lift-out is acceptable.
- Avoid prolonged labour or prolonged second stage.
- A low threshold for caesarean section should be considered in prolonged labours.
- Haemostasis is essential when surgery is performed. Repair episiotomy or tears immediately.
- Infuse Syntocinon for 4–8 hours after delivery to ensure the uterus remains contracted.
- If shown to be useful before pregnancy, 1-deamino-8-arginine vasopressin (DDAVP) can be helpful for postpartum bleeds in haemophilia A carriers or type I and type IIa VWD.

- Clotting levels may require adjustment over 3–4 days (after vaginal delivery) or 4–5 days after caesarean section.
- Physiological low levels of factor IX at birth may complicate early diagnosis of haemophilia in the newborn.

Platelet disorders

Platelet disorders are usually due to platelet destruction or consumption, failure of production or splenic sequestration. The commonest problems encountered in pregnancy are due to destruction/consumption, e.g. gestational thrombocytopenia, autoimmune thrombocytopenia.

- Gestational thrombocytopenia accounts for 70% of this disorder. Normal non-pregnant counts range between 150 and $400 \times 10^9/l$. In gestational thrombocytopenia the counts are usually above $80 \times 10^9/l$ and return to normal by 7 days post partum. Diagnosis is by exclusion since aetiology is not known.

- Autoimmune thrombocytopenia (AITP) accounts for 3% of this complication and is often evident before pregnancy. The disorder can be primary (idiopathic) or secondary to systemic lupus erythematosus, antiphospholipid syndromes, drugs, lymphomas plus viral infections, e.g. human immunodeficiency virus (HIV).

- Non-immune causes include disseminated intravascular coagulation, pre-eclampsia, HELLP syndrome, acute fatty liver and heparin-induced thrombocytopenia.

Pregnancy
- Take a detailed history and perform clinical examination.

- Examine blood film and instigate other investigations as appropriate.

- A platelet count $<20 \times 10^9/l$ in early pregnancy or below $50 \times 10^9/l$ in late pregnancy requires treatment. Start with prednisolone 30 mg daily for a week. If no response, try intravenous immunoglobin. Reserve platelet transfusion for bleeding episodes. In autoimmune thrombocytopenia the risk to the fetus is small. In second pregnancies the best guide of severity is the platelet count of the last baby.

Labour
- Anticipate vaginal delivery unless contraindicated.

- Elective caesarean section is not necessary purely for thrombocytopenia.
- Epidural anaesthesia is acceptable when the platelet count is above $80 \times 10^9/l$.
- Prescribe prophylactic antibodies if the woman has had a splenectomy.
- Ensure adequate haemostasis during surgery and prompt repair of episiotomies or tears is mandatory.
- Check cord sample for platelet count.
- Neonatal platelet count is lowest 2–5 days after birth. If count at birth is low monitor daily until platelet numbers increase. Severe thrombocytopenia requires treatment.

RESPIRATORY PROBLEMS

Respiratory function during labour may be compromised when there is asthma, infection such as pneumonia or tuberculosis, cystic fibrosis or restrictive lung disease.

Asthma

- Most common pre-existing lung condition affecting pregnant women.
- Continue medication during pregnancy.
- Give hydrocortisone 100 mg intravenously (6 hourly till restart of oral medication, if there has been prolonged or recent oral steroid use).
- Epidural anaesthesia is safe. General anaesthesia requires experienced anaesthetist.
- Prostaglandin E_2 is safe. Prostaglandin $F_2\alpha$ is a potent bronchoconstrictor.
- For acute severe attacks in labour (tachypnoea, tachycardia more than 120 beats per minute, severe wheezing and difficulty with speech)
  - administer 100% oxygen by mask
  - nebulise β-agonist
  - give hydrocortisone 100 mg intravenously.
- Intravenous aminophylline or β-agonist may be needed in severe attacks.
- Consider ventilatory support if the woman is very ill.

Respiratory problems

The fetus is likely to be affected if severe infection causes maternal oxygen saturation to fall below 90% (8 kPa). Infection can precipitate preterm labour. When infection is diagnosed:

- Take blood for full blood count, urea and electrolytes, blood cultures, viral titres and serological test to exclude atypical organisms such as mycoplasma or legionella.
- Collect sputum for culture and sensitivity and to exclude acid-fast bacilli.
- Chest radiology. This is not contraindicated as there is little risk to the fetus.
- Initiate antibiotics (usually intravenous if infection is severe). Isolation procedures, for example for tuberculosis, may be appropriate. For women with tuberculosis, the baby should be separated after birth and treated with isoniazid and vaccinated (bacille Calmette Guérin (BCG)). If mother has been recently treated and cured the baby only requires vaccination.
- An experienced anaesthetist is required if surgical delivery is necessary.

NEUROLOGICAL CONDITIONS

The following are the more usual neurological conditions relevant to labour.

Epilepsy

- This condition affects 0.5–1% of childbearing women.
- Increase renal and liver clearance of anticonvulsant drugs in pregnancy will lower the pregnancy levels by 10–25%. If fits increase, check drug levels and correct dosage accordingly. Ensure medication is continued during labour.
- Avoid sleep deprivation which results in increased frequency of fits.
- Epileptic women have a lower threshold to fit if pre-eclampsia supervenes. Anti-epileptic drugs can potentiate effects of magnesium sulphate. Rule out eclampsia if fits occur during labour.
- Vaginal delivery with epidural anaesthesia is acceptable.
- Lorazepam and diazepam can be used to control fits during labour.
- Anticonvulsants decrease maternal (not significant) and fetal vitamin K levels. It is essential to give baby vitamin K after delivery.
- Maternal phenobarbital can accumulate in baby through breastfeeding.
- Advise women against sleep deprivation. Baths should be no more than 7.5 cm (3 inches) deep. If fits are frequent advise the woman to sit on the floor for breastfeeding to avoid dropping baby.

Raised intracranial pressure

This may be benign (benign intracranial hypertension) or secondary to space-occupying lesions, cerebral oedema, infection, impaired cerebral spinal fluid absorption or drugs.

- Manage secondary raised intracranial pressure with neurologist or neurosurgeon.

- Benign intracranial hypertension is rare but can present for the first time in pregnancy (usually between 8 and 20 weeks). Diagnosis is by exclusion after a normal brain scan and lumbar puncture shows raised intracranial pressure (above 271.9 cmH$_2$O (200 mmHg)). Presentation includes headaches with or without visual disturbance, bilateral papilloedema and sometimes sixth nerve palsy (inability to abduct eye, with convergent squint and diplopia maximum on lateral gaze to the affected side). Spontaneous resolution in a few months is usual but visual changes can persist. Treatment is to protect visual function.

- Prescribe acetazolamide to reduce cerebrospinal fluid production.

- Repeated lumbar puncture can be performed to drain cerebrospinal fluid.

- Advise weight reduction as condition often occurs in very obese women.

- Vaginal delivery with epidural anaesthesia is acceptable. Pushing does not exacerbate the problem.

Neuromuscular disease

Multiple sclerosis, myasthenia gravis and myotonic dystrophy affect women of childbearing age with implications in labour.

Multiple sclerosis
- Pregnancy does not alter course of the disease. Relapse in pregnancy is half that expected but relapse rates are increased post partum. Relapse is also increased after elective termination of pregnancy and is possibly reduced by use of intravenous immune globin.

- Manage labour as normal.

- Regional anaesthesia was previously avoided but contemporary lower dose bupivacaine/fentanyl combinations and peridural techniques suggests no increase relapse risk.

Myasthenia gravis
An autoimmune disorder of acetylcholine receptors with resultant muscle fatigue, visual disturbance, coughing and speech difficulty. Effect of pregnancy on disease is uncertain. During pregnancy treatment is usually with steroid, anticholinesterase, immunosuppression and plasmapheresis for life-threatening exacerbations. Thymectomy can also be considered if diagnosed before pregnancy.

- Vaginal delivery is safe.
- Administer hydrocortisone 100 mg 6 hourly for 48–72 hours if the woman has had recent steroid usage.
- Assisted vaginal delivery is usual to overcome muscle fatigue.
- Use regional anaesthesia for caesarean section. Avoid muscle relaxants and opioids. Respiratory function must be carefully monitored post operatively.
- Magnesium sulphate and gentamicin (neuromuscular blocking properties) are contraindicated.
- Transplacental antibodies cause transient muscle weakness in 20% of newborns. Support is needed for neonatal hypotonia, feeding and respiratory difficulties. Resolution is usually complete by 1 month.
- Breastfeeding is not contraindicated even if women are on steroids or immunosuppressives.

Myotonic dystrophy
Autosomal dominant condition with progressive distal muscle weakness, wasting and impaired muscle relaxation leading to loss of facial expression. Frontal balding and cardiovascular complications, which are often evident before 40 years of age can occur.

- Diagnosis is often made for the first time in early pregnancy. Congenital muscular dystrophy is more common if the mother is affected (rather than the father) as the gene undergoes rapid expansion when passed through the maternal line.
- Perform an electrocardiogram to define cardiovascular status when women are admitted to the labour ward if this has not been done.
- Affected fetuses present with polyhydramnios, positional talipes and reduced movement. Preterm labour, stillbirth and neonatal death rates are increased.
- Prescribe Syntocinon, as labour is often dysfunctional.
- Assisted vaginal delivery is usual for maternal weakness.
- Regional anaesthesia is the preference for analgesia and for caesarean section. Avoid opioids, which potentiate respiratory compromise. Neuromuscular blockade can be difficult to reverse.
- Postpartum haemorrhage is increased. Infuse oxytocin (Syntocinon) for 4–8 hours after delivery.

Bibliography

Arulkumaran S, Rauff M, Ingemarsson I et al 1986 Uterine activity in myotonia dystrophica. Case Report. British Journal of Obstetrics and Gynaecology 93:634–636

Batocchi AP, Majolini L, Evoli A et al 1999 Course and treatment of myasthenia gravis during pregnancy. Neurology 52:447–452

Confavreux C, Hutchinson M, Hours MM et al 1998 Rate of pregnancy-related relapse in multiple sclerosis. Pregnancy in Multiple Sclerosis Group. New England Journal of Medicine 339:285–291

George JN, Woolf SH, Raskob GE et al 1996 Idiopathic thrombocytopenic purpura – practice guideline developed by explicit methods for the American Society of Hematology. Blood 8:3–40

Howard RJ. Management of sickling conditions in pregnancy 1996 British Journal of Hospital Medicine 56:7–10

Jaffe R, Mock M, Abramowicz J et al 1986 Myotonic dystrophy and pregnancy: a review. Obstetrical and Gynecological Survey 41:272–278

Lusher JM, McMillan CW 1978 Severe factor VIII and factor IX deficiency in females. American Journal of Medicine 65:637–648

Orvieto R, Achiron R, Rotstein Z et al 1999 Pregnancy and multiple sclerosis: a 2 year experience. European Journal of Obstetrics, Gynecology and Reproductive Biology 82:191–194

Ramsahoye BH, Davies SV, Dasani H et al 1995 Obstetric management in von Willebrand's disease: a report of 24 pregnancies and a review of the literature. Hemophilia 1:140–144

Weisberg LA 1975 Benign intracranial hypertension. Medicine 54:197–207

Yerby MS, Freil PN, McCormick K 1992 Antiepileptic drug disposition during pregnancy. Neurology 42(Suppl):12–16

(ii) ENDOCRINE DISORDERS

Renée Page

ADRENAL INSUFFICIENCY

Labour and delivery

In response to the stress of labour or surgery the adrenal gland will increase production of corticosteroids. Major stress leads to the secretion of up to 300 mg of cortisol in 24 hours with gradual reduction to usual levels once the stress has been removed. In women with adrenal insufficiency additional corticosteroid therapy is required. This should be considered in:

- Primary adrenal failure, e.g. Addison's disease
- Secondary adrenal failure, e.g. pituitary disease
- Previous cortisol therapy – within 1 year
- Chronic steroid therapy for other conditions, e.g. asthma

Various regimens include hydrocortisone 50 mg (usually sodium succinate) parenterally at the start of labour or with premedication in elective caesarean section. Repeat 8 hourly. In the absence of complications halve the dose daily and switch to oral therapy until maintenance dose is reached.

Fetus

It is unlikely that the short term increase in dosage at the time of delivery will have any effect on the newborn.

THYROID

Hypothyroid

Thyroxine therapy is often increased during pregnancy. No change in thyroxine therapy is required during labour. After birth, reduce thyroxine therapy to pre-pregnancy dose.

Thyrotoxicosis

During pregnancy women with thyrotoxicosis should be on the lowest possible dose of propylthiouracil or carbimazole. Propylthiouracil is the preferred therapy. Block and replace therapy should not be used. Maintain thyroid function at the upper end of the normal range. Many women become euthyroid and able to discontinue therapy.

Labour and delivery

In well-controlled women problems are unlikely.

Thyroid storm

Thyroid storm is rare but can occur in a poorly controlled or undiagnosed women subjected to stress or surgery. Clinical features include: fever, tachycardia (out of proportion to fever) and other features of thyrotoxicosis, e.g. tremor, restlessness, frequent bowel motions, eye signs.

Management
This is a medical emergency.

- Start treatment while waiting for thyroid function assessment to confirm diagnosis.

- Intravenous fluids are needed.

- Give propranolol to block β-adrenergic reactions and conversion of T4 to T3. Recommended oral doses vary from 160 mg to 320 mg/day in divided doses. Intravenous administration should be used if necessary (1–10 mg).

- Propylthiouracil blocks further synthesis of thyroid hormone and T4 to T3 conversion. Give 600 mg orally daily (if necessary via a nasogastric tube). If unavailable use carbimazole.

- Aqueous iodine oral solution (Lugol's iodine) has traditionally been used to inhibit thyroid secretion. Start 1–2 hours after the propylthiouracil. Some recommend the cholecystographic agents iopanoate or ipodate, which in addition to inhibiting thyroid secretion, also block T4 to T3 conversion. These agents are unlicensed in the UK but can be used on a named patient basis.

- Give intravenous hydrocortisone (100 mg 6 hourly) or dexamethasone orally.

- Add supportive therapy – digoxin, oxygen, diuretics and antipyretics as required.

Fetus

Transient neonatal thyrotoxicosis is uncommon. It occurs due to the transplacental passage of maternal immunoglobins. The mother will usually have had a history of thyrotoxicosis but does not have to be hyperthyroid. It is self-limiting but requires treatment as mortality can be high. Maternal thyroid receptor stimulating antibodies can be measured to predict the risk in the newborn. Close intrapartum and post partum monitoring is required.

DIABETES

All women regardless of type of diabetes, requiring therapy other than diet during pregnancy will have been treated with insulin. Insulin usage therefore cannot be used to define type of diabetes. Studies of oral therapies in pregnancy are taking place.

Labour and delivery

- Women with diabetes are no longer induced early unless for obstetric reasons. However, most obstetricians advise delivery at 39–40 weeks.

- Aim to maintain a steady glucose level with neither hypoglycaemia nor hyperglycaemia.

- There are many regimens to regulate glucose levels. It is important to become familiar with one to minimise errors in management. For example: management of the woman taking short-acting insulin pre-meal and intermediate at night during labour.

Induction of labour
- The day before continue with normal meals and insulin doses.

- On the morning, if prostaglandin pessaries or gel are to be used and it is thought labour will be slow to proceed, normal meals and insulin should be given (usually breakfast and morning dose of insulin).

- Measure blood glucose hourly.

- At artificial rupture of membranes/spontaneous rupture of membranes control glucose by glucose infusion at a constant rate and insulin at a variable rate to maintain a normal blood glucose (4–7 mmol/l):
  - infuse 5% glucose at a rate of 100 ml/h controlled by an infusion pump (5 gm glucose every hour)
  - make up 50 units of short-acting soluble insulin (e.g. Actrapid) to a volume of 50 ml with normal saline in a 50 ml syringe, to be infused by pump (1 unit of insulin per ml)
  - monitor blood glucose half hourly to hourly. It is advisable to send a venous sample to the laboratory at the start of labour to double check the accuracy of the meter being used
  - adjust infusion rate of insulin according to blood glucose measurements. One to two units of insulin per hour are usually required.

- Test all urine samples for ketones.

- Check electrolytes. It may be necessary to add potassium to the infusion.

- Encourage use of epidural anaesthesia for pain and metabolic control. If it is required, infuse Syntocinon in normal saline not glucose.

Other common insulin regimens
The use of twice-daily intermediate insulin or once-daily long-acting insulin as background insulin, with short-acting insulin pre meal is becoming more common. These women may need less intravenous insulin and/or more dextrose, e.g. 10% dextrose during delivery. We recommend that women on large doses of once daily long-acting insulin (e.g. glargine) change to a twice daily regimen near delivery.

Table 22.1 Guide for insulin infusion with 30 minutes blood sugar monitoring

Blood glucose (mmol/l)	Insulin infusion (ml/h)
Below 4.0	Stop insulin. Check infusion system Consider oral or parental glucose (10% dextrose)
4.0–6.0	1 unit of insulin/h
6.0–8.0	2 units of insulin/h
Above 8.0	3 units of insulin/h
More than 12.0	3 units of insulin/h. Stop glucose

This helps to avoid profound hypoglycaemia after delivery.

Spontaneous labour

- Check food intake and insulin usage. Test for ketones.
- Manage as for induction of labour (see Table 22.1). If blood sugar levels are high omit glucose until control achieved.

Caesarean section

- In consultation with anaesthetist start infusion of glucose/insulin before anaesthesia and continue in theatre. Elective caesarean sections are ideally performed in the morning. Ensure blood sugar levels are between 5.0 mmol/l and 7.0 mmol/l before surgery.

- After delivery continue glucose/insulin infusion over night with regular, e.g. 2-hourly, blood glucose monitoring. Due to decreased insulin requirements a change to 10% glucose and/or decrease in insulin infusion rate may be required. Discontinue infusion and return to pre-pregnancy insulin dose when the woman is eating and drinking. Continue 4-hourly blood glucose monitoring.

- Women with gestational diabetes treated with insulin can sometimes be managed without an insulin infusion during a caesarean section. Individual assessment is required.

Management of women not requiring insulin

- Take hourly blood tests. Consider starting infusion of glucose and insulin when blood glucose rises above 7 mmol/l.

- It should be remembered that the following are more common:
  - large for dates babies
  - assisted delivery
  - fetal hypoglycaemia
  - congenital abnormality in offspring of women with pre-existing diabetes.

Post delivery

- Gestational diabetes: Stop insulin and monitor blood glucose twice daily for a few days. At 6 weeks after birth perform glucose tolerance test. Remember, although uncommon, women may have had newly diagnosed type 1 diabetes.

- Type 2 diabetes: Return to previous pre-pregnancy therapy. Oral hypoglycaemics are not recommended for those who are breastfeeding. If therapy is required insulin can be used, often at a greatly reduced dosage from that during pregnancy.

- Type 1 diabetes: After delivery insulin requirements return to pre-pregnancy levels. Decrease glucose/insulin infusion rate. Once eating use pre-pregnancy insulin doses. Further dosage reduction may be required:
  - during the first 24 hours, particularly for women who have taken a recent large dosage of long-acting insulin. Splitting the dose of long-acting insulin near the time of delivery can help to prevent problems with hypoglycaemia
  - if breastfeeding
  - when pre-pregnancy control was very tight.

- After normal delivery:
  - for delivery before midday give quick-acting insulin with lunch and normal regimen before evening meal
  - for delivery after evening meal give medium-acting insulin that night and normal pre-pregnancy regimen next day.

Fetus

Complications, especially hypoglycaemia, are more common. Close monitoring of blood sugar is required.

MEDICAL EMERGENCIES

Diabetic ketoacidosis and hypoglycaemic coma should be treated along conventional lines.

Bibliography

British National Formulary 2006 51, Section 6 Endocrine system. BMJ Publishing Group and RPS Publishing

Burger AG, Philippe J 1992 Thyroid emergencies. Balliere's Clinical Endocrinology and Metabolism 6:77–93

Lazarus JH 2003 Thyroid disease in pregnancy: a case for screening? Editorial Trends in Urology Gynaecology and Sexual Health September/October, 6
Livanou T, Ferriman D, James VHT 1967 Recovery of hypothalamo-pituitary adrenal function after corticosteroid therapy. Lancet 2:856–859
Muller AF, Drexhage HA, Berhout A 2001 Postpartum thyroiditis and autoimmune thyroiditis in women of

childbearing age: recent insights and consequences for antenatal and postnatal care. Endocrine Reviews 22:650–30
Report of the Pregnancy and Neonatal Group, Saint Vincent and Improving Diabetes Care Specialist UK 1994 Workgroup Reports. S43-S53 Diabetic Medicine Supplement 4, 13

(iii) CARDIAC DISEASE

Philip Baker

Common disorders include rheumatic heart disease (with or without prosthetic heart valves), congenital anomalies (for example the tetralogy of Fallot, Eisenmenger's syndrome) and cardiomyopathies of varying severity. The incidence of congenital heart disease in pregnancy is increasing because women with more severe defects can have corrective surgery as children and are now able to have children themselves.

Women with cardiac disease or defects are at risk of:

- Pulmonary oedema (precipitated by anxiety, pain, exertion, infection and tachycardia) when there is obstruction to cardiac outflow, as in mitral or aortic stenosis.

- Cardiac syncope and cyanosis. Follows hypertension, excessive blood loss, or any cause of poor venous return in women with defects such as the tetralogy of Fallot.

- Bacterial endocarditis. This infection is usually associated with *Streptococcus* (principally S. *viridans* and *faecalis*), *Staphylococcus* (*albus* and *aureus*) or Gram-negative organisms. Prevention by prophylactic antibiotics is essential.

- Arrhythmia.

LABOUR

- With the onset of labour or 1–2 hours before elective caesarean section, give amoxicillin 1 g intravenous/intramuscularly and gentamicin (120 mg intravenous/intramuscularly). When penicillin allergy is present, use vancomycin 1 g intravenously, or teicoplanin 400 mg intravenously.

- Ensure comfortable labour, avoid hypotension.

- Use the semi-recumbent or lateral position. The supine and, especially, lithotomy position should

be avoided as much as possible to minimise the risk of pulmonary oedema.

- Apply continuous electrocardiogram and monitor oxygen saturation. Full resuscitation facilities must be available.

- Beware of vasodilatation and hypotension with epidural blocks in women with limited stroke volume and left ventricular outlet flow obstruction (eg aortic stenosis, hypertrophic cardiomyopathy (HOCM)).

- If a pudendal block is required, lidocaine without adrenaline should be used.

Delivery

There should be a low threshold for assisted delivery if birth is not achieved within 20 minutes after onset of second stage. Reserve caesarean section for the usual indications. Avoid ergometrine, give oxytocin (Syntocinon) 10 units intramuscularly and by subsequent intravenous infusion to control post partum bleeding. All women must be observed carefully for at least 24 hours after delivery. Transfer to a high dependency or intensive care unit may be appropriate.

FETUS

The fetus suffers as a consequence of maternal hypoxia and hypertension. Continuous fetal heart rate monitoring should be employed throughout labour.

ACUTE PULMONARY OEDEMA

- The woman experiences acute dyspnoea with frothy sputum. Characteristic moist sounds are audible at the lung basis. Hypoxaemia and increased vascular markings are present.
- Confirm diagnosis.

- Chest X-ray, pulse oximetry and arterial blood gases (acute acidosis with consequent decreased pH and increased pCO_2 but only slight alteration in base excess).

Management

- Involve cardiologist to provide team care.

- Provide supportive measures. These include oxygen administration via facemask and nursing with head elevation above the level of the right atrium. Measure oxygen saturation of the circulating blood via pulse oximetry.

- Maintain fluid balance by careful monitoring of intake and output. Serum electrolytes must be closely monitored especially in women receiving diuretics. The use of a pulmonary artery catheter will help distinguish between fluid overload, left ventricular dysfunction, and pulmonary oedema associated with vascular bed injury.

- Perform frequent arterial blood gas measurements to assess the underlying respiratory status.

- Administer furosemide (10–40 mg) intravenously over 1–2 minutes. Larger doses may be required if diuresis does not ensue.

- If left ventricular failure is suspected, reduction in preload by agents such as glycerol trinitrate may help. Likewise, hydralazine may be employed to reduce the after load.

- Treat arrhythmia if present (paroxysmal supraventricular tachycardia and atrial fibrillation are more common in pregnancy).

- Involve an anaesthetist; hypoxia may persist despite treatment and mechanical ventilation may be required.

MYOCARDIAL INFARCTION

See Box 22.2.

HYPERTENSION

This is diagnosed where a blood pressure (BP) of 140/90 mmHg or more is recorded on two separate occasions at least 6 hours apart. Causes include chronic hypertension, chronic renal disease, endocrine disorders (phaeochromocytoma) and coarctation of the aorta, in addition to pregnancy-induced hypertension (patients are normotensive prior to twentieth week of pregnancy). If presenting in labour:

Box 22.2   Points to note in myocardial infarction at term

- Rare but will present more frequently as older women and those with pre-existing heart disorders are becoming pregnant.

- Incident of 1 in 10 000 maternities with 45% maternal mortality and 34% fetal loss.

- Present with classic symptoms of chest tightness, pain and shortness of breath. Aetiology is usually structural pathology or coronary artery thrombosis with a transmural rather than subendocardial infarct.

- Occurrence is usually during labour or immediately following delivery.

- Team care with cardiologist and anaesthetist is mandatory.

- Maternal mortality is higher if delivery is within 2 weeks of an acute myocardial infarction.

- Cardiac output increases 50% in the second stage of labour. Each contraction pushes 300–500 ml of blood into the general circulation causing increase in stroke volume, cardiac output (up by 15%) and increased arterial pressure. Vaginal delivery if appropriate necessitates:
  - electrocardiographic monitoring
  - epidural analgesia (pain increases release of catecholamines)
  - elective assisted instrumental vaginal delivery
  - cardiotocograph monitoring of the fetus
  - avoiding ergometrine. Oxytocin reduces coronary blood flow and levels above 4 MU/l may not be safe.

- Elective caesarean section is the preferred mode of delivery but cardiac output still increases by 50%.

- check blood pressure at 15-minute intervals to confirm diagnosis.
- test urine for protein.
- engage care team when diagnosis is made.

See Box 22.3 for management of hypertensive crises.

PRE-ECLAMPSIA

Defined as: confirmed blood pressure of more than 140/90 mmHg, proteinuria: 2 pluses or more than 300 mg urinary protein in 24 hours.

Box 22.3   Management of hypertensive crisis

- Defined as blood pressure of 170/110 mmHg or more.

- Labetalol (see below) is a first line therapy. Give 20 mg bolus intravenously followed by infusion of 40 mg/h (max 60 mg/h).

- Alternatively give intravenously hydralazine 5–10 mg in 10 ml of normal saline over 10 minutes. Monitor BP every 5 minutes until level is between 140/80 and 160/100 mmHg. Note BP may drop 20 minutes after this bolus dose.

- Use 50 mg hydralazine in 50 ml normal saline to give 1 mg/ml and deliver by syringe pump for subsequent control of hypertension. Note side effects which include tachycardia, hot flushes, facial erythema, headaches.

This multi-systemic disorder of pre-eclampsia is pregnancy-induced hypertension with the addition of significant proteinuria. In pregnancy, protein excretion may be considerably increased but up to 300 mg of total protein per 24 hours is accepted as normal. A 24-hour measurement of urinary protein should confirm the diagnosis. When this is not possible, alternative approaches include setting a high limit for diagnosis such as 2 pluses protein on dipstick testing or a concentration of 1 g protein/l in a random sample.

Management of pre–eclampsia: investigation and assessment

- Obtain detailed obstetric history and perform clinical examination. Both mother and fetus are affected by this condition. Carry out neurological examination noting the presence or absence of hyper-reflexia, clonus (more than three beats), focal neurological defects and papilloedema. On abdominal examination, epigastric tenderness and hepatic tenderness indicate subcapsular liver haemorrhages. Note non-dependent oedema.

- Haematological: take blood for group and save, platelet count, clotting screen and biochemical tests.

- Biochemical: check urea and electrolytes. An elevated plasma uric acid is used as an indicator of impaired renal function and renal blood flow. (Note other conditions which increase plasma uric

acid). Abnormal liver function tests (increase in lactate dehydrogenase and transaminase) relate to altered liver perfusion or hepatic congestion. Note HELLP syndrome.

- General care include: obstetric assessment, ultrasound scan if appropriate, continuous heart rate monitoring, regular pulse and blood pressure check (every 15 minutes) and monitor hourly urinary output with an indwelling catheter. Adjust degree of surveillance to severity of pre-eclampsia.

Antihypertensive therapy

Aim is to protect the woman by minimising the risks of cerebral haemorrhage, cardiac failure or myocardial infarct and placental abruption. Although there is no specific threshold for such events, the risks are significant when the blood pressure exceeds 170/110 mmHg – commence treatment at this level. Treatment does not prevent disease progression – there is no place for complacency. Treatment must induce a smooth sustained fall in blood pressure. Hydralazine and labetalol are drugs which can fulfil this requirement. Typical regimens are hydralazine: bolus 5–10 mg intravenously followed by 10 mg per hour (max 40 mg per hour) doubling every 30 minutes until a satisfactory response is achieved (diastolic blood pressure 90 mmHg ± 5 mmHg), or labetalol: bolus 20 mg intravenously followed by infusion of 40 mg/h (max 60 mg/h) doubling every 30 minutes until satisfactory response is achieved.

Anticonvulsant therapy

Magnesium sulphate ($MgSO_4$) reduces the incidence of recurrent convulsions after an eclamptic fit. The benefits of prophylactic therapy in severe pre-eclampsia have yet to be established.

- Magnesium sulphate is dispensed as 50% w/v solution with 1 g in 2 ml.

- Suggested regimen is 4 g loading dose (8 ml 50% w/v $MgSO_4$ in 20 ml 5% dextrose) intravenously over 20 minutes, then maintenance dose of 1 g/h. The infusion should be continued for 24 hours after delivery or until a maternal diuresis (>100 ml of urine for 2 consecutive hours) has commenced. For fits during infusion add 2 mg $MgSO_4$ intravenously over 2–3 minutes if drug levels are low.

- Contraindications include cardiac disease (digoxin therapy) and acute renal failure (less than 30 ml of urine per hour over 2 hours). $MgSO_4$ will potentiate neuromuscular blocking agents.

- Monitor by clinical observations (deep tendon reflexes, electrocardiogram/pulse oximetry), and by plasma levels (therapeutic range 2–3 mmol/l). At 4–5 mmol/l there is loss of patella reflex, weakness, nausea, flushing, double vision, slurred speech, hypotension and hypothermia. At 6–7.5 mmol/l the women experiences muscle paralysis and respiratory arrest. At >12 mmol/l there is cardiac arrest.

- Fetal side effects include flaccidity, hyporeflexia and respiratory depression.

- Hypermagnesaemia in the woman also results in flushing, sweating, hypotension, depressed reflexes, cardiac, respiratory and neurological function, hypothermia, flaccid paralysis and collapse.

- The antidote is 10–20 ml of 10% calcium gluconate intravenously.

Fluid balance

- Hypovolaemia associated with pre-eclampsia necessitates close attention to fluid balance to protect the kidneys and prevent pulmonary oedema.
- Urine output is best monitored by siting an indwelling urethral catheter and taking measurements hourly.
- Fluid input should be no more than 1 ml/kg per hour (normal saline is the fluid of choice).
- Delivery quickly reverses the effects of pre-eclampsia on renal function. If not, invasive monitoring with central venous pressure (CVP) lines, or more accurately by pulmonary capillary wedge pressure readings, should be considered.

General management

- Involve haematologist for multidisciplinary management if there is evidence of coagulopathy.

- There are few contraindications to use of epidural anaesthesia. Thrombocytopenia (platelet count $<50 \times 10^9/l$) is an absolute contraindication.

- Delivery is mandatory when pre-eclampsia is diagnosed at term. The dilemma occurs in women with early onset of pre-eclampsia between 24 weeks' and 34 weeks' gestation. If the severity of the disease necessitates antihypertensive and anticonvulsant therapy as detailed above, deliver once the woman's condition is stabilised. Mode of delivery depends on the gestational age and severity of disease.

- The fetus is at risk of hypoxia if there is associated growth restriction or placental insufficiency. Close intrapartum surveillance is mandatory.

- Second stage should be short. Assisted instrumental delivery is recommended for delay (more than 30 minutes).

- Ergometrine should be avoided in the third stage as it may precipitate eclampsia – Syntocinon 10 units should be administered.

- Observe the woman closely for 24 hours after delivery.

ECLAMPSIA

Eclampsia (flashing lights) is the occurrence of convulsions, not attributable to other cerebral causes, in association with the signs and symptoms of pre-eclampsia. The risk of eclampsia is low (1%) even if there is severe pre-eclampsia.

The initial eclamptic fit should be controlled by either an intravenous bolus of 4 mg of magnesium sulphate over 20 minutes or an intravenous bolus of diazepam (10 mg intravenously over 1 minute). Thereafter a magnesium sulphate infusion should be commenced.

RENAL FAILURE

Renal failure is a rare complication of pre-eclampsia and usually follows acute blood loss, when there has been inadequate transfusion, or after profound hypotension. Oliguria without rising urea or creatinine is a manifestation of severe pre-eclampsia and not of incipient renal failure.

Procedure

- Oliguria (<400 ml/24 hours) is not an indication for treatment if women are well perfused.
- Loop diuretic (furosemide) or osmotic diuretic (mannitol) administration temporarily improves urine output but further decreases circulating blood volume and disturbs electrolyte balance.
- Consult a renal physician if renal failure is suspected.
- Without invasive monitoring, repetitive fluid challenges should be avoided.
- If there is no response to therapeutic measures suspect occurrence of acute cortical necrosis.

Bibliography

Altman D, Carroli G, Duley L et al 2002 Do women with pre-eclampsia, and their babies, benefit from magnesium sulphate? The Magpie Trial: a randomised placebo-controlled trial. Lancet 359:1877–1890

Chua S, Redman CW 1991 Are prophylactic anticonvulsants required in severe pre-eclampsia? Lancet 337:250–251

Duley L, Gulmezoglu AM, Henderson-Smart DJ 1999 Anticonvulsants for women with pre-eclampsia. In Cochrane Collaboration. Cochrane Library Issue 1, Oxford

Duley L, Henderson-Smart DJ 2001 Drugs for rapid treatment of very high blood pressure during pregnancy (Cochrane Review). In: The Cochrane Library, Issue 2, 2001. Update Software, Oxford

Gulmezoglu M, Duley L 1998 Use of anticonvulsants in eclampsia and pre-eclampsia: survey of obstetricians in the United Kingdom and the Republic of Ireland. BMJ 316:975–976

Hayman RG, Baker PN 2000 Labour ward management of pre-eclampsia In: Kean LH, Baker PN, Edlestone DI (eds) Best Practice in Labour Ward Management. WB Saunders, Edinburgh pp 253–294

Lipsite PJ 1971 The clinical and biochemical effects of excess magnesium in the newborn. Paediatrics 47:501–509

The Eclamptic Trial Collaborative Group 1995 Which anticonvulsant for women with eclampsia? Evidence from the collaborative eclampsia trial. Lancet 345:1455–1463

Tucker D, Liu DTY, Ramoutar O 1996 Myocardial infarction at term: a case report to consider management options. Journal of Obstetrics and Gynaecology 16:522–524

(iv) INFECTIONS

Christine A Bowman

BACTERIAL

Amniotic fluid may become infected. Women with diabetes, prolonged membrane rupture or repeated catheterisation of the bladder are more prone to infection.

Maternal signs

Pyrexia (the temperature may be normal or subnormal with Gram-negative infections) and tachycardia are usual.

Fetal signs

Persistent tachycardia and evidence of fetal distress (fetal heart rate pattern changes and fetal acidosis) are present.

Bacteraemia and septic shock

Organisms

Escherichia coli, other Gram-negative bacilli, *Staphylococcus aureus*, anaerobic infections including *Bacteroides* spp, group B streptococcus, *Listeria monocytogenes*.

Symptoms

High fever (temperature may be low or normal in Gram-negative septicaemia) nausea, vomiting, malaise, tachycardia (sometimes). Symptoms from infection source, e.g. dysuria.

Septic shock

Profound hypotension, cold clammy skin, tachycardia, tachypnoea, oliguria.

Management

- Collect two sets of blood cultures.
- Urine for microscopy and culture (other samples as indicated, e.g. cerebrospinal fluid (CSF) if signs of meningism).
- Administer broad-spectrum antibiotics intravenously chosen on the basis of likely source, local antibiotic resistance patterns and severity of illness, e.g. ampicillin, gentamicin and metronidazole or cefotaxime plus metronidazole.
- Give appropriate loading doses and monitor gentamicin levels subsequently.
- Consult on-call microbiologist for advice.
- Give treatment for shock including careful fluid maintenance, electrolyte balance, blood sugar monitoring. If severe may require immediate admission to intensive care.

Labour and delivery

- Locate the cause of infection.
- Maternal infection can interfere with uterine activity.
- Fetal infection results in fetal tachycardia and early onset of fetal distress. Consider a caesarean section if delivery is not expected in 1–2 hours or if fetal distress is evident.

- Obtain blood, urine and amniotic fluid for culture. Administer antibiotics as described.
- An experienced paediatrician should attend the delivery.
- Obtain samples from the placenta for culture.
- Take samples for bacteriological screening of the newborn.

Haemolytic streptococcus group B

A major cause of maternal bacteraemia, premature labour, postpartum endometritis and neonatal bacteraemia and meningitis.

- Group B streptococcus is a normal commensal of the vagina or intestinal tract in 15–30% of women. Women can be chronic, transient or intermittent carriers. Some 40–73% of babies are colonised but only 1–2% develop disease within 7 days after vaginal delivery. In 80% disease onset is within 48 hours. Mortality rate of infected babies is 10–20%.
- Positive culture is most likely from the rectum and vaginal swabs. Note 50% of carriers can be missed. A positive urinary culture sometimes indicates vaginal colonisation.

Management
- Population screening is of little value.
- Women at risk include those with:
  - previous infected baby (10 times increased risk)
  - positive cultures (four times increased risk if group B streptococcus detected in urine or recto-vaginal area)
  - positive culture and preterm labour (before 37 weeks)
  - ruptured membranes more than 18 hours (intravenous antibiotics for 24 hours followed by treatment for 10 days or until delivery. Repeat swabs and continue treatment if group B streptococcus infection persists). Augment labour if at term. Metronidazole (500 mg intravenously 8 hourly) if there is clinical evidence of infection (fever, uterine tenderness, the woman's heart rate is more than 100 beats per minute, fetal tachycardia is more than 160 beats per minute). If <34 weeks betamethasone is not contraindicated
  - intrapartum pyrexia of 38°C or more and evidence of infection (tender uterus or fetal tachycardia).
- Intrapartum prophylactic antibiotics include:
  - intravenous loading dose of penicillin, e.g. intravenous benzylpenicillin 3 g followed by 1.5 g 4 hourly until delivery

- clindamycin (900 mg intravenously 8 hourly) or erythromycin (500 mg intravenously 6 hourly) if allergic to penicillin
- if carrier state proven start intravenous antibiotics at onset of labour. Ideally start treatment at least 2 hours before delivery
- for emergency or elective caesarean section give intravenous Augmentin 1.2 g or cefuroxime 1.5 g plus metronidazole 500 mg if allergic to penicillin

Note 1: 10% women will have a mild allergic reaction to penicillin, 1 in 1000 will develop anaphylaxis and this anaphylaxis proves fatal in 1 in 100 000 of those affected.

Note 2: The Royal College of Obstetricians and Gynaecologists Clinical Green Top Guidelines recommend that broad-spectrum antibiotics such as ampicillin should be avoided if possible, as concerns have been raised regarding increased rates of neonatal Gram-negative sepsis.

Newborn infants with clinical signs of early-onset group B streptococcus disease should be treated promptly with the necessary antibiotics (blood cultures and CSF taken from the sick newborn).

Listerosis (*Listeria monocytogenes*)

Listeria monocytogenes gains access to the amniotic cavity through haematogenous spread and may cause bacteraemia, preterm labour, severe sepsis meningo-encephalitis and fetal death. Infection is usually acquired by eating pate and unpasteurised milk products.

Maternal symptoms
- Fever
- Headaches
- Myalgia
- Flu-like symptoms
- Evidence of chorioamnionitis

Diagnosis
- Blood cultures from mother and newborn
- Neonate CSF, tracheal/gastric aspirates; meconium specimens

Management
High-dose intravenous ampicillin plus gentamicin.

Chlamydia trachomatis

- Endocervical infection is common in 15–25-year-olds (10–15%).

- Genital infection in the woman may be asymptomatic.
- Vertical transmission in labour may cause conjunctivitis, pneumonia and otitis media.
- Postpartum complication includes pelvic inflammatory disease, endometritis and cervicitis.

Diagnosis

Nucleic acid amplification tests (NAAT) are now the investigations of choice. Endocervical samples are most reliable in women. Some NAAT tests perform well on vaginal swabs and first-catch urine samples. (Some also detect gonorrhoea.) If NAAT unavailable use enzyme immunoassays (EIA) test from endocervical swab. In about 20% of infected women gonorrhoea is also present.

Management

- Treat the mother with erythromycin 500 mg four times daily for 7 days (or twice daily for 14 days) or azithromycin 1 g stat (Amoxil may be used if she is intolerant of erythromycin).
- Neonatal infection requires systemic erythromycin.
- Refer the mother to genitourinary medicine for follow-up and contact tracing. Fifty per cent of babies with infected mothers develop conjunctivitis. Babies need oral erythromycin.

If gonorrhoea also isolated on culture give ceftriaxone 250 mg stat intramuscularly or cefixime 400 mg stat by mouth. If gonorrhoea is found by NAAT, take swab for culture and antibiotic sensitivities before giving the above. Refer to genitourinary medicine for follow-up and contact tracing.

Syphilis

Infectious syphilis is increasing rapidly in the UK. The woman may be asymptomatic, have painless anogenital or oral ulcers (chancres) with non-tender regional lymphadenopathy (in primary syphilis) or generalised rash, oro-genital mucous lesions and lymphadenopathy (secondary syphilis).

Congenital syphilis may cause intra- and peripartum death, early signs (including snuffles, vesiculobullous lesions, condylomata lata, lymphadenopathy and hepatosplenomegaly) or late signs (neurological deficits, tooth and bone and cartilage deformities).

Diagnosis

Syphilis serology (may be negative in early primary syphilis). Dark ground microscopy of exudate from genital ulcers (genitourinary medicine clinic only).

Management

- Refer to genitourinary medicine for treatment, follow-up and contact tracing
- Treatment of infectious syphilis is with daily procaine penicillin 750 mg intramuscularly for 10 days or an injection of benzathine penicillin 2.4 MU intramuscularly weekly × 2 (day 1 and 8). If allergic to penicillin hospital inpatient based desensitisation must be given immediately prior to treatment (seek advise from genitourinary medicine first)
- Liaise with paediatrician. Take neonatal bloods for syphilis serology including fluorescent treponemal antibody absorption test IgM and treat baby with intravenous benzylpenicillin if mother not treated earlier than 6 weeks pre-delivery or signs of congenital syphilis
- Note highly infectious nature of baby's mucocutaneous lesions.

VIRAL

Genital herpes

- May be caused by either herpes simplex type I or II (incubation period 2–10 days).
- Women who acquire genital herpes during the last trimester of pregnancy have a significant risk of vertical transmission to their babies. Some 5% neonatal infections are intrauterine following transplacental or ascending transmembrane spread.
- The risk of neonatal herpes is extremely low if the woman acquired her genital herpes before conception. The risk is 40–50% with primary but less than 5% with recurrent infection.

Diagnosis

- 75% of herpes simplex infections in women are asymptomatic hence there is no warning history in 60% of neonatal infections.
- Clinical appearance (confirm with culture or PCR). Women may experience burning or pain. Vesicles, ulcers and lymphadenopathy are present. Rarely neuropathy and meningitis
- Culture or polymerase chain reaction for herpes simplex virus from herpetic ulcer or blister. Send swabs immediately to virology laboratory or keep in refrigerator then send as soon as possible.

Management

- Examine vulva and cervix for ulcers. Allow vaginal delivery for recurrent genital herpes if there are no genital lesions.

- Deliver fetus by caesarean section if active infection during labour. This is advised even if membranes have ruptured more than 6 hours.

- For women who develop their first episode of genital herpes in the third trimester of pregnancy, delivery should be by elective caesarean section. If vaginal delivery is unavoidable, aciclovir should be given to the mother and baby to prevent vertical transmission. Aciclovir, however, may not prevent viral shedding. Likewise caesarean section is not completely protective against neonatal herpes.

- Avoid invasive procedures if vaginal delivery is unavoidable as this will reduce transmission of infection.

Chronic bloodborne viruses

General measures
- Prevention of nosocomial infection by standard infection control procedures, e.g. safe disposal of sharps, use of disposable items where possible (e.g. plastic specula), decontamination of spillage's etc.

- Prevention of occupational infection:
  - appropriate use of gloves, eye protection, gowns, covering of minor cuts/abrasions
  - vaccination for hepatitis B.

- Follow local post exposure prophylaxis guidelines if needlestick injury occurs.

All pregnant women should be encouraged to have HIV testing at antenatal booking as part of routine care. Women at high risk for viral hepatitis (e.g. injecting drug users, those from high prevalence areas) should be screened for hepatitis B and C.

Hepatitis B
- Caused by a hepatitis B virus. Incubation period 50–180 days.

- Virus is present in all body secretions and fluid. Infection results in neonatal morbidity and mortality.

- Infectivity and risk of vertical transmission depends on both HBsAg and eAg status. HBsAg and e antigen positive patients are most infectious. Ten per cent vertical transmission if mother positive for only HBsAg – 90% if both HBsAg and HBeAg positive.

- Deliver according to usual obstetric indications.

- Following delivery baby should be vaccinated for hepatitis B and given hepatitis B immuno-

globulin in the other thigh if the mother is either eAg positive or lacking any 'e' markers (babies of women with antibody to HBe are given vaccine only).

- Breastfeeding is not contraindicated.

Hepatitis C
- Prevalence of 1–2% in women. Transfusion and drug misuse are risk factors.
- Vertical transmission can occur but risks are much less than for hepatitis B (2–5%).
- No vaccine or passive immunoglobulin currently available.
- Avoid intervention which breach fetal skin, e.g. scalp electrodes.
- Breastfeeding is not contraindicated.

Human immunodeficiency virus
- Virus is present in all body fluids. Antibodies appear 3–6 months after initial infection. Maternal viral load affects risks of transmission. Viral load is highest at seroconversion and in untreated significantly immunocompromised patients.

- The risk of vertical transmission can be reduced from 15–40% to 1% by the appropriate use of anti-retroviral drugs and caesarean section. In utero infection can occur.

- Zidovudine (antiretroviral therapy) alone can reduce transmission (by more than 60%) to 5–8% of neonatal infection. If not treated previously administer zidovudine 2 mg/kg bodyweight intravenously over 1 hour then 1 mg/kg bodyweight hourly until cord clamped.

- Pregnancy, labour and neonatal care should be carefully managed by close liaison between obstetrician, HIV physician and neonatologist.

- If the mother is on anti-HIV drugs these should be continued during labour and post partum. The woman's HIV physician will advise on the need for additional zidovudine during labour.

- The newborn should receive zidovudine syrup 2 mg/kg every 6 hours starting within 12 hours of delivery. Zidovudine is continued for 6 weeks in the newborn. Septrin prophylaxis may be started at 3 weeks.

- Delivery by elective caesarean section is usually recommended. Intravenous zidovudine should be started 4 hours before surgery and continued until the cord is clamped. Note however an increasing trend to vaginal delivery in women with undetectable viral loads on triple antiretroviral therapy.

- Breastfeeding should be avoided in developed countries (transmission rate 10–20%).

- Combination of antiretroviral therapy, caesarean section and avoidance of breastfeeding reduce vertical transmission to less than 1%.

Varicella zoster (chicken pox)

- Incubation period 10–24 days. Infectious 48 hours before rash until crusting of vesicles.

- 85–90% women are seropositive. Primary attack with maternal pneumonitis (10%) is associated with 1% mortality. Risk of pneumonia increases in later gestation.

- If maternal infection occurs at term there is a high risk of neonatal varicella with a 20–30% mortality. Severe neonatal infection is most likely if baby is born within 5 days of onset of mother's rash. If practical, consider delaying delivery until 5 days after onset of maternal illness to allow passive transfer of antibodies. If delivery occurs within 5 days of maternal infection, or if mother develops chickenpox within 2 days of giving birth, give the newborn varicella zoster immune globulin. Consider prophylactic aciclovir.

- Varicella zoster infection before 20 weeks gestation does not cause miscarriage. Fetal varicella syndrome (eye problems, limb hypoplasia, microencephaly, mental retardation, bowel and bladder sphincter dysfunction) complicates 1–2% if mother is infected before 20 weeks pregnancy. Viral complication is unlikely after 20 weeks of pregnancy.

- Immunoglobulin is effective up to 10 days after contact. If mother is not sure of immunity and was in contact, check immunity status before giving immunoglobins. Neonatal risk is minimal if mother was immunised, because of acquired maternal antibodies. This is not always the case if delivery is before 28 weeks' gestation.

- At the viraemic phase delivery is extremely hazardous because the mother is at risk of bleeding, thrombocytopenia, disseminated intravascular coagulopathy and hepatitis. Neonatal varicella is likely with significant morbidity and mortality. Intravenous aciclovir is recommended.

- Ensure neonatal ophthalmic examination and check for varicella IgM.

Bibliography

Brown ZA, Benedetti J, Ashley R et al 1991 Neonatal herpes simplex virus infection in relation to asymptomatic maternal infection at the time of labor. New England Journal of Medicine 324:1247–1252

Centers for Disease Control and Prevention. Prevention of varicella: recommendations of the Advisory Committee on Immunization Practices. Morbidity and Mortality Weekly Reports 45:1–36

Connor EM, Sperling RS, Gelber R et al 1994 Reduction of maternal-infant transmission of human immunodeficiency virus type 1 with zidovudine treatment. New England Journal of Medicine 331:173–80

Crowley P 2003 Prophylactic corticosteroids for preterm birth. Cochrane Database of Systematic Reviews, CD000065

Dillon HC, Khare S, Gray BM 1987 Group β streptococcal carriage and disease: A 6 year prospective study. Journal of Paediatrics 110:31–36

Dunn DT, Newell ML, Mayaux MJ et al 1994 Mode of delivery and vertical transmission of HIV-1: a review of prospective studies. Journal of AIDS 7:1064–1066

Enders G, Miller E, Cradock-Watson J et al 1994 Consequences of varicella and herpes zoster in pregnancy: prospective study of 1739 cases. Lancet 343:1548–51

European Collaborative Study 1994 Caesarean section and risk of vertical transmission of HIV-1 infection. Lancet 343:1464–1467

Fast P, Newell M-L, Mofenson L et al 1995 Strategies for prevention of perinatal transmission of HIV infection. Report of a Consensus Workshop (II), Sienna, Italy 3–6 June 1993. AIDS and Research and Human Retroviruses 8:161–175

Flenady V, King J 2002 Antibiotics for prelabour rupture of membranes at or near term (Cochrane Review). In: The Cochrane Library, Issue 4. Update Software, Oxford.

Gilbert RE, Pike K, Kenyon SL et al 2005 The effect of prepartum antibiotics on the type of neonatal bacteraemia: insights from the MRC ORACLE trials. British Journal of Obstetrics and Gynaecology 112:830–832

Hurtig A-K, Nicoll A, Carne C et al 1998 Syphilis in pregnant women and their children in the United Kingdom:results from national clinician reporting surveys 1994–7. BMJ 317:1617–1619

Kenyon SL, Taylor DJ, Tarnow-Mordi W 2001 Broad spectrum antibiotics for spontaneous preterm labour: The Oracle II Randomise Trial. Lancet 357:989–994

Kim KS 1985 Antimicrobial susceptibility of GBS. Antibiotics and Chemotherapy 35:83–89

Lin TY, Huang YC, Nin HC et al 1997 Oral acyclovir prophylaxis of varicella after intimate contact. Pediatric Infectious Diseases 16:1162–1165

Minkoff H, Mofenson LM 1994 The role of obstetric interventions in the prevention of pediatric human immunodeficiency virus infection. American Journal of Obstetrics and Gynecology 171:1167–1175

Moore MR, Schrag SJ, Schuchat A 2003 Effects of intrapartum antimicrobial prophylaxis for prevention of group B streptococcal disease on the incidence and ecology of early-onset neonatal sepsis. Lancet Infectious Diseases 3:201–213

Oddie S, Embleton ND 2002 Risk factors for early onset neonatal group B streptococcal sepsis: case control study. BMJ 325:308

O'Reilly GC, Hitti JE, Benedetti TJ 1999 Group β streptococcus infection in pregnancy: an update. Fetal and Maternal Medicine Review 11:31–39

Randolph AG, Hartshorn RM, Washington AE 1996 Acyclovir prophylaxis in late pregnancy to prevent neonatal herpes: a cost effectiveness analysis. Obstetrics and Gynecology 88:603–610

Royal College of Obstetricians and Gynecologists 2003 Clinical Green Top Guidelines. Prevention of Early Onset Neonatal Group B Streptococcal Disease. London, RCOG

Scott LL, Sanchez PJ, Jackson GL et al 1996 Acyclovir suppression to prevent Caesarean delivery after first-episode genital herpes. Obstetrics and Gynecology 87:69–73

Siegel JD 1998 Prophylaxis for neonatal Group β streptococcus infection. Seminars in Perinatology 22:33–49

Taylor GP, Hermione Lyall EG, Mercey D et al 1999 British HIV Association Guideline for prescribing antiretroviral therapy in pregnancy Sexually Transmitted Infections 75:90–97

Royal College of Obstetricians and Gynaecologists 2001 Guideline No. 13. Chickenpox in Pregnancy. London, RCOG pp 1–8

Wallace MR, Bowler WA, Murray NB et al 1992 Treatment of adult varicella with oral acyclovir. A randomized placebo-controlled trial. Annals of Internal Medicine 117:358–363

World Health Organization 1992 Consensus statement from the WHO/UNICEF: Consultation on HIV transmission and breast feeding. Weekly Epidemiological Record 67:177–179

(v) PSYCHIATRIC ILLNESS

David Liu

- 10–20% of newly delivered mothers will develop a depressive illness with 3–5% of them being severely depressed. Suicide ranks high although it is not the most common cause of maternal death in the year following delivery. Some 1–2 per 1000 women develop a psychotic illness after delivery.

- 2 per 1000 women will have a relapse of their pre-existing psychotic and affective disorders.

- At-risk women include:
  - those with a personal or close family history of affective disorder, severe depression or puerperal psychosis
  - those with panic disorder, severe anxiety or schizophrenia.

- After delivery watch out for obsessive or psychotic symptoms, severe anxiety, expression of guilt, suicidal intent and feelings of unworthiness.

DRUG MISUSER

- There is no typical misuser and non-disclosure is common because of fear that their lifestyle will be scrutinised or their baby may be taken away into care.

- Take full history, ask about withdrawal symptoms and psychological symptoms. Obtain consent for urinary analysis, e.g. Micro-Line, SureStep.

- Drug users encounter a high incidence of preterm labour, fetal growth retardation, intrauterine fetal death and cot deaths. Close fetal monitoring in labour is essential.

- Do not withdraw drugs suddenly.

- Watch out for infections such as bacterial endocarditis, hepatitis B and C or HIV.

- Encourage contact between mother and baby to maximise bonding.

- Protect confidentiality of the mother as a drug user. Her relatives may not be aware of her habits.

Opioid user

- Prescribe methadone 20–30 mg daily as substitute.

- Treat as if infection may be present.

- Opioid receptors are saturated hence these women will need large doses of drugs for analgesia. Do not use opioids if the woman has been weaned from her habit. Epidural anaesthesia for pain relief is recommended.

- Risk of placental insufficiency is increased. Avoid use of fetal scalp clips. Continuous external cardiotocographic monitoring for the fetus is essential but note opiates can interfere with interpretation of fetal heart rate patterns.
- There is no evidence of long-term organ damage in the baby.
- Do not give Narcan to baby after baby is born if mother has been using opioids.
- Withdrawal symptoms start in the baby within 24–48 hours after delivery. There is usually a high pitched cry, tachycardia, restlessness, sweating, fever, vomiting, diarrhoea or fits.
- Encourage breastfeeding.

Cocaine user

- This vasoconstrictor can cause maternal hypertension, tachycardia and placental abruption. The hypertension can confuse diagnosis of pre-eclampsia.
- Levels of protein C and antithrombin III are reduced hence an increased risk of thrombosis. On the other hand thrombocytopenia may be encountered so

- platelets must be checked before insertion of epidural anaesthesia.
- Monitor fetus during labour as placental insufficiency and fetal growth retardation are likely.
- Use phenylephrine or methoxamine for treatment of hypotension associated with epidural usage.

User of benzodiapines (temazepam or diazepam)

- There is increased risk of cleft palate.
- Babies with withdrawal symptoms may have low temperatures, poor muscle tone with poor sucking and respiratory difficulties.
- Breastfeeding is not recommended.

Amfetamine user

- Women may be malnourished and complain of tiredness.
- Intrauterine growth retardation is common.

Cannabis user

- No specific harmful side effects for mother.
- Intrauterine growth retardation is common.

Bibliography

American Academy of Paediatrics 2001 Transfer of drugs and other chemicals into human milk. Paediatrics 108(3)
Confidential Enquiry into Maternal Deaths in the UK 1998 Why Mothers Die (1994–1996). HMSO, London.
Cox JL, Murray P, Chapman E 1993 A controlled study of the onset, duration and prevalence of postnatal depression. British Journal of Psychiatry 163:27–31
Department of Health (DoH) 2002 Models of care for substance misuse treatment. National Treatment Agency (NTA), London

English National Board 1997 Substance Misuse – Guidelines for Good Practice
Kendell RE, Chalmers JC, Platz C 1987 Epidemiology of puerperal psychosis. British Journal of Psychiatry. 150:662–672
Royal College of Psychiatrists 2000 Recommendations for the Provision of Mental Health Services for Child Bearing Women. Royal College of Psychiatrists Report. London, RCP

Chapter **23**

Fetal and maternal misadventure

David T Y Liu
Mentor: Charles Rodeck

CHAPTER CONTENTS

Fetal abnormalities   207
Fetal trauma   208
    Procedure   208
Fetal death   208
Death of a co-twin   208
    Management   208
        Dichorionic twins – more than 34 weeks   208
        Dichorionic twins – before 34 weeks   208
        Monochorionic twins   208
Fetal/neonatal death at margin of viability   211
Maternal trauma   211
    Procedure   211
Maternal death   211
    Procedure   212

It is a sad but undeniable fact that, despite the best intentions, fetal and maternal damage or death occasionally complicate labour. The maternal mortality rate in England and Wales is around 1 per 10 000 live births (see Chapter 3). This can mean a tragedy about every two years in an obstetric department subserving 5000 pregnancies annually. The corrected perinatal mortality of around 1 per 100 births is 100 times higher than the maternal mortality rate. When misfortune presents itself appropriate counselling is essential. In most units a risk management form must be completed.

FETAL ABNORMALITIES

- The mother and her partner should be informed at the earliest opportunity of any major abnormality found at birth. Minor defects, which are detected, can be discussed later, at an appropriate time. Monstrosities are best not shown to parents unless explicitly requested and only after sensitive preparation.

- Discuss fully the likely cause and consequence of the abnormality. If appropriate arrange paediatric and genetic counselling for the couple.

- 3% of births are associated with an abnormality of some sort. Parents naturally want to identify a possible cause. Discuss all queries or suggestions and discourage any feelings of guilt.

- Rejection of the abnormal baby is a natural first reaction. Frequent discussion and counselling in the postnatal period is essential.

- All congenital abnormalities incompatible with life should be photographed, X-rayed and karyotyped to enhance subsequent genetic counselling.

- In contemporary practice most abnormalities are detected antenatally by ultrasound scan to allow proper care after birth.

FETAL TRAUMA

Fetal injuries can range from minor trauma, such as bruising or forceps marks, to major damage, such as fractures.

Procedure

- Inform the parents.
- Attend to the trauma if necessary.
- Discuss fully the likely cause and consequence of the trauma. Where appropriate offer an apology when the cause is clearly iatrogenic (e.g. skin incision to baby at caesarean section).
- Investigate fully where the cause is uncertain and inform the parents of the direction of the enquiry and its subsequent verdict.
- Document all proceedings in detail for medicolegal reasons.

FETAL DEATH

The stillbirth rate is around 5 per 1000 total births. Most stillbirths (80%) are unexplained fetal deaths where antepartum asphyxia is considered a direct cause (80%). In some 20% there may be a history of antepartum haemorrhage. Bleeding after 20 weeks and hypertensive disease remain as fetal risk factors.

Intrapartum asphyxia or trauma accounts for 10–15% of stillbirths. Failure to recognise a problem, inappropriate management and poor communication contribute to the adverse outcome.

Apart from the obvious disappointment facing all concerned, the response evoked in an individual can only be fully appreciated when the psychological background is considered. Medical personnel involved and a senior obstetrician should interview the couple jointly or on planned separate occasions. A tragedy such as this can greatly distress the staff as well as the couple concerned. Before counselling we must examine:

- our attitudes towards fetal loss
- our sense of guilt in terms of personal failure and the reasons why the obstetric system may have failed
- our ability to assess the aetiology objectively and identify avoidable factors
- our ability to detect pathological grief in the parents necessitating referral for psychiatric or social support
- our competency to conduct counselling.

Do not discourage discussion of the death or over-reassure and gloss over the tragedy. Too often clinicians have been viewed by parents as insensitive, unsympathetic and unconcerned. A suggested approach is shown in Box 23.1.

DEATH OF A CO-TWIN

Both counselling of parents and management of complication are challenging due to risk of preterm birth and fetal brain damage.

- There is up to 30% of vanishing twin in first trimester with up to 4% death of a co-twin after 20 weeks. For monochorionic twin pregnancies this complication may be as high as 25%.
- After fetal death onset of labour occurs within a few weeks (usually three weeks).
- Monochorionic twins share their circulation. Hypotension and thrombotic episodes following death of a co-twin result in death (25%) and varying degrees of cerebral damage (25%) in the remaining twin. Leukomalacia is detectable 2–5 weeks after a hypotensive episode.

Management

Dichorionic twins – more than 34 weeks
- Discuss delivery with parents.
- Give steroids if not full term.
- Consider abdominal delivery if the lead twin is dead. Otherwise manage according to usual practice.

Dichorionic twins – before 34 weeks
- Negotiate with parents to delay delivery to gain fetal maturity.
- Monitor surviving twin by Doppler and cardiotocography.
- Monitor mother's clotting factors, e.g. fibrinogen, platelets, thrombophilia screen at least weekly. Changes usually not obvious for 4 weeks after intrauterine death.

Monochorionic twins
- In addition to above management some 50% of remaining twins may die or suffer brain damage (porencephaly observed by ultrasound or magnetic resonance five weeks after death).
- Damage more likely if survivor is anaemic.
- Delay delivery if possible to allow examination of the fetal brain by weekly ultrasound scans.

Box 23.1   Stillbirth or fetal death protocol

- Confirm fetal death or stillbirth has occurred – inform the mother immediately.

- Allow ample time for both the mother and her partner to ventilate their feelings and seek causes.

- Do not make excuses. Adopt an accepting attitude. Guilt feelings in mothers are common. Expression of anger is therapeutic, allowing a mother to offload some of her guilt feelings.

- Remember fetal death or stillbirth may be viewed by the mother as further evidence of her failings and inadequacies. It can also be felt as the loss of part of herself and stimulate fantasies analogous to that of phantom limbs after amputation. The birth of a child may hold symbolic significance as a means of redeeming some of the mother's shortcomings in life. Search for these background factors in the discussion to understand the mother's responses and to assist in subsequent counselling. Existing children can be affected by the tragedy and may need help and counsel. Support for the couple must extend into the next pregnancy and next birth.

Management
- Confirm suspicion of fetal death by auscultation, cardiotocography and ultrasound scanning.

- Obtain detailed history. This may help determine the cause and is important for the management of subsequent pregnancies.

- Note condition of the mother, clinical assessment, blood pressure, urinalysis, vaginal bleeding.

- Take blood from the mother for haemoglobin, full blood count, cross-matching, clotting screen and Kleihauer count.

- Consider delivery. Women seldom wish to continue pregnancy once fetal death is confirmed. A quarter to a third may develop disseminated intravascular coagulation if the fetus is not delivered within 3–4 weeks.

- Transfusion or resuscitation may be necessary if fetal death followed placental separation. Problems with clotting may need to be corrected.

- Avoid caesarean section unless there are mechanical problems such as transverse lie. Aim for a delivery with minimum intervention, discomfort or surgical intervention.

- Allow labour to continue if contractions are present; otherwise if there is no contraindication induce labour at a time acceptable to the mother. The most effective method is the combination of the anti-progesterone agent mifepristone (600 mg) followed 36–48 hours later by oral or vaginal misoprostol (50 µg).

- Intravenous oxytocin (Syntocinon) can be used to augment labour.

- Leave membranes intact until labour is advanced (5 cm cervical dilatation) and delivery is assured. Prolonged rupture of membranes increases risk of intrauterine infection.

- Use analgesia (morphine or diamorphine) liberally. Discuss with the woman the degree of sedation she requires. An epidural block can be given provided there is no clotting defect.

- Keep delivery as uncomplicated as possible.

Following stillbirth
- Encourage the parents to see and hold the baby. If there is reluctance a photograph should be taken and kept for future reference. This practice will help identify the dead baby as an entity and facilitate parental mourning. The mother and father must be warned if there is gross abnormality or maceration. Display the baby to show as much normality as possible.

- Interview the couple on at least three occasions to provide opportunities for repeated discussion, to express empathy and to assess the couple's psychological status. Grief and the usual reactions to loss such as denial, guilt and aggression are normal responses but inappropriate behaviour indicates the need for psychiatric counselling.

Documentation
- Obtain consent.

- Conduct detailed inspection for malformations, deformities, infection and trauma.

- Photograph abnormal or dysmorphic features.

- Skeletal radiography is mandatory to assist subsequent genetic counselling.

- Record occipitofrontal circumference, crown–heel length, limb length, etc.

- Conduct detailed inspection of the placenta, record weight, take swabs for culture and dispatch for pathological examination.

- At an appropriate time broach the sensitive question of post mortem or histology. Emphasise the value of

Box 23.1 *Continued*

this investigation to determine aetiology of fetal death and for subsequent care. If full autopsy is not allowed seek permission for limited biopsy of skin, lung and liver. Make sure the consent form is signed and full ethical details are on the request form. See Box 23.2.

Investigation

- Obtain parental consent.
- Maternal blood should be screened for infection (TORCH, parvovirus, etc) Kleihauer count, liver and thyroid function, anti-cardiolipin antibodies, blood sugar, urea, liver function and bile salts.
- Take swabs from vagina, placenta and baby.
- Take fetal blood (cardiac puncture) for infection screen and examination of fetal chromosomes. Fetal skin (from the axilla so as not to disfigure) can be used for karyotyping (if no maceration otherwise use muscle or cartilage).
- Dispense placenta (in formalin) for histological examination.

Administration

- Inform as soon as possible all relevant people such as general practitioners, community midwives, health visitors and other involved colleagues to avoid unnecessary or inadvertent comments. This will allow early arrangements for after care following discharge from hospital.
- Allocate a family room so the partner can stay. The baby, cleaned and dressed, is left with the couple to allow time to grieve in privacy. Notify religious advisor if this is requested.
- When gestation is more than 24 weeks a stillbirth certificate (issued by the obstetricians) and a certificate of burial or cremation (issued by a registrar of births and deaths) is required. Unless mothers request otherwise the law does not require burial or cremation for gestations before 24 weeks. If burial of the baby is intended, a certificate stating that the fetus was stillborn is required.
- In the United Kingdom, a maternity grant allowance is payable for fetal death after 24 weeks.
- All women must be given a postnatal follow-up appointment at the gynaecological clinic (away from an obstetric environment) to allow further discussion and counselling with the consultant obstetrician. Where appropriate refer for genetic counselling or psychiatric support.

Box 23.2 Post-mortem request

- Consent for post-mortem examination should be by a senior member of the obstetric team able to understand the sensitivity of the task; discuss reasons for the request; identify where and who performs the examination and provide comprehensive information.
- Parents should know value of the post mortem for identifying time and cause/causes of death; to confirm or elicit structural abnormalities and search for placental pathology.
- Information should include how the post mortem is performed (usually incision over back of the head to examine the brain and a midline neck to pelvis cut for access to relevant organs) and if organs (e.g. brain or heart) or tissues are likely to be retained.
- Consent for organ retention must be specifically notated. This will include use for teaching, research or dispense for tests, e.g. metabolic and any additional consultation. If there is doubt consult the perinatal pathologist.
- Parents must be told when results are available and the length of time organs/tissues are retained (usually 3 weeks to 3 months).
- Where full post mortem is declined approach parents for a limited post mortem to answer specific questions or confirm diagnosis, e.g. heart lesion. In certain circumstances, e.g. metabolic disorders, tissue samples may need to be taken early (within hours).
- Parental consent is not needed for a coroner's autopsy.
- Fill in the structured post-mortem request form. This will include a detailed history. A copy will be kept by the parents.
- A father can countersign to support consent but usually cannot give consent by himself, i.e. without the mother's consent.

Post mortem: specific steps

- *Placenta*: take appropriate samples (e.g. for genetics and microbiology) then place in formalin and send with baby to the pathologist.
- *Obtain consent for*: chromosome analysis (skin, blood, placenta, radiological examination and photographs).
- *Document*: clinical assessment of baby and placenta; record weight and measurements. Take photographs and x-ray if indicated. All these steps will help geneticist even if post mortem is refused.

Box 23.3   Maternal death

The Government requires all involved health professionals to provide full and accurate information for the CEMACH, which is a work remit for the National Institute of Health and Clinical Excellence (NICE). This allows audit of cases and trends in maternal deaths. Avoidable or substandard factors are identified to improve care of future expectant women.

Definition
- Maternal death is defined as death occurring during or within 1 year of pregnancy, childbirth, miscarriage or termination of pregnancy.
- Direct maternal death – death due to complications or management of pregnancy, labour and puerperium.
- Indirect maternal death – death due to pre-existing disease, disease developed during pregnancy or disease compromised by the physiological changes of pregnancy.
- Fortuitous maternal death – death not related to the woman being pregnant.
- Late maternal death – death between 42 days and 1 year due to direct or indirect causes of pregnancy.

Process
- Appoint a coordinator to review medical records, institute internal investigation, collate documentation, list names of all involved and obtain their reports. An untoward incident form is generated. The coordinator is tasked to inform relevant personnel involved (in the United Kingdom this will involve notifying regional midwife assessor, regional coordinator for CEMACH and the mortuary department for the post mortem).
- Appoint a supporter for the mother's family to provide a point of contact and relay of consistent available information.
- Photocopy of medical records for relevant personnel.
- Arrange support for involved medical personnel, e.g. chaplain, occupational health department or mentor.
- Arrange contact with the family's religious leaders, e.g. priest or rabbi.
- Arrange further meeting with consultant to ensure findings can be discussed comprehensively.

FETAL/NEONATAL DEATH AT MARGIN OF VIABILITY

Babies delivered at known gestation of 23 weeks or less are previable (physical appearance, fused eyelids, etc). Heart activity and gasping movements may be evident at birth.

- Discuss fully with mother and partner to ensure appreciation of situation and obtain indication of their feelings and wishes (e.g. question of resuscitation, holding baby after birth, request for neonatal death certificate despite gestation; baby will be classified as neonatal death if there is sustained breathing and heart activity).
- When appropriate or at parents' request, a neonatologist should attend to support staff and parents.

MATERNAL TRAUMA

Maternal trauma in the pelvic region can occur spontaneously during labour and delivery or as a consequence of operative delivery. Where possible minimise long term damage to urethral and anal sphincter.

Procedure
- Elicit the nature and the extent of damage.
- Explain and discuss any requirements for surgical repair and prognosis.
- If the cause is iatrogenic, offer an apology, explain the reason for the damage and adopt a neutral accepting role during any discussion.
- Document all proceedings fully for medicolegal reasons.

The medical profession is not taught to dispense harm or damage, but accidents can happen. An objective appraisal of the situation is instructive and experience gained can be used to benefit others. In current practice untoward incidence forms must be completed for audit and action to avoid a recurrence.

MATERNAL DEATH

The death of any young person as a result of a natural function, which usually brings happiness, is a catastrophe. The fact that it occurs is a constant reminder of Nature's capriciousness, our need for further knowledge of obstetrics and, above all, a reminder that events may be difficult to predict and that constant vigilance is necessary in the care of our expectant women.

Procedure

- The most senior person should inform, console and interview the husband/partner and relatives. Discuss fully all possible aetiologies.
- Notify the relevant staff and personnel, e.g. community midwives and general practitioners.

- Document fully all the proceedings for medicolegal reasons.
- Complete a death certificate.
- A post mortem is usually mandatory.
- A thorough investigation is always necessary.
- Adopt the same attitude as suggested for other misadventures during interviews.

Box 23.3 describes how maternal deaths are defined by the Confidential Enquiry into Maternal and Child Health (CEMACH) and the process involved in reporting a maternal death.

Bibliography

CESDI 2000 Report focusing on stillbirths etc, project 27/28. London, Maternal and Child Health Research Consortium, London

Fisk NM, Bennett PR 1995 Prenatal determination of chorionicity and zygosity. In: Wald RH, Whittle MJ (eds). Multiple Pregnancy. London, RCOG Press pp 56–67

Maternal and Child Health Consortium 2002 Confidential enquiry into stillbirths and deaths in infancy. Maternal and Child Health Consortium, London

Murphy KW 1995 Intrauterine death in a twin: implications for the survivor. In: Wald RH, Whittle MJ

(eds). Multiple Pregnancy. London, RCOG Press pp 218–230

Pharaoh POD, Adi Y 2000 Consequences of in utero death in a twin pregnancy. Lancet 355:1597–1602

Hughes P, Riches S 2003 Psychological aspects of perinatal loss. Current Opinions in Obstetrics and Gynaecology 15:107–111

Roger MW, Baird DT 1990 Pre treatment with Mifepristone (RU 486) reduces the interval between prostaglandin administration and expulsion in second trimester abortion. British Journal of Obstetrics and Gynaecology 97:41–45

Chapter **24**

Obstetric emergencies: training with skills drills

Andrew Simm

CHAPTER CONTENTS

Guidelines 214
Training in acute obstetric emergencies 214
    Formats 214
        National courses 214
        Local courses 214
        Debriefing after incidents or real
            emergencies 214
    Fire drill 214
    Efficacy of training 215
    Example of fire drill for major obstetric
        haemorrhage 215
        Planning 215
        Running the scenario 216
        Feedback 217
    Learning from the drill 217
        Team working and communication 217
        Contacting emergency teams 217
        Equipment 217

Local clinical governance, reinforced by various national structures, now underpins the functioning of the National Health Service (NHS). It requires the establishment of systems and ways of working that result in an improved standard of care for patients (Chief Medical Officer 2000).

Within obstetrics it is recognised that many untoward outcomes are unpredictable and unpreventable, but many reports have highlighted substandard care as being contributory to adverse outcomes (Confidential Enquiry into Stillbirths and Deaths in Infancy (CESDI) (1999), Chief Medical Officer (2000) Confidential Enquiry into Maternal and Child Health (CEMACH) (2004)).

As a result litigation costs are high, as often is the human cost. Rarely is one factor alone responsible, and investigation of such incidents has now moved from a culture of blame to one of analysing systems that have contributed to the event, and seeking to establish measures that will help prevent a recurrence (Chief Medical Officer 2000).

- Adverse outcomes are now systematically investigated at a local level (as part of a risk management strategy) and national level, the latter most notably portrayed by CEMACH (2004).

- The Clinical Negligence Scheme for Trusts (CNST) (2005) requires evidence of strategies in place to identify and minimise risk, and so hopefully reduce litigation.

- Both CEMACH and CNST highlight the need for establishing guidelines for the management of various clinical conditions, and rehearsing these in the form of a 'fire drill'. The Royal College of Obstetricians and Gynaecologists (RCOG) and Royal College of Midwives endorse this.

This is driven by the notion that although many complications of childbirth are infrequently encountered, they have a propensity to be catastrophic. Prompt appropriate management endeavours to reduce serious morbidity and mortality.

GUIDELINES

- Guidelines are established to provide an evidence base for management of specific conditions. Evidence is graded according to its quality and applicability (RCOG 2000). Where good evidence is lacking, expert opinion is utilised.
- They are produced at a national level, most notably by the RCOG and the National Institute of Health and Clinical Excellence (NICE).
- They are usually adapted by individual institutions in the recognition that they must be workable within the organisation of that hospital.
- The danger in guidelines is that they are adopted as policy that must not be breached. By their nature they are there to 'guide', and must be individualised to suit the needs of each patient.

Nonetheless, the usefulness of guidelines cannot be understated. They provide an easy source of reference for those on the 'shop floor' where uncertainty regarding management exists. They also provide some uniformity to management.

Some regions have adopted regional guidelines for conditions such as severe pre-eclampsia, thus facilitating audit of management of a condition infrequently encountered within individual institutions. This also allows familiarisation and uniformity for junior medical staff rotating within a region, when previously individual units adopted different guidelines.

TRAINING IN ACUTE OBSTETRIC EMERGENCIES

Formats

National courses
The two most established courses in the UK are:

- Advanced Life Support in Obstetrics (ALSO) course
- Managing Obstetric Emergencies and Trauma (MOET) course.

These combine lectures and skills practice to train candidates in a wide variety of clinical scenarios relevant to obstetric practice. Experienced instructors give standardised teaching. A uniform way to tackling a given scenario is provided. Feedback from participants regarding the courses is very positive.

Local courses
These usually take the form of scenario-based classroom teaching. Many have been based on the national courses described.

Debriefing after incidents or real emergencies
Fire drills These have been cited by CEMACH and CNST and are discussed further below.

Fire drill

Various names have been given to these, e.g. skills drill, emergency drill, and fire drill. The term is imprecisely defined, and takes numerous formats. A survey of practice in 2003 assessed what format of drill individual units were undertaking, and how these drills were being organised and evaluated. The authors proposed the term 'fire drill' should imply the drill is conducted in the normal working environment (most commonly the labour ward) without prior knowledge of the staff involved (Anderson et al 2005). This has the following advantages:

- testing local systems and guidelines for given clinical scenarios
- testing multidisciplinary teamwork among professionals who usually work together in the same unit, as well as individual skills and knowledge.

A 'fire drill' has additional benefits to training from that undertaken in the classroom or at a site distant from one's usual workplace and work colleagues.

At the time of the survey half of the responding units were conducting 'fire drills' as defined above. Many units were undertaking other forms of training in obstetric emergencies in addition to or in place of fire drills.

The positive aspects of fire drills as reported in the survey are:

- Increased confidence in emergency teamwork.
- Better multidisciplinary working.
- Improved physical organisation e.g. of emergency equipment.
- Use of a written report to make learning points available to a wider audience.
- Use of a volunteer to play the patient and/or relative; this enhances the value of the exercise. This had been recognised in national courses, and actors/actresses are used on the MOET course.

Difficulties in running fire drills as reported in the survey are:

- Threatening to staff.
- Unable to reach a large volume of staff.

- Problems in arranging multidisciplinary training because of time constraints, historical factors, lack of interest, and differences in study time allowed for separate professional groups.
- Business of unit sometimes meant the drill could not go ahead.
- Substantial time and energy in organising a drill.
- Distractions from other workload when drill being run.

Thus even where drills are run, units often utilise additional formats of training in obstetric emergencies.

Efficacy of training

Unfortunately there is little published evidence on the efficacy of different training strategies in terms of improved outcome for mothers and babies. There is recent evidence from Bristol that training in cardiotocograph interpretation, in addition to training in acute obstetric emergencies (not skills drills as defined here) has led to a reduction in the incidence of low Apgar scores at 5 minutes and cases of hypoxic ischaemic encephalopathy within the unit where the training is conducted (Draycott et al 2006). Prior to this it had only been shown that training produced softer outcome measures in terms of a perceived greater confidence in handling emergencies (Johanson et al 1999). A current study looking at evaluation of fire drills is in progress in the South West of England.

Assessing the impact of the training on outcomes is usually difficult given that adverse outcomes are fortunately rare. As an example, let us look at skills drills for shoulder dystocia:

- Shoulder dystocia is essentially unpredictable, and thus unpreventable, so one cannot anticipate a reduction in prevalence.
- However, it would be reasonable to anticipate that with improved handling of the shoulder dystocia there will be less adverse sequelae, most notably brachial plexus injury, fetal bone fracture and encephalopathy.
- Given the infrequent occurrence of these, it may take a long time to notice an improvement in outcomes.

Crofts et al (2005) looked instead at different outcome measures that should lead to less adverse sequelae, utilising a birth training mannequin. This showed a trend toward reduction in head-to-body delivery interval and reduced delivery force. In our own unit there has been a noticeable improvement in documentation, with an appreciation by those reviewing the incidents that the recorded management has been appropriate and timely.

Example of fire drill for major obstetric haemorrhage

CNST defines four clinical scenarios for which all staff should participate in an annual 'rehearsal of emergency procedure'. These are:

- Cord prolapse
- Vaginal breech delivery
- Shoulder dystocia
- Antepartum haemorrhage/severe postpartum haemorrhage

They also stipulate requirements for evidence of training in cardiotocograph interpretation and basic adult and neonatal life support.

An example of a fire drill for major obstetric haemorrhage outlines the key points in planning, conducting and learning from the training. For an example on eclampsia see Thompson et al (2004).

Planning
- The scenario must be defined, with clarity regarding the endpoint, i.e. do you wish to pursue a major post-partum haemorrhage drill as far as transport into theatre, or progress on to a cardiac arrest and basic then advanced life support?

- The scenario should be sufficiently detailed to allow progression in a realistic way (e.g. blood pressure recordings that are consistent with the given blood loss at any point in time). However, it requires some adaptability given that responses from participants are not always predictable. Hence the need for an experienced practitioner to lead the scenario.

- Timing can be difficult as workload on the labour ward is unpredictable. It is useful to utilise a time when sufficient staff are available to take care of the existing workload. (A period of overlap of shifts can be useful for midwives.) If utilising the laboratories then daytime working is preferable so that other activity is not significantly disrupted.

- Roles must be defined.
  - Lead – it is important for one person to act as the lead in giving out information, guiding if the scenario goes 'off track', and calling an end at an appropriate time.
  - Observer(s) – an observer is necessary for keeping a note of activities in accordance with a proforma to aid evaluation. If the drill is being videoed such observation is not necessary within the room.

- Role player – the value of role play has already been alluded to. Usually actors play the role of the patient and/or relative. If not utilised, a mannequin will be necessary. Even with actors it is useful to have equipment such as a 'dummy arm' for cannulation, and a model pelvis for demonstration of bimanual compression technique.

- The equipment must be set up in advance without alerting staff working in the area that a drill is pending. Thus the assistance of the labour ward co-ordinator is invaluable.

- If the drill involves assessment of the blood transfusion laboratory (communication, ability to get group specific blood quickly etc) it must be organised in conjunction with the chief medical laboratory scientific officer. In our own unit we set up in advance a 'dummy patient' with a factitious name and hospital number, and utilised blood from one of the organisers for grouping and antibody status (as would have occurred for any patient booked to deliver in our unit). Blood will then need to be taken during the scenario from the same person and sent to the laboratory as an urgent cross-match. This usefully tests labelling procedures too.

- An assessment proforma is useful to draw up beforehand so that the observer can tick off actions with timings as they occur (Box 24.1).

Running the scenario

- To commence the drill it is useful for the organiser or actor to request assistance in the room. The first person to attend is then briefed on arrival regarding the clinical scenario and instructed to treat the scenario as a real situation. Our own experience is that in this situation help is summoned from all quarters before it would have been in reality, and it can be useful to temper this with an instruction to the effect of 'medical staff are currently tied up with another emergency; you may request them again if your initial procedures do not effect a satisfactory response form the patient.'

- There should be clear instruction as to the roles of the leader and observer so that they are not expected to assist in the drill. Instructions may require repetition as more people enter the room.

- Requests for information should only be given if the relevant procedure for obtaining the information has been undertaken, e.g. the sphygmomanometer should be utilised before a blood pressure reading is given.

> **Box 24.1   Checklist for drill**
>
> **Expected actions – initial**
> - Communication with patient (assesses airway and breathing).
> - Communication with relative.
> - Measurement of pulse and blood pressure (assessment of circulation).
> - Estimation of blood loss.
> - Request for midwifery assistance.
> - Emptying of bladder.
> - Palpation of uterus and rubbing up of contraction.
>
> **Expected actions – subsequent (the order is approximate and not precise)**
> - Regular assessment of pulse and blood pressure.
> - Rechecking of uterine tone.
> - Request for assistance from obstetrician and anaesthetist.
> - Siting of intravenous cannula.
> - Administration of intravenous normal saline or Hartmann's solution.
> - Sending of bloods for full blood count, coagulation screen.
> - Request for cross-match of 4 units (group and save sent in labour but need to send request form).
> - Commencement of intravenous oxytocin infusion.
> - Administration of facial oxygen.
> - Commencement of bimanual compression (having established placenta complete and episiotomy wound dry).
> - Request for further uterotonic agents (e.g. Syntometrine, misoprostol, Hemabate).
> - Insertion of Foley catheter if not already in situ.
> - Request for type specific blood and O-negative blood from fridge.
> - Consultant obstetrician informed.
> - Transfer to theatre arranged.

- Equipment and drugs required should be sought by the participants and placed by the patient or mannequin. It must be decided in planning whether drugs should be drawn up or merely positioned by the patient.

- It useful to request participants to explain their actions as they go along so that actions do not go unnoticed.

- The participants should communicate with the patient or mannequin.

- If phone calls or bleeps to other staff members or services are required, these should be undertaken. In cases utilising the transfusion laboratory, it may be useful once the specific request has been clarified to have that information relayed by one of the organisers so that confusion regarding the patient does not hamper the events.

- An end-point should have been agreed before the scenario began, and the scenario terminated when this is reached. It may still be appropriate to continue timing if further communication with the laboratory is anticipated.

Feedback

- It needs to be agreed on what format the debriefing will take afterwards. It is always useful to provide an immediate debrief, but this may be supported by a written report. If a video is used it will be useful to run this back in order to provide feedback.

- Positive aspects of performance should always be highlighted before any criticisms are expressed.

Learning from the drill

The drill will almost certainly highlight systems or practices that can be improved. Examples of this from our own experience, with actions taken, are given.

Team working and communication

Frequently there was no clear lead participant overseeing the drill, and handovers of this role to a more experienced person were implied rather than clarified. Instructions were often not directed to specific people, so some tasks were duplicated and some not done.

Action: Feedback with examples, including running a demonstration 'drill'.

Contacting emergency teams

Bleep systems were incorrectly utilised resulting in inappropriate staff attending.

Action: Placement of a laminated sheet by telephones to clarify the process for contacting emergency teams, and clarification of communication with the switchboard.

Equipment

Valuable time was wasted searching for necessary equipment and drugs.

Action: Establishment of a 'Major haemorrhage box'.

It is important to run the drill again to establish that changes have been successful in their purpose.

References

Anderson ER, Black R, Brocklehurst P 2005 Acute obstetric emergency drill in England and Wales: a survey of practice. British Journal of Obstetrics and Gynaecology 112:372–375

Chief Medical Officer 2000 An organisation with a memory. Report of an expert group on learning from adverse events in the NHS. HMSO, London

Clinical Negligence Scheme for Trusts 2005 Maternity Clinical Risk Management Standards. NHS Litigation Authority, London

Confidential Enquiry into Maternal and Child Health 2004 Why Mothers Die 2000–2002. London, RCOG Press (www.cemach.org.uk/publications.htm)

Confidential Enquiry into Stillbirths and Deaths in Infancy 1999 6th Annual Report Focusing on The '1 in 10' Enquiries 1996–7, The '4 kg and over' Enquiries 1997, Perinatal Pathology, Record Keeping and Developing the Enquiries. Maternal and Child Health Research Consortium, London (www.cemach.org.uk/publications.htm)

Crofts FC, Attilakos G, Read M et al 2005 Shoulder dystocia training using a new birth mannequin. British Journal of Obstetrics and Gynaecology 112:997–999

Draycott T, Sibanda, T, Owen L et al 2006 Does training in obstetric emergencies improve neonatal outcome? British Journal of Obstetrics and Gynaecology 113(2):177–182

Johanson R, Cox C, O'Donnell E et al 1999 Managing Obstetric Emergencies and Trauma (MOET). The Obstetrician and Gynaecologist 1:46–52

Royal College of Obstetricians and Gynaecologists 2000 Clinical Governance Advice No 1. Guidance for the development of RCOG green-top guidelines. RCOG Press, London

Thompson S, Neal S, Clark V 2004 Clinical risk management in obstetrics: eclampsia drills. BMJ 328:269–271

Bibliography

Black R, Brocklehurst P 2003 A systematic review of training in acute obstetric emergencies. British Journal of Obstetrics and Gynaecology 110:837–841

Index

Note: Page references in italics refer to pictures/diagrams.

A

Abdominal examination, 25–7
Abdominal incisions, caesarean section, 146–7, *146*
Abnormal labour, 109–15
    abnormal uterine activity, 109–10
    false labour, 109–10
    precipitate labour, 110
    prolonged labour, 110–14
    sudden cessation of labour, 110
    trial of labour, 114–15
    trial of scar or vaginal delivery, 115
Abortion, 9
Abortion Act 1967, 9
Abscess, after regional analgesia, 62
Acceleration of heart rate, transient, 76, *76*
Acidaemia
    fetal, 80, 82
    maternal lactic, 82
    metabolic, 75
Acid–base
    fetus, 80–2
    newborn, 92
Acidosis, metabolic
    fetal, 75
    maternal, 55
Actin, 45
Adenosine triphosphate, 45
Adherent placenta, pathologically, 160
Admission emergencies, 35–44
    see also specific condition
Admission to labour ward, 23–32
Adrenal insufficiency, 192
Advanced directives, 6
Advanced Life Support in Obstetrics (ALSO) course, 214

Air embolism, 156
Alexandra unit, 47
Alkalosis, respiratory, 55
American College of Obstetricians and Gynaecologists (ACOG)
    classification of forceps deliveries 2000, 132
Amnion, 46
Amniotic fluid
    embolism, 15, 156
    meconium in, 82–3, 93
Amfetamine user, 205
Anaesthesia
    caesarean section, 65–7
    combined spinal–epidural, 67
    criteria for referral, 70
    drug depression in newborns, 94
    eclampsia, 69–70
    epidural, 66–7
    general, 67–8
    maternal mortality, 14, 66
    oxytocics, 68
    placenta praevia, 69
    pre-assessment, 69
    pre-eclampsia, 69
    spinal, 65
    tocolysis, 68
Analgesia, 59–65
    inhalation, 59–60
    parenteral opioids, 60
    postoperative, 68–9
    pre-eclampsia, 68
    regional *see* Regional analgesia
    transcutaneous electrical nerve stimulation (TENS), 60
Android pelvis, 28, *28*, 31
    occipitoposterior positions, 165, *166*
Aneurysms, 155

Anoxia, 82
Antepartum fetal death of a twin, 185
Antepartum haemorrhage, 37–8, 40
Anterior asynclitism, 168, *169*
Anthropoid pelvis *see* Ellipsoid pelvis
Antibiotics in preterm labour, 103–4
Anticonvulsant therapy, 197–8
Antidiuretic hormone (ADH), 56
Antihypertensive therapy
    in eclampsia, 41–3
    in pre-eclampsia, 197
Antiretroviral therapy, 202
Apgar scores, 82, 93
Arachidonic acid, 46
Artificial rupture of membranes, 120–1
Aseptic conditions, 48
Asphyxia, 208
Asphyxia pallida, 94
Aspiration pneumonia, 56
Assisted breech delivery, 175–6, *175–6*
Assisted vaginal delivery, 127–40
    forces operating in second stage of labour, 128
    indications for instrumental, 127–8
    maternal complications, 139
    medicolegal issues, 139–40
    neonatal complications, 139
    requirements for, 128
    rotational procedures, 135–9
    symphysiotomy, 140
    traction procedures, 132–4
Asthma, 190
Asynclitism, 136, 168, *169*
Attitudes, 1–3
Augmentation of labour, 124
Auscultation, 25, 26

Autoimmune thrombocytopenia (AITP), 189

B

Bacterial endocarditis, 195
Bacterial infections, 199–11
Bacterial vaginosis, 103–4
Bacteriuria, 197–200
Bag and mask ventilation, 95
Benign intracranial hypertension, 191
Benzodiazepines user, 205
β-adrenergic agonists, 103, 105–6
β-haemolytic streptococcus group B, 200
β-sympathomimetics, 56, 105
Bimanual compression of the uterus, 158, 158
Binovular twins, 180
Birth defects, 207–8
Birthing environment, 19–22
  home births, 21
  hospital birthing rooms, 19–20
  support in labour, 20
  water births, 20–21
Birthing rooms, hospital, 19–20
Birth plans, 3
Birth registration, 10
Birth trauma see Trauma
Birthweight, low, 94
Bishop's score, 28, 118, 119–20
Bladder function after assisted delivery, 141–2
Bleeding
  severity of in placental separation, 39
  see also Haemorrhage; Vaginal bleeding
Bloodborne viruses, chronic, 202
Blood component therapy, 38
Blood gas analyser, 81
Blood sampling, fetal, 81, 81–2, 184
Blood transfusion, women who refuse, 158
Body, delivery of the, 50, 50
Body temperature of newborns, 92
Brachial plexus palsy, 99
Bradycardia, 75
Braxton Hicks contractions, 109
Breathing, newborns, 92
Breech, 172, 174
  antenatal assessment, 172
  assisted delivery, 175–6, 175–6
  classification of, 172
  delivery by caesarean section, 177–8
  diagnosis of, 170
  dos and don'ts, 177

induction of labour, 123
in the second twin or triplet, 176–7
special situations, 178–9
spontaneous breech delivery, 173–6
twins, 176–7, 183
Brow presentation, 168, 168
Bupivacaine, 64
Burns-Marshall technique, 176, 176, 178

C

Caesarean hysterectomy, 151–2
Caesarean section, 2, 145–52
  after intrauterine fetal death, 150–1
  anaesthesia for, 65–8
  breech delivery, 177–8
  classical, 147, 147, 152
  combined spinal–epidural anaesthesia, 67
  diabetic mothers, 194
  dos and don'ts of, 150
  eclampsia, 69–70
  epidural anaesthesia for, 66–7
  general anaesthesia for, 67–8
  indications for, 145–6
  induction of labour following previous, 121–2
  operative steps for, 148, 149
  placenta praevia, 69
  postoperative care, 146
  pre-eclampsia, 69
  pre-operative care/preparation, 65–6, 146
  specific issues, 148–52
  spinal anaesthesia for, 66
  twins, 183–4
  types of incision, 146–8
  uterine scar rupture, 149–50
  vaginal delivery after previous, 115
Calcium ions, 46
Calmodulin, 45
Cannabis user, 205
Capacity test, 6
Caput succedaneum, 98, 99
Cardiac arrest in the obstetric woman, 43
Cardiac compressions, 96
Cardiac disease, 195–8
Cardiac output, fetal, 73–4
Cardiac syncope, 195
Cardiopulmonary resuscitation of the obstetric woman, 43
Cardiotocograms (CTGs), 74

Cardiovascular system of newborns, 92
Care
  assisted delivery, 141–2
  quality of, 24
  satisfaction with, 3, 22
Catheter-transducer system, 80
Cephalhaematoma, 98, 99, 129, 139
Cephalic presentation, 28
Cerclage, cervical, 103, 103
Cerebral palsy, 75
Cerebrospinal fluid (CSF), 65
  distinction between saline and, 64
Cervical cerclage, 103, 103
Cervix
  dilatation of, 27, 27
    deficient/delayed, 114
    manual, 159, 159
  effacement of, 27, 27, 48, 119
  effect of uterine activity on
    before labour, 47
    during labour, 48
  examination of, 27
  incisions, 114, 114
  ripening of, 119
Cessation of labour, sudden, 110
Chicken pox, 203
Chignon, 139
Children, consent, 6
Chlamydia trachomatis, 200–1
Choanal atresia, 95–7
Chorioamnionitis, 104
Chorion, 45, 46
Circulation, newborn, 96
Classical caesarean section, 147, 147, 152
Clinical governance, 11
Clinical Negligence Scheme for Trusts (CNST), 213
Clomethiazole, 95
Coagulation disorders, inherited, 189
Cocaine user, 205
Collapse in the obstetric patient, 63
Communication, caesarean section, 148
Complete breech presentation, 172, 172
Complications, medical, 187–205
  see also specific problem
Compound presentation, 168
Conduct, 1–3
Confidential Enquiries into Maternal Deaths in the UK, 13
Confidential Enquiry into Maternal and Child Health (CEMACH), 213
Confidential Enquiry into Stillbirths and Deaths in Infancy (CESDI), 213

Confidentiality, 10
Conjoined twins, 183
Connexin-43, 45
Consent, 5–9
    see also Informed consent
Contracted pelvis, 28–30
Contractions, 46, 46, 45, 47
    abnormal, 110–11
    assisted delivery, 128
    Braxton Hicks, 109
    complications of strong, 155, 156
    display of, 78–9
    frequent strong (hypertonic),
        110–11
    incoordinate uterine activity, 111
    infrequent weak (hypotonic), 110
    measurements of, 79–80
    recording methods, 74
Convulsions, 40
Cord see Umbilical cord
Corticosteroids, 102–3
Corticotrophin-releasing hormone, 46
Cortisol, fetal, 45–6
Court applications for medical
    treatment, 8
Cryoprecipitate, 38
Cusco's speculum, 26, 26
Cutting bevel tip spinal needles, 60,
    61
Cyanosis, 195

D

Data Protection Act, 10
Deceleration of heart rate, 76–7, 77,
    78
Deflexed head, 164, 165–6
Dehydroepiandrosterone (DHEAS),
    45
Delivery
    of the body see Body, delivery of
        the
    breech see Breech
    of the head see Head, delivery of
        the
    management of, 48–51
    normal, 49–52
    of the placenta, 51, 51
    position, 48
    preterm see Preterm delivery
    of the shoulders, 49, 50, 50
    umbilical cord, 49–51
Depressive illness, 204–5
Dermatomes, 64, 67
    perineal, 87
Descent, abnormal, 112–14
Diabetes, 193–4
Diabetic ketoacidosis, 194

Diaphragmatic hernia, 97
Diazepam, 94, 207
Dichorionic twins, 208
Diclofenac, contraindications to, 68
Dilatation, cervical see Cervix,
    dilatation of
Direct occipitoposterior, 164, 165
Disproportion, 112–13, 178
    inlet, 113
    mid-pelvic, 113
    outlet, 115
Diving reflex, 74
Dizygotic twins, 181, 182
Doppler fetal heart rate detector, 25,
    26, 26, 74, 77
Doyen retractor, 148
Drug depression in newborns, 94–5
Drugs
    effect on fetal heart rate, 74
    misusers of, 204–5
    see also specific drug
Dural tap, 62, 64–5

E

Early deceleration of heart rate, 76, 77
Eclampsia, 40, 41–3, 198
    anaesthesia, 69–70
Effacement, cervical, 27, 27, 48, 119
Efficacy of training, 215
Electrolytes, intrapartum, 55–6
Electronic FHR monitoring, 77–8
Ellipsoid pelvis, 28, 28, 31
    occipitoposterior positions, 165
Embolism
    air, 155
    amniotic fluid, 155
Emergencies
    admission, 35–44
    drill for, 213, 214–15
    in immediate puerperium, 153–61
        acute uterine inversion, 160–1
        postpartum haemorrhage,
            155–8
        retained placenta, 158–60
    training for obstetric, 213–17
Endocarditis, bacterial, 195
Endocrine disorders, 192–4
Endotracheal intubation, 96
Engagement, 25, 25
Entonox, 52, 59–60
Environment, birthing see Birthing
    environment
Enzyme immunoassays (EIA),
    201
Epidural anaesthesia
    for caesarean section, 66–7
    pre-eclampsia, 198

Epidural analgesia, 60, 60–5
    counselling before, 62
    drug regimen for, 64
    see also Regional analgesia
Epidural blood patch, 65
Epidural space, 60
Epidural venous engorgement,
    63
Epilepsy, 40, 190
Episiotomy
    dos and don'ts, 87–8
    repair of an, 88, 88
    restructuring an, 88–9
    technique, 86, 86
    timing, 86–7
    types of incision, 85–6, 86
Equanox, 59–60
Equipment
    birthing room, 19–20
    home births, 21
    water births, 21
Erect lateral pelvimetry (ELP), 31,
    31–2
Ergometrine, 44
European Convention on Human
    Rights, 11
Examination in theatre, 40
Expectations, 2–3
Extended breech presentation, 172,
    172
External cephalic version (ECV), 172,
    173

F

Face presentation, 166, 166–7, 167
Face to pubes breech position,
    179
Facial palsy, 98
Factor IX deficiency, 189
Faecal incontinence after third degree
    tears, 90
False labour, 109–10
Fentanyl, epidural, 67
Fetal acid–base balance
    blood sampling, 81–2
    fetal pH, 80–1
    management of abnormal FHR
        trace, 82
Fetal death, 208
    caesarean section after
        intrauterine, 150–1
    of a co-twin, 208
    intrauterine, 123–4, 150–1
    at margin of viability, 211
    protocol, 209–10
    suspected, 43
    of a twin antepartum, 185

Fetal heart rate (FHR)
  baseline, 75–6
  effect of drugs on, 74
  late deceleration of, 77, 78
  management of abnormal trace, 82
  monitoring see Fetal surveillance,
    heart rate
  pattern changes, 78
  transient changes in, 76–7
Fetal surveillance, 73–83
  acidaemia, 82
  acid–base balance, 80–2
  Apgar scores, 82
  heart rate
    background, 74–5
    electronic, 77–8
    improving recording of, 77–80
    management of abnormal trace,
      82
    requirements for, 77–8
    types, 75–7
  meconium, 82–3
  multiple deliveries, 184
  neurological outcome, 82
  physiology and pathophysiology,
    73–4
Fetal varicella syndrome, 203
Fetus
  abnormalities of, 207–8
  acid–base, 80–2
  assessment equipment, birthing
    room, 20
  blood glucose levels, 55
  blood sampling, 81, 81–2, 184
  cardiac output, 73–4
  causes of shoulder presentation
    due to, 169
  complications with assisted
    vaginal delivery, 139
  consequences of prolonged labour,
    114
  death of see Fetal death
  effect of uterine activity on the, 48
  fibronectin testing, 104
  heart rate see Fetal heart rate
    (FHR)
  indications for assisted vaginal
    deliveries due to, 128
  indications for induction due to,
    117–18
  movements of, 83
  pH, 80–1
  presentation of, 24, 182 (see also
    Malposition; Malpresentation)
  problems causing prolonged
    labour due to, 112
  surveillance of see Fetal
    surveillance
  trauma to, 208

Fire drill, 213, 214–15
First degree tears, 89
First stage of labour, effect of uterine
    activity on cervix, 48
Fits, 40
Flat trace, 76, 77, 78
Flexed breech presentation, 172, 172
Flexed occipitoposterior, 164
Fluid balance
  in eclampsia, 41
  pre-eclampsia, 198
Footling breech presentation, 172, 172
Forceps, 129, 130, 133
  caesarean section, 151, 151
  rotational procedures, 137, 137–8
  traction procedures, 133, 134, 134,
    135
  trial of, 138–9
Forewater rupture, 120, 120–1
Fourchette, unyielding posterior, 87,
    88
Fourth degree tears, 89
Fractures, 99
Frank breech presentation, 172, 172
Fresh frozen plasma (FPP), 38
Full breech presentation, 172, 172
Fundal height, 25, 25
Fundal pressure, assisted delivery,
    128, 129
Furosemide, 198

G

Gardnerella vaginalis, 103–4
General anaesthesia, 67–8
  pre-eclampsia, 69
Genital herpes, 201–2
Genital trauma, maternal mortality
    following, 16
Gestational diabetes, 194
Gestational thrombocytopenia, 189
Gillick competence, 6
Gluconeogenesis, 55
Glucose, 55
Glyceryl trinitrate (GTN), 68
Gonorrhoea, 201
Groin traction, 175, 175
Gynaecoid pelvis, 28, 28, 31
  occipitoposterior positions, 165

H

Haematological problems, 188–90
Haematoma
  after assisted delivery, 141
  after regional analgesia, 62
  vaginal, 139

Haemophilia, 189
Haemorrhage
  antepartum, 37–8, 40
  example fire drill for major
    obstetric, 215–17
  intracranial, 98
  major obstetric, 37, 215–17
  maternal mortality, 15
  postpartum see Postpartum
    haemorrhage
  pulmonary (newborn), 97
  subdural, 98
Handicap incidence for preterm
    babies, 102–3
Head, deflexed, 164
  occipitoposterior positions,
    165–6
Head, delivery of the
  difficulty in caesarean section, 151,
    151
  forceps, 135
  normal, 49, 50, 50
Healthcare proxies, 7
Heart rate monitoring, fetal see Fetal
    surveillance, heart rate
Heart sound, fetal, 26
Heminevrin, 95
Hepatitis B, 202
Hepatitis C, 202
Hernia, diaphragmatic, 97
Herpes, genital, 201–2
Holding stitch, caesarean section, 152,
    152
Home births, 21
Hospital birthing rooms, 19–20
Hospital infection, 202
Human immunodeficiency virus
    (HIV), 202–3
Human Rights Act, 10
Husbands, 2
Hydralazine treatment, 42, 197
Hydrostatic balloon, 158
15-hydroxyprostaglandin
    dehydrogenase, 46
Hypermagnesaemia, 198
Hypertension, 191, 196
Hypertensive crisis management,
    197
Hypertensive disorders, maternal
    mortality, 15
Hypertonic contractions, 110–11
Hypoglycaemic coma, 194
Hypothyroid, 192
Hypotonic uterine activity, 110
Hypovolaemia, 198
Hypovolaemic shock in newborns,
    94
Hypoxaemia, 75
Hypoxia, 80–1

Hypoxic ischaemic encephalopathy, 98
Hysterectomy, caesarean, 151–2

I

Identical twins, 181
Imminent delivery, 35
Immunoglobulins, 203
Implied consent, 6
Incision types
    caesarean section, 146–8
    episiotomy, 85–6
Incomplete breech presentation, 172, 172
Incontinence after third degree tears, faecal, 90
Induction of labour
    contraindications to, 118
    diabetics, 193
    general considerations, 118
    indications for, 117–18
    key points in, 124
    process of, 119–21
    as prophylaxis, 118
    requirements before, 118–19
    risks of, 121–2
    special situations, 121–4
    as therapy, 117
Infection
    bacterial, 199–201
    intrauterine following induction, 122
    preterm labour, 103–4
    viral, 201–3
Informed consent, 3, 5, 129
Infusion pump, 121, 122
Inhalation analgesia, 59–60
Inherited disorders of coagulation, 189
Instruments for assisted delivery, 129–32, 130, 131
Insulin, 193–4
Internal podalic version, 177, 178
Intertuberous diameter, 31, 31
Intracranial haemorrhage, 98
Intracranial pressure, raised, 191
Intrapartum fetal surveillance see Fetal surveillance
Intrapartum nutrition and electrolytes, 55–6
Intrauterine fetal death, 123–4
    caesarean section after, 150–1
Intrauterine growth restriction, 113
Intrauterine pressure, 46–7, 47, 74
Invasive positive pressure ventilation (IPPV), 96
Ischial spine, 30, 30, 87, 87

J

Jehovah's Witnesses, 6
J-shaped incision, episiotomy, 85–6, 86

K

Ketoacidosis, diabetic, 194
Ketonuria, 55
Kilopascals, 46
Kjelland's rotational forceps, 129, 130, 131, 137, 137–8
    inherent dangers of, 138
Knee breech presentation, 172, 172
Kocher's forceps, 120, 120
Krönig–Gellhorn–Beck incision, 147, 147–8, 178

L

Labetalol treatment, 42, 197
Labour
    abnormal see Abnormal labour
    augmentation of, 124
    false, 109–10
    first stage, 48
    induction of see Induction of labour
    mechanism of, 50, 50
    myometrial activity in, 46–52
    preterm see Preterm labour
    second stage, 48, 128
    third stage, 51, 51
Labour ward admission, 23–32
Lactic acid, 80
Late deceleration of heart rate, 77, 78
Left occipitoposterior (LOP), 164, 165
Legal considerations, 5–12
    instrumental vaginal delivery, 139–40
Levobupivacaine, 64
Lie of fetus, 24, 24
Listeria monocytogenes, 103–4, 200
Listeriosis, 200
Living wills, 6–7
Locked twins, 184–5
Loop diuretic administration, 198
Lovset's manoeuvre, 175, 175–6, 178
Low ARM, 120, 120–1
Low birthweight infants, 94
Lower segment caesarean section, 147, 147
Low molecular weight heparins (LMWHs), 62
Lung liquid in newborns, 92
Lungs of newborns, 92

M

Macrosomia, 112
Magnesium sulphate, 197
    drug depression in newborns, 95
    in eclampsia, 41
Major obstetric haemorrhage, 37, 215–17
Malposition, 112, 163–6
    definition of, 163
    twins, 182
Malpresentation, 112, 166–70
    definition of, 163–4
    twins, 182
Managing Obstetric Emergencies and Trauma (MOET) course, 214
Mannitol, 198
Manual rotation, 136, 136
Maternal expulsive effort, assisted delivery, 128
Maternal mortality, 13–16, 211–12
    attributable to anaesthesia, 66
    cause of, 14
    rate of, 207
Mauriceau–Smellie–Veit manoeuvre, 176, 176
Mazzanati's procedure, 141
McRoberts' manoeuvre, 141
Meconium, 82–3
    in amniotic fluid, 82–3, 93
    aspiration, 83
Medial incision, episiotomy, 85, 86
Medical attendants, 48–9
Medical complications, 187–205
    see also specific problem
Medical records, 11
Medicolegal issues, instrumental vaginal delivery, 139–40
Mediolateral incision, episiotomy, 85, 86
Membranes
    artificial rupture of, 120–1
    pre-labour rupture of, 123
    preterm premature rupture of, 104–5
    reduction of bulging, 103, 103
    vaginal examination of, 27
Mendelson's syndrome, 56
Mental Health Act, 6
Mental illness, 6, 204–5
Mentoanterior position, 166, 166, 167
Mentolateral position, 166, 167
Mentoposterior position, 166, 167
Metabolic acidaemia, 75
Metabolic acidosis
    fetal, 75
    maternal, 55
Misoprostol, 157–8
Modern technology, 2

Modesty, 1
Monochorionic twins, 181, 208
Monovular twins, 181
Monozygotic twins, 181, *182*
Montevideo units, 46, *47*
Mortality
    maternal *see* Maternal mortality
    multiple birth/pregnancies, 182–3
    perinatal, 16 (*see also* Fetal death;
        Stillbirths)
    preterm babies, 102–3
Mother
    birthing room resuscitation
        equipment for, 20
    causes of shoulder presentation
        due to, 169
    complications with assisted
        vaginal delivery, 139
    consequences of prolonged labour,
        114
    death of *see* Maternal mortality
    indications for assisted vaginal
        deliveries, 127
    indications for induction due to,
        117–18
    refusal of blood transfusion, 169
    trauma to, 211
Moulding, severe, 83
Movements, fetal, 83
Multiple pregnancies, 182, 185
    breech delivery, 176–7
    see also Twin pregnancies
Multiple sclerosis, 191
Myasthenia gravis, 191
Myocardial infarction, 43–4, 196
Myometrial activity
    labour, 46–9, 46–52
    pregnancy, 45–6
    see also Contractions; Uterine
        activity
Myometrial parathyroid hormone-
    related peptide, 45
Myosin light-chain kinase, 45
Myotonic dystrophy, 191

N

Naloxone, 60, 94
National Institute of Health and
    Clinical Excellence (NICE), 214
Negligence, 10–11
Neonatal resuscitation equipment in
    birthing room, 20
Neurological conditions, 190–1
Neuromuscular disease, 191
Newborn, 91–9
    birth trauma, 99
    death of, 16, 207

emergencies due to congenital
    abnormalities, 95–9
physiological considerations, 92
resuscitation at birth, 92–3, 94, 95,
    96
special situations, 93–5
Nitric oxide, 45
Nitrous oxide and oxygen, 52, 59–60
Non-identical twins, 181
Normal delivery, 49–52
Nosocomial infection, 202
Nucleic acid amplification tests
    (NAAT), 201
Nutrition, intrapartum, 55–6

O

Oblique lie, 169–70
Obstetric emergencies training,
    213–17
    acute, 214–17
    guidelines, 214
Obstruction to descent, 112–14
Occipitoposterior positions, 164–6,
    165, *166*
Occupational infection, 202
Oedema, pulmonary, 156, 195–6
Oliguria, 198
Opioids
    adverse reactions to, 155
    drug depression in newborns, 94
    epidural anaesthesia, 67
    parenteral, 60
    users of, 204–5
Osmotic diuretic administration, 198
O'Sullivan's technique, 161
Oxygen and nitrous oxide, 52, 59–60
Oxytocics, 68, 110
    adverse reactions to, 155
Oxytocin, 44, 45, 46
    regimen for induction of labour,
        121

P

Pajot's manoeuvre, 138, *138*
Palisade patterns, FHR, 78
Parenteral opioids, 60
Parietal presentation, 168
Partners, 2
Partogram example, *49*
Passage, assisted delivery, 128
Passenger *see* Fetus
Pathologically adherent placenta,
    160
Patient information, confidentiality,
    10

Pelvic planes, 28, 29, *29*
Pelvis
    average diameter of normal, 30
    contracted, 28–30
    examination of, 25–7, 28–32
        routine for, 30–1
    magnetic resonance image of,
        31–2, *32*
    types of, 28, *28*, 31
Pencil point spinal needles, 60, *61*
Penicillin, 200
Perinatal mortality, 16, 207
    see also Fetal death; Stillbirths
Perineum, tears in the *see* Tears,
        perineal
Pethidine, 60
Pfannenstiel's incision, 147, *147*, 148
Phenothiazines, 94
pH of fetus, 80–1
Phospholipase, 46
Pinard stethoscope, 25, *25*, 26, 74
Placenta
    delivery of the, 51, *51*
    inspection of, 52
    manual removal of, 159–60, *159–60*
    pathologically adherent, 160
    retained, 158–60
Placental separation (abruption), 37,
        38–9
    consequences of, 39
    presentation, 39
    severity of bleeding in, 39
Placenta praevia, 37, 40
    anaesthesia, 69
    grading of, 40
    low ARM, 120, *120*
    management of, 40
Platelet disorders, 189–90
Platelet packs, 38
Platypelloid pelvis, 28, *28*, 31
Pneumonia, aspiration, 56
Pneumothorax, 97–9
Podalic version, internal, 177, *178*
Position, delivery, 48
Post-dural puncture headache
    (PDPH), 62
Posterior asynclitism, 168, *169*
Post-mortem request, 210
Postoperative analgesia, 68–9
Postpartum haemorrhage, 155–8,
        182
    alternative procedures, 158
    bimanual compression, 158
    diagnosis, 156
    management, 157–8
    predisposing factors, 156–7
    results of, 157
Powers, assisted delivery, 128
Precipitate labour and delivery, 110

Pre-eclampsia, 40, 196–8
    anaesthesia, 69
    analgesia, 69
    management of, 197–8
    see also Eclampsia
Preferences for labour, 2
Pregnancy
    myometrial activity during, 45–6
    termination of, 9
Presentation of fetus
    assessment of, 24
    twins, 182
    see also Malposition;
        Malpresentation
Presenting part distance, 27–8, *28*
Pressure-tipped catheter, 80, *80*
Preterm delivery, 106
    breech, 172, 178
    twins, 182
Preterm labour, 101–4
    antibiotics and infection, 103–4
    at 23–26 completed weeks, 102–3
    cervical cerclage, 103
    definition of, 101
    general statements, 101–2
    guidelines for management of, 102
    management of, 105
    and tocolytics, 105–6
Preterm premature rupture of
    membranes (PPROM), 104–5
Primary brow presentation, 168
Primary face presentation, 167
Progesterone, 45
Prolonged labour, 110–14
    abnormal contractions, 110–11
    abnormal descent, 112–14
    consequences of, 114
    deficient/delayed cervical
        dilatation, 114
    fetal problems, 112
Prophylaxis, induction of labour as,
    118
Prostacyclins, 45
Prostaglandins, 45, 46, 119
Prostaglandin synthase antagonists,
    105–6
Psychiatric illness, 204–5
Psychiatric patients, consent, 6
Psychological requirements for place
    of birth, 22
Psychotic illness, 204–5
Pudendal artery, *87*
Pudendal canal, 87
Pudendal nerve, 87, *87*
    block, 65, 87
Puerperal sepsis, maternal mortality,
    15–16
Pulmonary haemorrhage, newborn,
    97

Pulmonary oedema, 156, 195–6
Pulmonary thromboembolism, 14–15,
    156, 157

R

Raised intracranial pressure, 191
Regional analgesia, 60–5
    complications of, 63
    consent, 62
    contraindications to, 62
    counselling before, 62
    establishing, 63–4
    pre-eclampsia, 69
    resources for treatment of
        complications, 61
    symptoms of toxicity, 63
Registration of births/stillbirths, 10
Relaxin, 45
Renal failure, 198
Respiratory alkalosis, 55
Respiratory problems, 190
Resuscitation
    birthing room equipment, 20
    newborn at birth, 92–3, 94, 95, 96
    of the obstetric woman, 43
Retained placenta, 158–60
Right occipitoposterior (ROP), 164,
    165
Rigid cups, vacuum extractors, 129
Risk management, essentials of, 11
Ritodrine, 103
Rotational procedures, 135–9, *136, 138*
Royal College of Obstetricians and
    Gynaecologists (RCOG), 213,
    215

S

Sacrosciatic notch, 30, *30*
Sacrospinous ligament, 30, *30*
Saline, distinction between CSF and,
    64
Satisfaction with care, 3, 24
Scalp clip, 27, 74, 75, 77
    application of, 79, *79*
Secondary brow presentation, 168
Secondary face presentation, 167
Second degree tears, 89
Second stage of labour
    effect of uterine activity on cervix,
        48
    forces operating in the, 128
Seizures, 41
Sepsis, maternal mortality, 15–16
Septic shock, 199–200
Sheehan's syndrome, 156, 157

Shock, 157
    hypovolaemic, 94
    septic, 199–200
Shoulder dystocia, 140–1
Shoulder presentation, 169–70
    causes of, 169
Shoulders, normal delivery of, 49, 50,
    50
Sickle cell disease, 188
Sickling crisis, 188
Silent trace, 76
Sim's speculum, 26, *26*
Skills drill, 213, 214–15
Skull fractures, 98
Sodium retention, 56
Soft cups, vacuum extractors, 129
Special requirements, women with,
    3
Speculum examination, 26, *26*
Spinal anaesthesia
    for caesarean section, 66
    pre-eclampsia, 69
    total, 62, 63
Spinal–epidural anaesthesia, 67
Spinal–epidural analgesia, 71
Spinal needles, 60, *60*, 61
Sponge forceps, 103
Spontaneous breech delivery, 173–6
Spurious labour, 109–10
Sterilisation, 152
Sternomastoid tumour, 98
Stillbirths, 16, 208
    protocol, 209–10
    registration of, 10
    see also Fetal death
Streptococci, group B, 103–4, 200
Subarachnoid space, 60
Subdural haemorrhage, 98
Subpubic angle, 30, *30*
Substitute head (caput succedaneum),
    98, *99*
Subumbilical midline incision, 146–7,
    147
Suicide, 204
Superficial birth injuries, 98
Support in labour, 20
Surrogacy, 9
Suspected fetal death, 43
Symphysiotomy, 140
Syncope, cardiac, 195
Syntocinon, 68
    see also Oxytocin
Syphilis, 201

T

Tachycardia, 75, *78*
Tact, 2

Tears, perineal, 89–90
  consequences of, 90
  grading of, 89
  repair of, 89, *89*
Technology, 2
Temazepam, 205
Termination of pregnancy (TOP), 9–10
Thalassaemia, 188–9
Third degree tears, 89, *89*
  faecal incontinence after, 90
Third stage labour, 51, *51*
Thrombocytopenia, 189, 198
Thromboembolism, pulmonary, 14–
  15, 156, 157
Thrombosis, maternal mortality,
  14–15
Thyroid, 192–3
Thyroid storm, 192–3
Thyrotoxicosis, 192, 193
Tocodynamometer, 75
Tocolysis, 68
Tocolytics, 103
  preterm labour and, 105–6
Tocometer, 78–9, 79–80, *80*
Total spinal anaesthesia, 62, 63
Tracheo-oesophageal fistula, 97, *97*
Traction forceps, 129, *130*
Traction procedures, 132–4, *134, 135,*
  138
Training in acute obstetric
  emergencies, 214–17
Transcutaneous electrical nerve
  stimulation (TENS), 60
Transient acceleration of heart rate,
  76, *76*
Transient neonatal thyrotoxicosis, 193
Transverse incision, 147, *147*
Transverse lie, 169–70
Trauma
  fetal, 98–9, 208
  maternal, 15, 211
Trial of labour, 114–15
Trial of scar, 115
Triennia audit
  1994–1996, 13
  2000–2002, 13
Triplets, 185
Tuohy needles, 60, *60, 61*
Twin pregnancies
  breech delivery, 176–7
  complications of, 182–3
  death of a co-twin, 208
  delivery of, 183–4
  diagnosis, 182

induction of labour, 123
labour surveillance, 184
presentation at delivery, 182
special problems, 184–5
types of, 181–2
vaginal delivery of caesarean
  section, 183
Type 1 diabetes, 194
Type 2 diabetes, 194

U

Umbilical cord
  delivery, 49–51
  presentation, 36, *36*
  prolapse, 36, 36–7
    following induction, 122
Umbilical vein compression, 74
Undiagnosed second twin, 184
Uniovular twins, 181
Upper airway obstruction, 97
Uterine activity
  effect on cervix
    before labour, 47
    during labour, 48
  effect on fetus, 48
  effect on mother, 52
  hypotonic, 110
  incoordinate, 111, *112*
  occipitoposterior positions,
    165
  see also Contractions
Uterine atony, 157
Uterine contractions *see* Contractions
Uterine inversion, acute, *160,* 160–1,
  161
Uterus
  abnormal activity during labour,
    109–10
  activity of *see* Uterine activity
  bimanual compression of, 158,
    158
  hyperstimulation following
    induction, 122
  incisions, caesarean section, *147,*
    147–8
  massage to encourage contraction,
    157, *157*
  during pregnancy, 45–6
  rupture of, 16, 111, 156
  scar rupture, 149–50, *151*
  work during labour, 46–7, *47*
  see also Myometrial activity

V

Vacuum delivery
  traction procedures, 133
  trial of, 138–9
Vacuum extractors, 129–32
Vaginal birth after caesarean section
  (VBAC), 148–9
Vaginal bleeding, 37–8
  important points about, 38
  see also Antepartum haemorrhage;
    Postpartum haemorrhage
Vaginal delivery
  after caesarean section,
    148–9
  assisted *see* Assisted vaginal
    delivery
  twins, 183–4
Vaginal examination, 27–8
  breech, 171
  occipitoposterior positions, 165
Vaginal haematoma, 139, 141
Vaginal lacerations, 139
Valium, 94, 205
Varicella zoster, 203
Vasa praevia, 37
Ventilation
  bag and mask, 95
  invasive positive pressure (IPPV),
    96
Ventouse extractor, 129, *131*
Ventouse rotation, 136, *136*
Verbal consent, 6
Viral infections, 201–3
Visceral damage, 99
Von Willebrand's disease, 189

W

Water immersion labour and birth,
  20–1
Woods cork screw manoeuvre,
  141
Wrigley's forceps, 151, 178
Written consent, 6

Z

Zavanelli's option, 141
Zidovudine, 202